Psychiatry observed

Psychiatry observed

Geoff Baruch
and
Andrew Treacher

Routledge & Kegan Paul
London, Henley and Boston

First published in 1978
by Routledge & Kegan Paul Ltd
39 Store Street,
London WC1E 7DD,
Broadway House,
Newtown Road,
Henley-on-Thames,
Oxon RG9 1EN and
9 Park Street,
Boston, Mass. 02108, USA
Printed in Great Britain by
Thomson Litho Ltd
East Kilbride, Scotland

British Library Cataloguing in Publication Data

Baruch, Geoff
  Psychiatry observed
  1. Psychiatry - Great Britain
  I. Title II. Treacher, Andrew
  616.8'9'00941   RC450.G7   77-30669

  ISBN 0 7100 8876 0

Contents

vi   Contents

Preface

For historically determined reasons, the psychiatric profession
still dominates decision-making in the field of mental health. The
changes that have occurred in the psychiatric services during the
last two decades have therefore largely reflected the 'expert'
opinion provided by the profession. Since 1962 successive govern-
ments have been committed to a policy of desegregating the mentally
disordered, and it has been proposed that psychiatric treatment
should take place in general hospitals and the community rather
than in the geographically isolated mental hospitals. In practice
this policy is nowhere near fruition. There has been a shift
towards providing psychiatric beds in general hospitals, but the
provision of community care remains vestigial.

The importance of this major change in mental health policy for
both the psychiatric profession and the mentally disordered cannot
be easily estimated. To begin with, mental health policy-makers
hoped that by changing the locus of treatment the mentally disordered would be viewed as 'ill' in the same way as the physically
ill and would therefore escape the stigma associated with being a
patient in a mental hospital. With the development of drug treatments it was assumed that patients would no longer have to undergo
lengthy hospital admissions. The new policy was therefore based on
the belief that patients would be returned to the community as soon
as possible and that the number of psychiatric beds in mental hospitals would be reduced accordingly. The number of NHS psychiatric
beds has indeed declined, but whether this decline reflects any
real improvement in psychiatric care remains an open question.
Indeed, we would argue that the latent function of the shift in
policy was to provide for the desegregation of the psychiatric
profession.

The introduction of psychiatric units into general hospitals has
contributed to the desegregation of the profession since it has
brought the profession closer to the mainstream of ordinary medicine and has conferred on it a similar status to that of other
branches of the medical profession. The introduction of such units
into general hospitals is the administrative expression of the 1959
Mental Health Act which removed the legal distinction between
psychiatric and other types of hospitals; but it is ironic that

this Act, which helped to desegregate psychiatry within the broader profession of medicine, served also to establish another form of segregation. Since the Act reasserted the hegemony of the psychiatric profession in relation to the treatment of the mentally disordered, other professionals (psychologists, social workers and nurses) were forced to retain their ancillary roles. It was equally ironic that this hegemony should be reasserted at a time when the medical model was being increasingly criticised. In the same period in America other mental health professionals were seeking more independent and powerful roles within the field of mental health and were able successfully to influence the terms of the new legislation that was being introduced by the Kennedy Administration.

In our view, anybody who seeks to explore the state of contemporary psychiatric practice must start from an understanding of the historical roots of the dominance exerted by the psychiatric profession. In the opening chapters of our book we therefore explore the social, economic and political conditions that have contributed to the dominance of the psychiatric profession. Briefly, we argue that the ideology of the profession, which has been firmly rooted in the traditions of 'scientific' medicine, is peculiarly appropriate to the economic and social conditions of capitalism in the twentieth century. We therefore regard the success of psychiatry in actually treating mental disorders as largely irrelevant to any arguments concerned with the possible objective basis for its domination. In this context we document the development of the medical model within psychiatry and explore the major forms of treatment derived from it in order to illustrate that the methods adopted have little or no proven efficacy and at best can be considered only palliative.

In the second part of the book we explore the historical origins of psychiatric units in general hospitals and examine the basis of their advocacy by mental health policy-makers.

The final section of the book consists of an analysis of the functioning of a psychiatric unit in a general hospital. In order to achieve this aim of exploring the decision-making, diagnostic and therapeutic activities of the unit we have elected to present the 'careers' of three patients who underwent treatment during the period of research.

The final part of the book attempts to draw together the historical and empirical material we have presented. We consider the issues that emerge from the study in terms of both the historical arguments that we advance in the first two sections of the book and the findings that emerge from the empirical study. In this chapter we also provide some tentative conclusions about the future of the psychiatric services.

Having outlined the contents of the book, it is necessary to make some specific points about the empirical study. First the judgements that we make about the running of the unit are concerned with the period during which the research took place. Since that time the unit has undergone changes independent of our study in order to correct certain deficiencies. We do not know what effect these have had on Porchester as a diagnostic and therapeutic setting.

Two factors have been of paramount importance in selecting the three cases we have documented in the book. To begin with they accurately reflect, in our opinion, the unit's approach to decision-making with respect to diagnosis and treatment as observed by the researcher (G.B.) during his eleven-month period of study. However, this is not to suggest that every case which was recorded in the unit during this time revealed exactly the same features. It must be stressed that we have not been concerned to evaluate the outcome or treatment of particular cases. We would argue that regardless of the efficacy of a treatment programme a successful case would present the same defects regarding decision-making and other factors as an unsuccessful one. A further consideration regarding selectivity has been to do with the themes that emerge from the study. They are not only pertinent to Porchester unit but are relevant to the practice of psychiatry generally and general hospital psychiatry in particular. On the basis of the study we have become preoccupied with the relationship between hierarchical treatment teams (and their division of labour) and the employment of a psycho-social approach to diagnosis and treatment. A further preoccupation has been concerned with the problems surrounding the training and practice of psychotherapy within the NHS. Also we have become interested in the value of a 'contract-making' approach in clinical practice. These issues and others to do with the empirical study are explored in those parts of the book not specifically devoted to the Porchester unit. Therefore we feel it is important that the reader should consider the material on the hospital itself within the context of our general critique.

We have given fictitious names to the hospital and to the people and places mentioned in the study in order that they should remain unidentified. Although we make many criticisms of the unit's functioning we do not seek to attack individuals in a personal sense - we see the inadequacies of the unit as being historically conditioned and in this sense we see individual members of staff trapped in role relationships which are largely not of their own making. That is not to argue that their behaviour is totally determined by social processes external to them but to argue that their actions and behaviour tend to be determined by such processes in the absence of concerted attempts to confront them.

This leads us to a more general point - throughout the book we are critical of psychiatry and psychiatrists and it may appear to some readers that we overstep the mark on this issue. In our defence we would quote Dr Henry Miller who, in attacking contemporary psychiatry (admittedly from a different standpoint), also pointed out that some of his best friends were psychiatrists. The same is true of us - we have the highest regard for individual psychiatrists whose skills and abilities are contributing to major innovations in psychiatry. Despite this we are not deterred from critically examining the profession as a whole.

It is also important for us to add a personal note about our own backgrounds. The perspective from which we have written this book has been largely determined by our training in the social sciences. Both of us have been trained in disciplines (sociology and psychology) that are considered ancillary within the area of mental health, but both of us are currently being trained as

psychotherapists. However, in seeking to achieve this aim and then
to go on to take responsibility for providing therapy for patients
is to confront a major historical anachronism. The profession of
psychiatry still bases itself upon reductionist models having their
origin in medicine, and yet it exerts its hegemony in the field of
therapy by effectively precluding other, differently trained
therapists from having primary responsibility for patient care.
It is hoped that our book will contribute to the movements that are
seeking to remove this anachronism.

One final point should be made concerning the writing of our
book. Although the book is a joint effort, there is a division of
labour within. Chapters 1 to 5 were written by one of us (A.T.)
while chapters 6 to 9 were the responsibility of the other (G.B.).
Chapter 10 is a joint effort in which we attempted to bring our
two approaches together.

It may well be that our readers will feel that we have been
over-ambitious in writing a book with this structure. That is a
risk we have been prepared to take because we feel that the issues
we seek to raise are of sufficient importance. Our book is therefore designed as a discussion document - we make no pretence that
our findings are definitive, but we do hope that the book succeeds
in contributing to the ongoing discussion of the best ways of
tackling mental health problems.

Part one

The psychiatric profession

Chapter 1

The rise of the psychiatric profession

In the introduction to his controversial book 'Medical Nemesis'
Illich (1975) attacks the medical profession on the grounds that
it is responsible for expropriating health:

> The medical establishment has become a major threat to health
> ... a professional and physician-based health care system which
> has grown beyond tolerable bounds is sickening for three reasons:
> it must produce clinical damages which outweigh its potential
> benefits; it cannot but obscure the political conditions which
> render society unhealthy; and it tends to expropriate the power
> of the individual to heal himself and to shape his or her
> environment.

In Britain the care and treatment of the mentally ill is still
largely the responsibility of the psychiatric profession, so the
obvious question arises - does the profession function in the way
that Illich suggests? In his own work Illich makes only passing
reference to the psychiatric profession, but it is obvious that he
would seek to include its activities within his general critique.
Our own critique of contemporary psychiatry has many parallels
with Illich's attack on the medical profession as a whole, but our
aims and interests are far more proscribed than his. We begin our
discussion by examining how the psychiatric profession was able to
establish its claim to be the main agency for treating the mentally
disordered.

PROBLEMS IN THE PRESENTATION OF THE HISTORY OF PSYCHIATRY

In practice this question is difficult to answer satisfactorily
because historians of the mental health services have not considered
it to be a problematic issue. For instance, Jones (1970), in her
much quoted book 'A History of the Mental Health Services', presents
the issue in a very simplistic way. In summarising the state of the
mental health services at the middle of the nineteenth century, she
says that there were three possible channels of development for
further reform:

> It could develop along the social and humanitarian lines; it
> could develop along purely medical lines, blurring the

distinction between mental and physical disorders, sharing in
the great developments which characterized general medicine in
the second half of the nineteenth century; or it could proceed
along legal lines, piling safeguard on safeguard to protect the
sane against illegal detention, delaying certification and
treatment until the person genuinely in need of care was
obviously (and probably incurably) insane. In the social
approach, the emphasis was on human relations; in the medical
approach, it was on physical treatment, in the legal approach,
it was on procedure.

But Jones insists that the actual developments that then took place
were determined by the activities of professional pressure groups
which, because of their particular histories, had greater or lesser
power:

The legal profession had been fully established for centuries.
Medicine was engaged in throwing off the shackles of a long
association with barbering and charlatanism, and did not achieve
full status until the passing of the Medical Registration Act of
1858, which set up a register of doctors who had passed prescribed examinations. Social work and social therapy were to
remain occupations for the compassionate amateur until well into
the twentieth century. It is therefore not surprising that the
legal approach took precedence, to be followed after 1890 by the
medical approach. It is only now, when the social services have
developed a comparable professional status, that the social
approach is coming into its own again.

In our view such an explanation is very one-sided, since it fails
to explore the major social, economic and political changes that
would facilitate a profession's ability to legitimate its claims
to influence and would even determine the structure of a country's
mental health services. Since we are concerned with the rise of
the psychiatric profession we shall not discuss the role of the
legal profession in the latter half of the nineteenth century.
Jones calls this era the triumph of legalism, but it is significant
that she does not label the next phase in the development of the
services 'the triumph of medicalisation'. The phrase is of course
clumsy, but Jones avoids using it not because of her sensitivity
for style but because she seems unable to clarify her own conceptualisation of the nature of mental disorders. Towards the end of
her book she pays lip service to non-medical conceptualisation,
but it is clear from other sections of the book that she tends to
adhere to the medically derived view that mental disorders are
indeed forms of illness.

We would argue that it is because Jones uncritically accepts
this view that she cannot at times distance herself from her
subject matter sufficiently. She therefore tends to present some
of the developments in the mental health services as natural, even
ordained, processes which are not open to dispute or discussion.
This tendency is well illustrated by her presentation of the
findings of the Royal Commission on Lunacy and Disorder (1924) and
the Mental Treatment Act of 1930 which followed in its wake.
Since both the Commission and the Act contributed crucially to the
strengthening of the medical profession's power to gain control
over the definition and treatment of mental disorders, we shall

discuss both in some detail.

The Commission owed its existence to a prolonged crisis in the
functioning of the asylums which had been starved of staff and
resources particularly during the First World War. The Commission
was charged with investigating the legal and administrative
machinery for certifying persons alleged to be of unsound mind,
and the possibilities of treating persons suffering from mental
disorders without certifying them. The majority of the Commission's
members were lawyers although there were two medical members (a
neurologist and a specialist in organic diseases), and it was the
latter's view of mental disorder that prevailed. The Commission
therefore adopted a definition of mental disorder that was clearly
medical:

It has become increasingly evident that there is no clear line
of demarcation between mental and physical illness. The distinction as commonly drawn is based on a difference of symptoms.
In ordinary parlance, a disease is described as mental if its
symptoms manifest themselves predominantly in derangement of
conduct, and as physical if its symptoms manifest themselves
predominantly in derangement of bodily function. A mental
illness may have physical concomitants; probably it always has,
though they may be difficult of detection. A physical illness
on the other hand, may have, and probably always has, mental
concomitants. And there are many cases in which it is a
question whether the physical or the mental symptoms predominate.

To many, such a definition may appear entirely reasonable and non-
controversial. For example, in her book Jones (1970) gives us an
interesting evaluation which is worth exploring in some detail:

These definitions were perhaps common place to psychiatrists;
but for many people, even in the medical profession, it involved
thinking of a new kind. Insanity had always been treated as a
subject bearing little relation to general medicine. This
statement, backed by two of the greatest medical brains of the
day, meant that a patient should no longer be regarded as a
'case' of peptic ulcer or dermatitis, schizophrenia or hysteria.
Here was a unique fusion of mind and body; and illness, whether
mental or physical in symptomatology, was something which
affected his whole nature. To the psychiatrist, this was not
new. Freud had demonstrated long before how many apparent
physical ailments could be the product of 'hysteria' and something was known about the effect of mental processes on skin
conditions and gastric disorders; but the authority of this
statement, and the wide publicity accorded to it, make it a
landmark in the development of the public attitude to mental
illness.

It never occurs to Jones that such an approach could indeed be
disastrous to a psychological and sociological approach. Her
citing of Freud is most intriguing - Freud did indeed take up such
a position in relation to hysteria, but that is beside the point.
Freud would have obviously advised a psychological form of treatment (psychoanalysis) for such cases, whereas a medically orientated
therapist would prescribe drugs or physical forms of treatment. In
fact, the treatment era opened up by the Mental Treatment Act (which
embodied many of the recommendations of the Royal Commission) was

an era in which physical treatments (insulin shock treatment,
electro-convulsive therapy, lobotomy and leucotomy) became
increasingly important. Jones in her enthusiasm fails to examine
the actual nature of such treatments in any detail - indeed, one
searches her index in vain to find any reference to them! And
yet if the contents of the 'Journal of Mental Science' (fore-
runner of the 'British Journal of Psychiatry') are examined during
this period, one can detect an explosion of psychiatric interest
in these new treatments, coupled with a declining interest in
psychoanalysis or psychotherapy.

THE ISSUE OF ECLECTICISM IN BRITISH PSYCHIATRY

In practice it is difficult to summarise the changes that occurred
in British psychiatry at this time. It is important to stress,
as Clare (1976) has done in his book 'Psychiatry in Dissent',
that British psychiatry has always been eclectic. Nevertheless
it is possible to discern some general trends within this eclecticism. As Russell Davis (1970) has pointed out, there was a
shift in psychiatric thinking during the 1930s and 1940s towards
faulty-machine models. The faulty-machine model, as its name
implies, is based on the assumption that some form of change at
a metabolic cellular or electro-physiological level is responsible
for causing the mental disorder. According to Russell Davis, it
traditionally drew upon an analogy with diabetes mellitus. The
discovery in 1889 that diabetes could be produced by removing the
pancreas led to the search for a chemical means for repairing the
fault. The introduction of insulin in the early 1920s ushered in
a new allegedly more 'scientific' era in medicine, and it was
inevitable that psychiatry should be profoundly influenced by
such an approach. The emergence of insulin shock treatment flows
naturally from this development, but it is important to stress
just how mechanical conceptualisation in psychiatry became.
Diabetic patients go on receiving insulin throughout their lives,
so it is logical (in terms of the model) that one would expect
psychiatric patients to take drugs on a long-term basis.
  Russell Davis (1970) argues that such a model has always had
an obvious appeal to psychiatrists:
  The (model) is highly attractive because it confirms their
  status as physicians in the new scientific tradition and
  indicates for them a role that they may regard as charac-
  teristically medical. This role prescribes for them a relationship with the patient similar to that they have learnt to adopt
  during their long apprenticeship in treating cases of organic
  disease. Moreover, the emphasis on specific endogenous factors,
  however obscure they may be ... weakens the tendency to identify
  with the patient, and helps them to preserve their professional
  detachment.
The significance of this point for our argument becomes clear when
it is related to research on the professional socialisation of
psychiatrists. As Russell Davis points out, psychiatrists in
academic posts in the United Kingdom have traditionally acquired
a higher qualification in internal medicine and therefore have

tended to adhere to a faulty-machine type of model. Research by
Walton and Drewery (1966) shows that they tend to focus on treatment of the individual patient and to avoid approaches that stress
the interactional nature of mental disorder. As teachers they
tend to create students in their own image, and it is not surprising
therefore that succeeding generations of psychiatrists have been
strongly influenced to accept the faulty-machine model.

THE IMPLICATIONS OF THE MENTAL TREATMENT ACT (1930)

But it is essential at this point to return to the main line of
our argument. The passing of the Mental Treatment Act and the
introduction of physical methods of treatment, which closely
followed it, had far more contradictory effects than Jones allows.
The overall effect was indeed to help to legitimate the medical
profession's claim to be the only body of practitioners capable
of treating the mentally disordered. However, it is important to
examine the types of treatment that emerged in the 1930s and 1940s.
They were largely antipathetic to the approaches that she assumes
were enshrined in the Act itself. They were almost exclusively
physical forms of treatment which were based on faulty-machine
models and which clearly contradicted psychologically and socio-
logically based approaches. In practice, the collapsing of the
boundary between physical illness and so-called 'mental' illness
led to psychiatry becoming increasingly narrow and 'technological'
in its approach to patients.

THE ISSUE OF PSYCHOTHERAPY

This point can also be established by considering the role of
psychotherapy in the training of psychiatrists. We would argue
that it is precisely because of the profession's historically
determined attachment to faulty-machine models and their associated
forms of treatment that training in psychotherapeutic skills has
never been considered an essential feature of a psychiatrist's
training; hence the recent irony of the National Association of
Mental Health actually calling for psychotherapy to be included
as an essential part of the training of psychiatrists (NAMH, 1974).
   But it is equally ironic that, although no specific formal
attention is yet paid to the training of psychiatrists in psychotherapy, the profession as a whole feels disposed to claim that
it has such skills. The position was made explicit in the British
Medical Association's reply to a recent DHSS circular concerning
the implications of the Foster Report (BMA, 1974). In this
document the BMA makes a calculated attempt to establish that
doctors are a special breed of mankind who naturally have psychotherapeutic skills, and thereby raises the issue of professional
dominance. The roots of the BMA's attitude can in fact be traced
back both to the 1959 Mental Health Act and to the 1930 Mental
Treatment Act that foreshadowed it. Both of the Acts contributed
to the emergence of the psychiatric profession which was able to
prevent other professions from establishing significant footholds
in the area of the treatment of the mentally disordered.

PROFESSIONAL DOMINANCE

In this context it is worth noting the comments of Smail (1973)
who, in acting as a spokesman for clinical psychologists, has
spelt out the full implications of the power wielded by the
medical profession. In reviewing the difficulties experienced
by clinical psychologists working within the National Health
Service, he comments that:

> (after the formation of the National Health Service in 1948)
> clinical psychologists were dwarfed by a medical guild whose
> powers, self-determination and freedom of action must be
> almost unique - the state of psychological knowledge ... did
> not permit psychologists to adopt anything but a secondary
> role. The physical methods of treatments appropriate to so-
> called mental illness obviously necessitated possession of a
> medical degree, and non-physical methods stemming, in this
> country, largely from the psychoanalytic school could only
> be practised by people (most usually doctors) who had under-
> gone a lengthy and expensive initiation ceremony. In other
> words, the licence to practise treatment was based on a system
> where authority was accorded to would-be healers on the basis
> of their belonging to the appropriate (medical) club rather
> than on the basis of a scientifically demonstrable ability to
> assist psychological change. Above all, psychologists in the
> National Health Service were, and still are, prevented from
> direct involvement with patients by statutory constraints.

Smail's statement requires no further elaboration at this point.
It is essential for us to attempt to explain how the medical
profession was able to gain its ascendancy. As we have already
noted, little specific attention has been paid to this issue by
historians, but fortunately some recent work by Ewins (1974) has
provided a challenging analysis of this process.

EWINS'S ANALYSIS OF THE RISE OF THE PSYCHIATRIC PROFESSION

Ewins's work is primarily concerned with analysing the origins
of the compulsory commitment provisions of the Mental Health Act
of 1959, but his analysis involves an examination of the provisions
both of the 1930 Mental Treatment Act and the 1959 Mental Health
Act and of the much earlier 1890 Lunacy Act. In covering much the
same ground as Jones, Ewins has attempted to document the complex
political and social changes that facilitated the acceptance of
medical explanations of mental disorders. However, Ewins is
preoccupied by the legal changes embodied in these Acts because
he sees these as important barometers of social attitudes towards
the mentally disordered. For example, his comparison of the terms
of the 1930 Mental Treatment Act and the 1959 Mental Health Act
reveals a remarkable shift in the basis upon which compulsory
detention in hospital can be made. Authority for detention, which
had to be established by medical opinion, was no longer subject to
a final judicial decision. As Ewins (1974) comments,

> the Act essentially replaced detention on the basis of legal
> certification (immediate legal authority) by detention on the

basis of medical opinion (medical authority). Lay intervention
as a safeguard in the process of detention is retained only
after hospitalization in the form of Mental Health Review
Tribunals; and the very limited powers of these tribunals serve
only to emphasise the dramatic change from the suspicious,
legalistic approach of the 1890 Act to the handing over of power
with regard to the detention and treatment of the mentally ill
to informal agencies of social control (primarily the medical
profession, in conjunction with local health authorities and
the relatives of patients) by the 1959 Act.
There has been little attempt to explain this remarkable change.
Ewins's own explanation begins with an analysis of some of
Foucault's work. Foucault (1967) in his book 'Madness and
Civilisation' argues that medical men originally gained control
over the definition and treatment of madness during the eighteenth
century because of the complex social role that they enacted
rather than because of any real development in scientific knowledge.
However, with the development of scientific discoveries during the
nineteenth century the doctor-patient relationship changed.
Foucault argues that patients came to view the doctor as a possessor
of esoteric knowledge who could unravel the complexities of insanity
(Foucault, 1967):

in the patient's eyes, the doctor becomes a thaumaturge; the
authority he has borrowed from order, morality and the family
now seem to derive from himself; it is because he is a doctor
that he is believed to possess these powers ... it was thought,
and by the patient first of all, that it was the esotericism of
his knowledge, in some almost daemonic secret of knowledge,
that the doctor had found power to unravel insanity.

Foucault's explanation illuminates some aspects of the growing
power of doctors in general, but it should be noted that in Britain
this power was amplified by the Medical Registration Act of 1858,
which gave medically trained practitioners a new status in treating
patients. In the early part of the nineteenth century doctors had
been largely ignored by the various parliamentary committees that
were set up to investigate the conditions of lunatics. In the
1840s some aspects of the medical view of insanity were becoming
more widely accepted, but the Report of the Select Committee on
Lunacy (1860) is an interesting milestone in the growing power of
the medical view. The report argued that in theory it was better
to lessen the legal procedure of certification in order to make
early treatment easier, but despite this it actually recommended
that legal safeguards should be strengthened in order to prevent
wrongful committal.
As Ewins (1974) comments,
The Report of this Committee clearly indicates the position of
medicine with regard to insanity in the second half of the
nineteenth century. Despite the growing prestige and power of
the medical profession its claim to sole responsibility for
the insane was as yet by no means recognised in practice -
indeed, medical treatment of the insane was increasingly con-
strained within detailed legal regulations and safeguards,
culminating in the Lunacy Act of 1890. Thus at the end of
the century the medical profession's role in relation to the

> mentally ill was paradoxical. The profession had consolidated
> its claim to be solely ... responsible for treating insanity
> but it could only carry out this function within the constraints
> of a complex legal and administrative framework.

What caused this framework to be changed, first by the Mental
Treatment Act of 1930 and then the far more radical Mental Health
Act of 1959? The explanation is to be found partly in the changing
social and political conditions and partly in developments within
medicine itself. These two factors were closely interrelated,
since developments within psychiatric medicine were peculiarly
appropriate to the changing social and political conditions in
the first half of the twentieth century. Once medical men had
gained authority in administering treatment in asylums they
naturally began to concretise the view that insanity was a medical
problem to be dealt with by medical means. This change from a
'moral' to a medical view of insanity was lubricated by the impact
of science in medicine. The dissolution of the distinction between
physical and mental illness led predictably to doctors attempting
to 'cure' the insane by using methods developed in relation to the
physically ill, but such attempts met with no success until the
beginning of the twentieth century, when some forms of general
paresis of the insane began to be effectively treated with drugs.

THE ISSUE OF THE EFFICACY OF THE NEW FORMS OF TREATMENT

The success of medicine in devising new and effective methods of
treating syphilitic patients created a climate of opinion that
facilitated the acceptance of the medical view of insanity as
'illness'. This in turn strengthened the medical profession's
claim to ultimate control over the detention and treatment of
the mentally ill without the restrictions of detailed legal
regulations and safeguards. But the success of the new methods
would not of itself have been decisive in determining the
ascendancy of the medical profession. Indeed, one has immediately
to question whether the new methods were in fact successful.

Ewins himself does not argue this point in sufficient detail,
but we feel it is more convincing to postulate that the important
point about the new methods of treatment was not that they were
demonstrably successful but that they were construed as being
successful. Ewins tends to lump the various forms of treatment
together and therefore does not pay close enough attention to the
chronology of their introduction. For example, the Royal Commission
on Lunacy (1924-7) and the Mental Treatment Act of 1930 accepted the
medical definition of mental disorder as 'illness' and yet, as we
have already noted, the only major success that medicine had
achieved in treating mental illness was specifically in relation
to general paresis of the insane. In 1909 Ehrlich had synthesised
an arsenical compound (Salvarsan 606) which proved effective in
killing syphilitic spirochaetes in the blood stream. Eight years
later Wagner Jauregg developed a bizarre method of treating
patients who were suffering from advanced forms of the disease.
He discovered that the inoculation of such patients with blood
taken from patients suffering from malaria could produce effective

cures. These discoveries were important in that they seemed to
provide undeniable evidence that mental disorders were illnesses,
but it is inconceivable that these limited successes were alone
decisive in determining the way that mental disorder would be
construed.

PSYCHIATRIC TREATMENTS AS METHODS OF SOCIAL CONTROL

We would argue that the medical view came to prevail largely
independently of its success in providing treatment because the
main reason for its acceptance relates to its ideological content.
This is the essence of Ewins's position since he assumes that the
categorisation of forms of deviant behaviours as mental illness
is an especially advantageous form of social control. Any threat
or potential threat to the existing political and social conditions
of society can be eliminated or greatly lessened by forcing the
deviant to enter the sick role. Once the sick role has been
accepted, the deviant's actions can be invalidated since they are
seen either as meaningless or as mere symptoms whose meaning is
to be deciphered by the psychiatrist. The deviant is no longer
held responsible for his own behaviour - his illness is simply
something that happened to him and over which he has no control.
Given this helplessness, the deviant is entirely in the control
of the doctor, who alone has the power to cure him, but he remains
isolated from other social contacts since the strength of the
doctor-patient relationship generally precludes the formation of
contacts between fellow deviants, so that there is no question of
a subculture of the sick forming.
    Ewins's argument may seem dogmatic and over-prescriptive on
first examination, but he points out that even some sections of
the medical profession have expressed anxiety at the increasing
tendency for forms of antisocial behaviours to be classified as
illness. For example, he cites a leading article in the 'British
Medical Journal' ('BMJ', 1968), which argued that
    there is a growing danger that society will use psychiatry to
    gloss over its own short-comings and ills by making its victims
    'patients'. Anti-social behaviour must not be confused with
    mental illness, and psychiatrists must be aware of having forced
    on them the role of controlling misfits or regarding it as their
    function to normalise the abnormal and non-conforming. The
    doctor's primary duty is to diagnose and treat his patients,
    not to enforce society's rules.
The editorial is concerned primarily with preventing the concept of
'mental illness' from becoming discredited by being applied in a
blanket way to forms of behaviour that can obviously be viewed as
rational and purposeful, given the contexts in which they occur.
But what is to be gained by defining other less disputed forms of
deviancy or mental illness? Here Ewins once again derives his
arguments from Foucault's work since he argues that forms of deviant
behaviour that are regarded by most people as unintelligible,
irrational and purposeless threaten the status quo more subtly and
more profoundly than overt and intelligible forms. Thus he says
that

however many 'alternative realities' there may be in society, irrational behaviour can be perceived to a greater or lesser extent as a threat to all of them. This threat is effectively countered by regarding the 'unintelligible' and 'irrational' person as ill.

Unfortunately, Ewins fails to spell out the nature of this threat in precise detail. He seems to have a romantic and yet essentially rationalistic conception that the mere existence within a society of people who transgress normally accepted ways of thinking is a source of potential threat to the dominant groups within a society. An alternative explanation would place less emphasis on the ideo- logical conflict between the deviant and the society that defines him as such and more emphasis on the economic and social conse- quences that flow from the behaviour of individuals who are judged deviant. It is precisely because they no longer function within culturally prescribed roles that deviants threaten (and are seen as threatening) the economic and social fabric of society. For example, failure of an individual to work (or to function effectively within a family by supporting the breadwinner) because of mental disorder is clearly a problem in a work-orientated society. Such individuals become incapable of supporting them- selves, and if sufficiently large numbers of people were involved then the efficient functioning of the society as a whole would be in question. Such forms of deviancy must clearly be 'regulated'.

Ewins argues that the power of medical explanations of such forms of deviant behaviour lies in their ability to divest them of any possible ideological content. If deviant behaviours are construed as pathological symptoms resulting from a disease process, there is no longer any question of conceptualising them in other ways. For example, there would be no question of examining the content of the symptoms to see whether they reflect the effects of having to cope with the alienating effects of living in a capitalist form of society. Ewins himself illustrates this point very graphically by utilising the analogy of industrial sabotage (Ewins, 1974):

while sabotage by production-line workers can often be explained as a perfectly intelligible reaction to a frustrating demora- lizing or dehumanizing situation, such behaviour is usually defined by the employers and social control agents either as 'irrational' or as being a result of 'illness'. These actions themselves do not in any case represent direct threats to the employers, but to recognise meanings of such actions would to some extent undermine the taken-for-granted 'rationality' and inevitability of the present system: it is this indirect and limited threat that is effectively countered by allocating such actions to the sphere of illness. It is more effective, however, to prevent such a threat even from arising, i.e. to persuade or force the potential saboteur to choose initially the sick role as a solution to the problems posed by his situation, rather than to attempt to fix the label of illness on him after he has chosen more aggressive (and threatening) solutions. The price paid in terms of the vast amount of absenteeism owing to 'mental disorder' is clearly more accept- able to the employers and authorities when compared to the alternatives.

PSYCHIATRIC ILLNESS AND THE SICK ROLE

Ewins's example is an excellent one, since it clearly demonstrates
the political implications of the sick role which Talcott Parsons
(1951) discusses in his own work. Parsons points out that
criminals, since they are labelled and extruded from the company
of upright citizens, must be prevented by coercion from joining
up with their fellow criminals. But there is no such problem
when the form of deviancy is illness rather than criminality. A
sick person's status is conditionally legitimated when he willingly
makes himself dependent upon other people (friends, family members,
doctors, etc.) who will support him. He therefore becomes
dependent on people who are not sick rather than on fellow
sufferers. This means there are real barriers to group formation
among the sick and little possibility of positive legitimation as
a consequence. As a result of these processes the sick role
functions not only to isolate and insulate the sick person but
also to expose him to very powerful forces which insist that he
should become reintegrated into society as a fully participating
member.

From Parsons's standpoint these processes are seen as natural.
He merely recognises entry into the sick role as one of several
deviant routes that individuals may take in response to personal
crises. But as Waitzin and Waterman (1974) have pointed out,
the sick role can be viewed as a particularly effective mechanism
of social control since it permits limited deviancy from occurring
but at the same time prevents the stability of the social system
from being threatened. It is for this reason that Ewins insists
that the medicalisation of mental disorder has to be understood
against the background of an emerging political consensus which
maintained that problems of health, and particularly mental illness, were not a matter for party politics. He correctly stresses
that the Labour Party played a crucial role in contributing and
shaping this consensus, but he fails to develop a sufficiently
detailed discussion of the relationship between developments in
capitalism and the development of the Labour Party as a vehicle
for reformist policies.

At this point our own argument is therefore based upon an
analysis put forward by Bernard Semmel (1960) in his book
'Imperialism and Social Reform'. Semmel is concerned primarily
with exploring the relationship between the development of
imperialism and changes in welfare policies between 1890 and the
First World War. In his analysis of the economic basis of social
reform he does not specifically discuss the provision of services
for the mentally disordered, but it is obvious that his general
analysis can be developed in order to provide a deeper understanding of the reasons for the changes that occurred in embryonic
form in the 1920s and 1930s and more strikingly after the Second
World War. However, in order to introduce this analysis it is
necessary to make some general comments about Semmel's approach.

Semmel views the provision of social and welfare reforms within
a specific historical context - one in which the ruling class in
Britain was faced with containing an increasingly sophisticated
and politically conscious working class (Semmel, 1960):

> Although the suffrage had been granted to the better part of
> the urban working classes in 1867, the working class had still
> not been admitted to power ... the 'depression' of the
> 'seventies', the revival of socialism in the 'eighties' the
> organisation of the unskilled workers in the 'nineties',
> combined to give the working class a new consciousness of both
> its strength and, at the same time, of its political helpless-
> ness. The working class had still to be 'satisfied'.... In
> the ... twentieth century ... international conflicts were
> going to be fought by mass national armies. Could the hundreds
> of thousands of able-bodied loyal soldiers, the mass armies
> required, be obtained from an unpatriotic and stunted working
> class? This seemed an especially serious problem to the fin-
> de-siecle statesmen who heard repeated warnings about war as
> a natural law of history, the struggle for existence, and the
> 'survival of the fittest' from the Social-Darwinists and who
> saw in Imperial Germany a 'rational organisation' determined
> to prove itself the fittest.

But what was to be done? Many politicians saw Bismarck's Germany
as the most suitable model to be emulated, since the 'state
socialism' he had introduced in the 1880s had been consciously
designed to stem social and political discontent in the working
class and to undermine the growing strength of the German socialist
movement. In the space of six years (1883-9) Bismarck secured the
passage of a major Sickness Insurance Law, an Accident Insurance
Law and an Old Age Insurance Law, and yet as part of his strategy
he also outlawed the Social Democratic Party and banned its newspapers. An alternative solution to the problem was suggested by
Cecil Rhodes, who argued that in order to avoid class conflicts
at home it was necessary to develop a policy of imperialist
domination. As he graphically put it, 'The Empire ... is a bread
and butter question. If you want to avoid civil war you must
become imperialists' (Semmel, 1960).

Semmel argues that British politics in the period prior to the
First World War were dominated by such discussions. In essence,
the majority of both Liberal and Tory politicians accepted that
imperialism was essential in order to provide the economic basis
for social reform in Britain; but it is also true that the
influential Fabian Society had developed a policy of advocating
imperialist policies. They therefore decided to support what
Semmel calls the liberal-imperialist wing of the Liberal Party
lead by Earl Rosebery. Rosebery's view of the relationship between
imperialism and social reform is summarised by the following
quotations cited by Semmel (1960):

> An Empire ... requires as its first condition an imperial
> race - a race vigorous and industrious and intrepid ... where
> you promote health and arrest disease, where you convert an
> unhealthy citizen into a healthy one, where you exercise your
> authority to promote sanitary conditions ... you in doing
> your duty are also working for the Empire.

Issues such as educational, housing and temperance reform were
linked by Rosebery to the idea of efficiency (Semmel, 1960):

> a condition of national fitness equal to the demands of our
> Empire - administrative, parliamentary, commercial, educational,

physical, moral, naval and military fitness - so that we should
make the best of our admirable raw material.

Since the Fabians believed that they could achieve their goals of
social reform by converting the leaders of the existing parties
(a policy of 'permeation'), they were naturally attracted to
Rosebery's view. In keeping with these political moves the Fabian
Society therefore preferred to drop references to socialism since
this term inevitably carried with it overtones of class-oriented
politics. The term 'collectivist' was used instead to describe
their policies which were primarily concerned with the promotion
of the national interest. The latter could be most efficiently
achieved by ensuring that the imperial economy (organised on a
collectivist basis) was directed by an elite of experts. The
efficiency of the economy would be the basis for improving the
conditions of the most depressed classes of the community.

The Fabians' corporatist ideas clearly influenced many groups
within the Labour Party, but Semmel demonstrates convincingly
that there was also a crucial ideological link between the Fabians
and the various political movements in which Sir Oswald Mosley
played a part. For Beatrice Webb Mosley was 'the perfect
politician ... (and) perfect gentleman' - her interest in him is
most remarkable since while still a Tory MP he had declared that
his policy was one of 'socialistic imperialism'. His rapid
political evolution was entirely consistent. From being a Tory
he became first an 'Independent', then a member of the Labour
Party (eventually with a Cabinet post) and finally the leader of
the British Union of Fascists. His corporatist doctrines were
often indistinguishable from policies put forward by the Fabians
whose basic authoritarianism is particularly clearly illustrated
in relation to their social welfare policies.

These policies have particular relevance to our arguments
concerning the provision of new forms of services for the mentally
disordered. For example, the Minority Report of the 1909 Royal
Commission on the Poor Laws (written by Sidney and Beatrice Webb)
contains some remarkably authoritarian recommendations. It
suggested that vigorous compaigns to improve the health of the
poor should be undertaken irrespective of the consent of the
people involved. These suggestions foreshadow the powers given
to doctors under the Mental Health Act in 1959 but other sections
of the recommendations are also significant since they argue in
favour of positive welfare legislation and attack notions of
laissez-faire.

Ewins in his analysis emphasises the role of the Fabians and
the policy-makers of the Labour Party in contributing to this
process, but they, of course, were not solely responsible for
formulating welfare policies. In practice the reforms (concerned
with working conditions, housing, health insurance and old age
pensioners) introduced by the Liberal Government from 1908 onwards
were formulated by the left-wingers in the party, who were not
influenced by the Fabians, although ironically their policies were
indistinguishable from those of the Fabians. Most sections of the
Conservative Party bitterly opposed such policies but the growing
power of the Labour Party, reflecting basic developments in the
working class, forced the Conservatives to accept and even endorse

many of the policies introduced originally by the Liberal Party
and later by the Labour Party as it inherited the mantle of the
Liberals. This consensus between the Conservative Party and the
Labour Party emerged most clearly during and after the Second
World War. The Beveridge programme for postwar reconstruction,
which included proposals for a national health service, had been
drawn up during a period of coalition; but the heavy defeat that
the Conservatives received at the hands of the Labour Party in
1945 made it clear to them that they had to accept the basic
tenets of the so-called 'welfare state'.

THE 1959 MENTAL HEALTH ACT AS AN EXAMPLE OF CONSENSUS POLITICS

In this context, the changes embodied in the 1930 Mental Treatment
Act but more crucially in the 1959 Mental Health Act must therefore
be seen as an example of the growing consensus over health and
welfare issues. Both parties were concerned with preserving the
existing political and economic system, so they were united in
seeking to eliminate or control any social phenomenon that
challenged the status quo. Both parties were also wedded to
policies designed to ameliorate social conditions under the present
system, and both placed a great stress on productivity and economic
growth. Since 'unproductiveness' was now viewed in much the same
spirit as pauperism, new forms of medical treatments (notably drug
therapy) which enabled the mentally ill to be returned to productive work were looked upon with great interest.
     But, as Ewins points out, these new forms of treatment had
wider implications: the development of community care was linked
closely to their success in preventing prolonged hospitalisation,
but such forms of treatment involve more effective methods of
social control. Psychiatric medicine could now not only return
patients to productiveness but could also resocialise them in
step with the norms and values of society.

THE SOCIAL FUNCTION OF COMMUNITY CARE

Ewins argues that these developments were particularly appropriate
from the reformist point of view of the Labour Party. Psychiatrists could now be viewed as performing a similar function to that
of social workers. But part of this function would necessarily
involve resocialising deviant members of society so that they would
accept the 'objective reality' which is dictated by the more
powerful groups in society. This essentially authoritarian aspect
of reformist thinking also stresses the importance of 'experts' in
deciding how people should regulate their lives. It is therefore
not surprising that the Minority Report on the Poor Law also
emphasised the importance of doctors in regulating the lives of
the poor. Clearly, psychiatrists can execute such a function in
very powerful ways, and in this context Ewins draws particular
attention to the use of mental welfare agencies as last resorts
for younger 'difficult' members of society who have been through
the hands of the educational and possibly also of the legal

authorities. He also insists that almost all contemporary
psychiatric practice operates in a similar way.

The recent extension of psychiatry to include community care
is therefore of fundamental importance. Indeed, Ewins (1974)
concludes that

as a result of the introduction of community care ... psychiatrists and mental welfare agencies could be increasingly integrated into the elaborate social welfare fabric (constructed
largely by the Labour Party with the increasing acquiescence
and support of the Conservative Party) behind which lay the
belief that social problems could be eradicated by positive
efforts to ameliorate social conditions.

The integration of the medical view of mental illness with the
notions of community care is clearly problematic, however.
Community care, with its emphasis on prevention, implies that
mental illness is at least partly caused by factors in the
individual's social environment. But as we have already noted
in relation to Russell Davis's argument, the medical view, reinforced by the supposed efficacy of purely physical or biochemical
methods of treatment, assumes that mental illness is a result of
pathological processes within the individual. This contradiction
is sometimes overcome by arguing that environmental factors are
significant but only because individuals are (genetically) pre-
disposed to be influenced by them; but generally the problem is
overlooked. In practice psychiatry continued to stress the
importance of individual pathology (since to argue otherwise
would have led to the weakening of the medical profession's own
claims for the exclusive right to treat mental illness) but at
the same time accepted the desirability of a move towards community
care.

Labour Party policy-makers reciprocated by emphasising the
necessity of moving towards community care but at the same time,
given their deference to expert opinion and their desire not to
antagonise the medical profession, accepted the diverse nature of
mental illness. Both sides benefited from this exchange - the
medical profession gained prestige and power while the Labour
Party was able effectively to remove discussions of mental illness
from the political arena since mental illness merely became a
'social problem' which could be ameliorated; no longer was it
construed as an endemic feature of a class society which only a
socialist reconstruction of society could attempt to eradicate
in any fundamental way.

THE NATURE OF THE EVIDENCE SUPPORTING EWINS'S ANALYSIS

Ewins's argument appears to be rather programmatic (particularly
as we have presented it here, owing to limitations on space), but
it is well supported by the analysis he makes of the political
background of the Mental Treatment Act and the Mental Health Act.
He clearly demonstrates the Labour Government's role in ensuring
that there was a radical break with the principles underlying
the 1890 Lunacy Act which had been preoccupied with defending
the rights of the individual against unlawful committal to a

mental asylum. For example, the Royal Commission on Lunacy and
Mental Disorder (1924-7) had stressed the need to move towards a
medical view of mental illness but had recommended the retention
of the judicial authority in all cases of the detention of the
mentally ill. The Labour Government, however, insisted on
including a provision whereby 'non-volitional' patients (i.e.
those judged to be incapable of expressing willingness to enter
a mental hospital) could be detained on medical authority alone
for a period of six months or a year. As the Minister of Health
of the time insisted, this provision was the heart of the Bill.
But it represented the first crucial move towards removing legal
constraints on the activities of the medical profession with
regard to detaining the mentally ill.

This provision was also important to Labour Party policy-makers
since it enshrined a crucial element of their reformist thinking.
The Government therefore not only ensured that any amendment that
threatened the central provision of the Bill was defeated, but
also effectively curtailed detailed discussion of many of its
provisions by using the technique of closure motions. The Labour
Government thus achieved its aim of granting increased power to
the medical profession, but the 1930 Act was clearly transitional.
As Ewins (1974) remarks,

   at the medical level ... there was still a marked tendency to
   regard many 'lunatics' as incurable and suitable only for
   detention ... at the political level there was still substantial
   opposition to this movement away from the legalistic approach
   to the detention of the mentally ill.

By 1959 changes in therapy combined with changes in political
attitudes so that the obstacles to the general acceptance of the
medical view of mental illness were removed. The establishment
of the National Health Service in 1948 contributed to these
developments since it resulted in the first steps towards the
integration of the mental health services with the general health
services - a process that tended to reinforce the acceptance of
the medical view of mental illness.

The Mental Health Act of 1959, like the Mental Treatment Act
of 1930, was preceded by a royal commission; but whereas the
previous commission had been composed mostly of lawyers with only
two medical representatives, this one was dominated by the medical
profession. Irrespective of their political and professional
background, the members of both commissions accepted the medical
view of mental disorder, but it is nevertheless obvious that the
commissions differed significantly as far as their actual functioning was concerned. The Report of the 1957 Commission shows
that opposition to granting the medical profession increased
powers was far more muted with only five organisations submitting
evidence to the Commission supporting the retention of judicial
powers. Significantly, the Medical Practitioners Union was one
of these organisations - it was afraid that the new powers given
to the medical profession would damage the relationship between
the general practitioner and his patients. But the MPU's opposition was swamped by the evidence submitted by the more pres-
tigious medical organisations, who were entirely in favour of
increasing the power of the medical profession.

Ewins also analyses the contributions that the legal profession made to the findings of the two royal commissions. He insists that the profession as a whole did not perceive its interests to be threatened by a movement towards medical rather than judicial control of the mentally disordered because of fundamental social and political changes. He argues that (Ewins, 1974):

> while the legal profession evinced great concern for the liberty of the subject with regard to the compulsory commitment of the insane in a period dominated by the ethics of individualism and laissez-faire ... it would not oppose the movement towards extending the powers of compulsory commitment in an era of increasing state intervention and social welfare, particularly since such opposition would become increasingly futile and inimical to the interests of the profession, as consensus between the political parties with regard to social welfare (including treatment of the mentally ill) became established.

The legal members of both commissions therefore typically accepted the medical view of mental disorder. This acceptance is most clearly demonstrated by the lack of opposition to the recommendations of the 1957 Commission which removed the necessity for the automatic review of the grounds upon which patients were detained in hospitals. The requirement for automatic review was replaced by the proposal that patients should only have a right of appeal to a tribunal, since it was argued that a formal procedure might harm the welfare of a patient. The same argument was used to justify two further recommendations of the Commission concerning the functions of the tribunals. These were concerned with whether continued detention was necessary, not whether the original period of detention was justified or not. They were also to be given discretionary powers, which meant that they could decide whether proceedings were to be publicly reported, whether medical reports would be made available to the patient, or whether the reasons for particular decisions would be made available to patients and their relatives.

The 1957 Royal Commission Report (and the 1959 Mental Health Act which translated its recommendations into law) can therefore be seen as reflecting the victory of the medical profession in establishing the legitimacy of its claims to regulate the mentally disordered. But what were the full implications of this victory? Ewins's verdict is that (Ewins, 1974):

> The Report emphasised that there should be a move from hospital treatment to community care, and, implicitly recognising the limitations (and functions) of the new physical (especially chemical) methods of treatment, suggested that in future the aim should be not only to 'cure' the mental patient, but also, where this was not possible, to 'strengthen his ability to regulate his social behaviour in spite of the underlying disorder'. The Commission thus implicitly recognised that the aim and function of treatment of the mentally ill was not so much to 'cure' them but rather to return them as soon as possible to a productive and conforming role in society. This underlying view is further indicated by the Report's brief mention of the importance of integrating mental welfare services with the other social welfare services. All treatment of the

mentally disordered, it was suggested, has the aim of social
rehabilitation, either by securing the patient's adjustment to
his social environment or by improving the environment itself.
The interwoven stress of Fabian ideology, the social control
functions of psychiatry and the developments within medicine
in the direction of comprehensive care are here clearly apparent;
it was these ... which essentially ... explain the unequivocal
acceptance by the Commission of the medical view of mental
illness.

THE SIGNIFICANCE OF EWINS'S ANALYSIS

Ewins's analysis of the rise of the psychiatric profession is an
integral part of our argument, but since we have presented it
largely uncritically it is essential at this point to raise some
issues that are likely to be disputed. Ewins bases much of his
argument on Parsons's conceptualisation of the sick role, but he
clearly parts company with Parsons when discussing its political
implications. Parsons sees entry into the sick role as benign
since it enables an individual who has an illness to be assisted
in such a way that he is able to return promptly to his normal
role functions. Both Ewins and we view the sick role as more
complex - we would place greater emphasis on the latent function
of the sick role in producing stabilising effects within society.
We therefore see the sick role as providing a controllable form
of deviance which mitigates potentially disruptive conflicts
between the personal needs of individuals and the role demands
placed upon individuals by the social system.
   We are also aware that such a straightforward functionalist
argument would be frowned upon by many sociologists but we share
Waitzin and Waterman's view (1974) that such forms of argument
are necessary in order to make sense of many forms of illness
behaviour. The essence of their argument is summed up in the
following quotation:

   In many functional analyses the (so-called) 'objective consequences (of deviant behaviour) have not been especially
   objective. The labeling of behavioural patterns as functional
   frequently becomes an interpretative exercise bearing a tenuous
   relation to empirical data. To invoke Popper's famous criterion, claims of functionality often lack the attribute of
   falsifiability; they cannot be disproved by data ... any
   behavioural pattern can become the object of functional interpretation; if it were not somehow functional, it would not
   persist. The largely speculative nature of many functional
   analyses may account for the present disrepute into which
   functionalism has fallen.

Ultimately Waitzin and Waterman accept that there is no wholly
satisfactory methodological solution to this problem. They
consider their own work on the latent functions of the sick role
as 'suggestive rather than conclusive', and we would accept that
our own ideas and those of Ewins are also of this nature. So
the attraction of Ewins's work to us lies mainly in its ability
to provide a coherent explanation of the rise and power of the

psychiatric profession. But having said this, there is an important addendum that must be established. Despite acknowledging the strength of Ewins's argument, we would maintain that it is one-sided. This chapter has been concerned partly with trying to establish the process whereby the sick role was extended to encompass individuals who were considered to be mentally disordered. Such a process, which Illich would see as an example of the medicalisation of life (or problems of living), is deeply significant.

As we have already argued, society at large gains a way of controlling deviance, but equally, and this is an issue not discussed by Ewins, the individuals involved (the mentally disordered) also gain the ability to exploit the sick role for their own benefit. We would argue that these aspects of the sick role (which are generally labelled 'secondary gains') are crucial to an understanding of the behaviour of 'mentally ill patients'. The sick role itself absolves the patient from responsibility for his 'illness' and hence carries with it the implication that the patient is no longer the agency determining the therapeutic changes that occur. It is the doctor who performs this function, but in doing so he tends to engineer passivity in his patients. This passivity can of course cause immense difficulties even when entrance to the sick role is the result of physical illness, but when entry occurs as a result of mental disorder the situation becomes much more problematical.

BECOMING MENTALLY ILL

Owing to intrinsic difficulties little research attention has been paid to this issue, but on the basis of available evidence (Mechanic, 1969) it is clear that the process of becoming mentally ill (i.e. of entering the sick role on the basis of being diagnosed as mentally ill) involves crucial personal and interpersonal adjustments which are clearly of a different order. Recent work in this country by R.D. Scott (which we will explore in greater detail in a later chapter) has provided many crucial insights into these processes. Scott, perhaps more clearly than any other theorist in this country, has attempted to demonstrate that many patients are able to use their 'madness' not only to control and influence their close relatives but also to manipulate the psychiatrists, social workers and other professionals they encounter. Scott's work therefore provides a rather different picture of the psychiatrist-patient relationship. The psychiatrist certainly has great power in this relationship - powers of detention, powers of providing compulsory treatment, etc. - but it should be acknowledged that the patient is often in a position to exploit the situation to his own advantage. Moreover, this ability to exploit some features of the sick role can turn into an inability ever to leave the role. The patient becomes trapped in the role and uses his manipulative skills to maintain the status quo. Any new therapeutic initiative taken by the psychiatrist or other member of staff is dislocated and eventually negated because neither the patient nor his family can tolerate any fundamental change.

Given this view of the patient-psychiatrist relationship, it becomes possible to see the psychiatrist more as a victim of a complex series of mechanisms which enables society to 'deal' with madness. Bott (1976), in a recent article exploring the relationship between a mental hospital and the community it serves, certainly comes to this conclusion - she assumes that therapeutic initiatives are in principle very limited because patients' motivations in entering the sick role by actually entering hospital do not conform to the generally accepted view that they are seeking to get better. Part of her position is summed up in the following passage taken from her paper:

Patients do not come to a mental hospital primarily to seek treatment or help. All the treatments available in hospital are available outside it. Admission is precipitated by a social crisis in which an unbearably destructive state of affairs between the patient and his relatives is redefined as an illness in the patient such that he is not responsible for his behaviour, behaviour for which he is thought to require control and care as well as medical treatment. By agreeing to admission, the hospital doctor tacitly agrees to define the trouble as a medical problem and to accept responsibility for its control and care as well as treatment. Relatives, with the tacit support of society, use the hospital to free themselves from madness. A mad relationship, or the mad aspects of it, are localized in the patient, who is sent away to be controlled, cared for and put right.

Organically oriented psychiatrists consider that chronic hospitalization occurs because the disease process involved in madness incapacitates patients and prevents them from occupying a social place outside hospital. In the 1950s and 1960s the popular psychiatric view was that mental hospitals 'institutionalized' patients and thus incapacitated them for ordinary social life outside hospital. Scott's work and to some extent that of Goffman, Szasz, Laing and others suggests that the crucial factor in chronic hospitalization is the nature of the relationship between the patient and society, especially his relatives. If the patient and his relatives are in a violently discordant but mutually dependent relationship, the patient is likely to end up permanently in hospital. For the patient the hospital is a refuge of sorts: for the relatives it acts as a place that contains and controls the madness and its destruction of their own sense of their identity as sane. In cases in which a patient is socially isolated, particularly if his relatives die or withdraw themselves from contact with him, a patient may use the hospital as a substitute for a world in which he feels he cannot make a place for himself. In brief, chronic hospitalization occurs when a hospital place is accessible and appears to the patient to offer a more viable social place than he could find outside.

In the final analysis Bott concludes that neither society nor its health services can eliminate either the mad aspects of familial relationships or madness in individuals - all that can be hoped for is the provision of better forms of asylum for mad individuals. These would be situated in the community rather than in hospitals

since the latter produce second-order effects usually summarised
under the rubric of 'institutionalisation'.

THE SIGNIFICANCE OF BOTT'S ANALYSIS

Much of Bott's analysis seems to us intrinsically correct, but we
feel that both she and Scott fail to analyse the historical role
of psychiatry in contributing to the current position of the mental
health services. Bott in particular assumes that the changes in
the pattern of hospitalisation of mental patients since the 1930s
(i.e. a pattern of increased hospitalisation but with shorter
periods of admission) can be explained in terms of changes in
family structure and social network formation causing families to
be more prepared to seek outside professional help for personal
difficulties. She also argues that the increased receptiveness
of the public was met by the provision of new physical and social
treatments that aroused hope that mental illness would become as
treatable and therefore as ordinary as physical illness.
However, her presentation of the reasons for these changes is
strangely bland - in practice she provides no concrete evidence
for her view, but she also fails to analyse both the full implications of the widening of the sick role to include the mentally
disordered and the role of the psychiatric profession in this
process. We would therefore argue that there is both a general
lack of concreteness in her argument and a failure to analyse the
full implications of the 'medicalisation' of mental disorder.
Ironically, despite being an anthropologist by training, she fails
to consider the possible changes in the belief systems about the
mentally disordered that occurred during this period.
These criticisms serve to take us back once more to the main
line of our own argument. We would acknowledge that Ewins's
argument is one-sided and requires expansion, but we would also
insist that, in order to understand the current state of the
mental health services, it is necessary to pay close attention
to the history of the psychiatric profession - and in particular
to consider the rise of the medical model as the main explanatory
framework used by the profession. In this chapter we have already
touched on this issue, but in the following chapters we seek to
explore it in much greater depth.

Chapter 2

Conceptual frameworks
in medicine and psychiatry

Kuhn's important work on the nature of scientific revolutions
provides a valuable starting-point for a discussion of the development of conceptual frameworks in medicine and psychiatry. In his
book 'The Structure of Scientific Revolutions' Kuhn (1962) dis-
tinguishes three basic stages in the development of science - the
first of these is a 'pre-paradigm' stage, in which several theories
compete (each theory is best suited to part of the data, but none
is completely adequate). This is followed by a 'normal science'
stage, in which a single paradigm has gained wide acceptance and
provides the primary structuring of the field. The final stage
is a 'crisis' stage, in which an accepted paradigm appears inadequate and a new one replaces it. In order to illustrate these
three stages Kuhn uses the example of Newtonian physics.

Prior to Newton, the field of physics was in a pre-paradigm
stage characterised by competing theories whose inadequacies were
well recognised. Newton provided the structure, the paradigm that
superceded all existing theories and provided the basic structure
for the 'normal' work of physics for the next two hundred years.
But by the end of the nineteenth century physics found itself in
a stage of crisis, which was eventually resolved by the emergence
of a new paradigm, that provided by Einstein and Bohr.

As Kuhn has argued (1970),
substantial innovations like those made by Newton served for
a time implicitly to define the legitimate problems and methods
of a research field for succeeding generations of practitioners.
They were able to do so because they shared two essential
characteristics. Their achievement was sufficiently unprece-
dented to attract an enduring group of adherents away from
competing modes of scientific activity. Simultaneously, it
was sufficiently open-ended to leave all sorts of problems for
the re-defined group of practitioners to resolve. Achievements
that share these two characteristics I shall henceforth refer
to as 'paradigms', a term that relates closely to 'normal
science'. By choosing it, I mean to suggest that some accepted
examples of actual scientific practice - examples which include,
law, theory, application, and instrumentation together - provide
models from which spring particular coherent traditions of

scientific research.... Men whose research is based on shared
paradigms are committed to the same rules and standards for
scientific practice. That commitment and the apparent consensus
it produces are prerequisites for normal science i.e. for the
genesis and continuation of a particular research tradition.
In our opinion, Kuhn's methods of analysis can also be applied to
the history of medicine and psychiatry, although he originally
developed his approach in order to explain developments in the
natural sciences. At this point in our argument we will turn to
George Rosen's work on the developments that occurred in nineteenth-
century medicine. Rosen has demonstrated that theories about the
nature and causation of physical illness underwent considerable
changes prior to the epoch-making discoveries of bacteriologists
like Koch and Pasteur. The success of the medical bacteriologists
in understanding and eventually treating infectious diseases
resulted in the establishment of a paradigm within medicine which
stressed the importance of pathological processes within the
individual while largely ignoring the social and economic factors
that inevitably influenced disease processes.

ROSEN'S ANALYSIS OF NINETEENTH-CENTURY MEDICINE

Rosen's approach is particularly important for our discussion
since he explores the impact of social and political changes on
the development of both medicine and the profession of medicine.
Significantly, he pays close attention to the impact of the
French Revolution on the development of the medical profession
in France and Germany. He sees the Revolution (Rosen, 1946)
   [as implanting] ideas of public service, public interest and
   social utility which provided the seedbed in which germinated
   views of the relation among health, medicine and society. The
   men of 1789 and 1793 could not foresee the consequences of
   their thoughts and acts. The triumph of the machine and the
   concentration of capital were still in the future, but it was
   in terms of the situation created by these developments that
   the men of 1848 endeavoured to apply the ideas of their pre-
   decessors. Social medicine, the idea of 1848, must be seen as
   the fruit of this historical process.
Rosen argues that the rapid industrialisation and urbanisation that
occurred in France between 1830 and 1870 imposed a series of
economic and social stresses that influenced the evolution of
French thought and action very profoundly. During this period
an energetic group of physicians and hygienists had been carrying
out surveys and statistical studies of living conditions among
workers in urban communities. Practical experience acquired during
the Revolutionary and Napoleonic Wars had made many French physicians alert to health problems. At the same time, political and
social theorists, such as Fourier, Saint-Simon, Comte, Proudhon
and many others, influenced French medicine, so that certain
sections of it were fermented with a spirit of social change.
Many doctors were in direct contact with the social realities of
indistrialisation and the profound effects it had on the lives
of the working class.

In 1838 Rochoux coined the term 'social hygiene' to describe a
category of social policy that would be concerned with establishing
a legal and administrative framework for providing minimum health
standards. Ten years later, at the height of the 1848 Revolution,
Guerin appealed to the French medical profession to develop a
social medicine that would enable the profession to contribute to
the good of society. According to Rosen, Guerin divided his social
medicine into four parts: social physiology, social pathology,
social hygiene and social therapy. These were to deal, respectively, with the relation between the physical and mental condition
of a population and its laws or other institutions; the study of
social problems in relation to health and disease; measures for
health promotion and disease prevention; and the provision of
medical and other measures to deal with social disintegration and
other conditions that societies may experience.

Guerin's idea of social medicine obviously awarded the medical
profession a key role in running society. Throughout Europe, the
profession was struggling to establish itself as a unified entity
(with uniform training and uniform payment for the services it
rendered) which would be able to provide more and better care for
the majority of the population. It is therefore not surprising
that the first proposals for a national medical service also began
to emerge in this period. But what became of this movement within
medicine?

In France the period of political reaction following the failure
of the 1848 revolution put paid to such proposals. Some German
physicians, such as Neumann, Virchow and Leubuscher, were profoundly influenced by the theories of social medicine in France.
In 1847 Neumann had issued a manifesto arguing that 'medical science
is intrinsically and essentially a social science, and as long as
this is not recognised in practice we shall have to be satisfied
with an empty shell and a sham'. Virchow formulated the idea
somewhat differently, stating that 'medicine is a social science
and politics nothing but medicine on a grand scale'. But, as
Rosen points out, the proponents of such ideas were not dreaming
of some utopian situation; they utilised their approach to formulate
definite principles from which a programme of action could be
derived. The exact details of such programmes are not our concern
here, but it is obvious that such physicians saw the task of
medicine in a much broader light than their biologically and
pathologically orientated colleagues.

THE FAILURE OF SOCIAL MEDICINE

The attempt of these men to turn medicine in a sociological and
preventative direction was abortive, since the failure of the
revolution in Germany created a political climate that was hostile
to social medicine. At the same time developments in other scientific disciplines (especially biology and physics) began to influence the future development of medicine. As Rosen (1946)
comments,

   The natural sciences developed rapidly and achieved enormous
   prestige in medicine, and the emergence of medical bacteriology

seemed to answer the problem of disease causation. Under these
conditions it was not difficult to overlook the significance of
the relationship between the patient and his environment.
As Emil Behring declared in 1893, the study of infectious diseases
could now be pursued unswervingly without being sidetracked by
social considerations and reflections on social policy.

Rosen's discussion of the developments within medicine concentrate mainly on France and Germany, but he does point out that
there were some developments towards an idea of social medicine in
Britain, although these were a pale imitation of the developments
on the Continent. Continental and British medicine became more
unified in their development precisely because of the successes
of medical bacteriology. It is important to stress that, as medicine became more scientific, more concerned with measurement and
classification, it became less humanistic and tended to treat the
patient as an object. Illich in his book 'Medical Nemesis' (1975)
has graphically argued this point. 'As the doctor's interest
shifted from the sick to sickness, the hospital became a museum
of sickness. The wards were full of indigent people who offered
their bodies as spectacles to any physician willing to treat them.'

ON THE HISTORY OF CLINICAL HISTORY-TAKING

In the same period, as Riese (1944) has shown, a basic shift
occurred in the way that medical case histories were taken. In
the Hippocratic tradition a clinical history was a history of a
human being who suffered and who had symptoms, but the type of
clinical history-taking that emerged in the second half of the
nineteenth century was very different. As pathology developed
as a science, doctors became more and more preoccupied with establishing the history of a particular disease process (historia
morbi). The individual, his social relations and his problems of
living, faded into insignificance when the doctor's concentration
was focused upon the symptoms and their bodily manifestations.

Illich has argued that this process became all the more powerful
and irresistible as the medical profession was able to develop
effective cures for a wide range of diseases. As a result of their
very real power, the medical profession increasingly gained control
over defining what is illness and what is health. Illich (1975)
argues therefore that
[there can be no solution to the present crisis in providing
health care without] a critical, scientifically sound, de-
medicalisation of the concept of disease. Medical epistemology
is much more important for the healthy solution of this crisis
than either medical biology or medical technology. Such an
epistemology will have to clarify the logical status and the
social nature of diagnosis and therapy, primarily in physical -
as opposed to medical - sickness. All disease is a socially
created reality. What it means and the response it evokes
have a history. The study of this history can enable us to
understand the degree to which we are prisoners of the medical
ideology in which we were brought up.

MEDICINE AND THE NATURAL SCIENCES

From the late nineteenth century onwards medicine increasingly
modelled itself on the natural sciences. It became progressively
more 'scientific', losing itself in discoveries in pathology,
physiology, bacteriology and biochemistry. The paradigm it adopted
was therefore a mechanistic one which ensured that medicine became
orientated towards attempting to correct individual pathology
rather than concentrating on changing the economic and social
factors that fundamentally influence illness and health. During
this period psychiatry became increasingly reductionist in its
approach to mental disorder, although earlier in the century
broader, more psychological and sociological approaches had been
in vogue. The minutiae of the so-called 'moral' treatment approach
have been explored by a number of previous researchers, but the
importance of this type of approach to our argument is immediately
obvious. When medicine became increasingly based on such natural
sciences as pathology and bacteriology, it can be assumed that it
entered Kuhn's 'normal science' phase. It became preoccupied with
processes within the individual and therefore considered processes
external to the individual as illegitimate or irrelevant to its
purposes. This holistic approach to the individual was considered
mystifying and antiquated.

MORAL TREATMENT

The moral treatment approach owed much more to older holistic
traditions in medicine since it was intimately concerned with the
relationship between the individual and his environment. It
developed in a different historical period. As Caplan (1969) has
pointed out, at the end of the eighteenth century a number of
factors had contributed to the formation of a new consensus concerning the nature of mental disorders. George III's insanity
gave rise to a rash of parliamentary inquiries which were widely
publicised. Fashionable doctors began to take an interest in
psychiatric cases, while a series of investigations documented
conditions of shocking abuse. The revolutionary events in France
also played a role in changing public attitudes. In September
1793 Pinel was appointed superintendent at the Bicetre Hospital
in Paris and within a few days of his appointment he had carried
out his famous act of liberating patients from their forest of
manacles. He owed his appointment to a group of newly influencial
philosophers and politicians which included Cabanis. Cabanis, a
doctor by training, was responsible for popularising the work of
de Condillac. The latter's philosophy was given the name of
'ideology' by its followers. Its starting point was the two major
premises that, first, sensations are the primary data of cognition
and that, second, all ideas and all faculties of human understanding are compounds of sensations that may be resolved by
analysis into their component parts. Experience was seen as the
basis for the formation and generation of ideas which were simply
representations of objects. This notion was identical with Locke's
conception of the brain as a tabula rasa which became etched with

life experiences, and it obviously had crucial implications for
the treatment of the mentally disordered.

As Caplan (1969) has argued,

the brain's outstanding characteristic was thought to be its
extreme sensitivity to environmental and somatic stimuli. Its
surface was thought to be highly malleable and in its convo-
lutions all powerful or habitual experiences, thought or
feelings became etched. What we would now consider psychological
forces were then felt to have a direct physical effect.

From birth onwards the brain was assumed to be susceptible to the
effects of all the sense impressions and emotions it encountered,
although it also had inherited tendencies to weakness or strength.
These latter hereditary tendencies could be modified by the effects
of education and experience so that features of the personality
might develop while others were overshadowed, just as the body's
natural propensities could be modified by exercise and diet. Thus
education, habits of thought, emotions, as well as traits and
general ways of living, could mould the structure of the brain and
hence determine the way an individual behaved.

These ideas led directly to particular notions about the nature
of treatments to be applied to the mentally disordered. Caplan
(1969) points out that:

The essence of moral treatment was the belief that because of
the great malleability of the brain's surface, because of its
susceptibility to environmental stimuli, pathological conditions
could be erased or modified by corrective experience. Therefore,
insanity, whether the result of direct or indirect injury or
disease, or of overwrought emotions or strained intellectual
faculties, would be cured in almost every case.

Two further crucial concepts contributed to the optimism of the
moral treatment approach. Firstly, under the influence of the
phrenologists, it was believed that the mind was divided into a
number of compartments, each controlling a faculty such as memory,
imagination, will, or even the sense of the divine. Damage to the
brain would affect only one or two of these faculties in most
cases, leaving the rest of the brain unharmed. The prevalent
notion of total insanity was therefore replaced by a far more
optimistic conception of monomania, or partial insanity. The
second source of optimism derived from the basic dualism adopted
by the practitioners of moral treatment. They believed that
intelligence, an attribute of the spiritual mind, would remain
unimpaired in spite of a diseased brain. So if the physical damage
could be repaired through appropriate treatment, intelligence could
be expected to re-emerge unscathed. In practice, this optimistic
view was modified by considering whether a given patient's illness
was a new one or a reoccurence of a pre-existing one. It was
assumed that in some cases damage had indeed become irreversible,
so asylum superintendents were careful to distinguish chronic from
acute cases.

The essence of the moral treatment era is well summarised by
Caplan (1969) in the following passage:

The belief that social and physical environments were critical
factors in moulding the surface of the brain and hence in
determining the individual's state of mental health or illness,

had far-reaching implications for prevention and care of
insanity, because it brought a major area of etiology within
reach of possible control and modification.

In practice this meant that the asylum superintendents were concerned with controlling facets of both extramural and institutional
life in order to ensure optimal conditions both for the prevention
and the early and rapid treatment of mental disorder.

The exact extent of the movement towards such methods of treatment is difficult to establish. In Britain, as Jones (1972) has
indicated, moral treatment is generally associated with the names
of Tuke (at the York Retreat), Charlesworth and Gardiner Hill (at
the Lincoln Asylum) and Connolly (at the Hanwell Asylum). Apart
from their general emphasis on attempting to avoid mechanically
constraining their patients, their approach to treatment was
essentially humanistic. They tended to avoid using the contemporary medical methods of treatment (bleeding, purging, spirates,
etc.) and relied more on education and occupational therapy as
means of rehabilitating their patients. Their approach assumed
that mental disorders were mostly curable and hence they created
a climate of opinion counteracting pessimistic popular conceptions
of insanity. Whether their methods actually were effective is
very difficult to establish as Bockoven (1956) has stressed, but
there is a crucial contrast between their viewpoint and the view
that emerged later in the century as psychiatry began to be
influenced more and more by the changes in medicine associated
with the development of bacteriology and pathology as powerful
new disciplines.

MENTAL DISORDER REDEFINED AS DISEASE

As Musto (1970) has pointed out,
   [a] new organic model of illness and function ... became over-
   applied ... psychiatry suffered most unfortunate effects.
   Mental illness and behavioural abnormality came to be considered an organic derangement of the brain. This led to
   therapeutic pessimism ... it also caused the virtual elimination
   of lay leadership. To understand the prevailing view of mental
   illness one had to have medical training and, when one was
   trained, the folly of cure by mere encouragement became obvious.
   There was no room for the layman in this new pathology of the
   mind.

Kraepelin's monumental work seeking to provide an all-embracing
classification of mental diseases was then published. This
endeavour owed its heritage to Linnaeus's attempt to provide a
definitive classification not only of plants and animals but also
of psychiatric cases. But as we have already noted, the most
crucial development occurred as a result of the painstaking work
that eventually resulted in the unravelling of the nature of
syphilis and general paresis of the insane.

MENTAL ILLNESS AND THE SURVIVAL OF THE FITTEST

Such discoveries were instrumental in establishing a paradigm of
mental disorder that insisted that mental disorders were strictly
comparable with physical illnesses. From 1860 onwards Darwin's
ideas concerning natural selection had begun to have a general
impact. Hofstadter (1965), in his book on social Darwinism, has
documented the role of British sociologists such as Spencer in
applying Darwinian ideas to human society, but there was a parallel
development in medicine, since notions of racial fitness and unfit-
ness became linked with the issue of susceptibility to disease.
     As an example of this approach it is worth citing a presidential
address to the British Medical Association given by Sir James Barr
in 1912. The address contained the following passage:
     If we could only abolish the tubercle bacillus in these islands
     we would get rid of tuberculosis disease but we should at the
     same time raise up a race peculiarly susceptible to this
     infection - a race of hothouse plants which would not flourish
     in any other environment. We would thus increase at an even
     greater rate than we are doing at present, nervous instability,
     the numbers of insane and feeble-minded. Nature, on the other
     hand, weeds out those who have not got the innate power of
     recovery from disease and by means of the tubercle bacillus
     and other pathogenic organisms she frequently does this before
     the reproductive age, so that a check is put on the multi-
     plication of idiots and the feeble-minded. Nature's methods
     are thus of advantage to the race rather than to the individual.
Ideas about mental subnormality and psychopathy were similarly
influenced by Darwinian ideas. Tredgold's famous 'Textbook of
Mental Deficiency', which was first published in 1908, contains
some bizarre examples of the extremes to which such thinking can
be carried. The following purple passage is to be found, still
unrevised, in the seventh edition of the book published in 1947
(Bury, 1974):
     Unfortunately, psychopaths (i.e. those 'stocks' which breed the
     'bulk of the inefficient members of the community') also inter-
     marry with the sound and normal members of the community. In
     so doing they drag fresh blood into the vortex of the disease
     and it is this which keeps the process alive, and which dilutes
     and reduces the aggregate mental vigour, stamina and efficiency
     of the nation. The immediate cause of a nation's downfall may
     be some violent social upheaval or political incapacity; but
     these, as has happened in past history, may well be the result
     of the mental instability and degeneracy of its people. As has
     been well said a nation has the government it deserves.
Tredgold's extreme views cannot be dismissed as idiosyncratic -
rather the reverse, for if the psychiatric textbooks of this
period are examined they show similar biases. For example,
Henderson and Gillespie's (1927) influential 'Textbook of
Psychiatry' (which we have already referred to) approvingly cites
Tredgold's work in the course of arguing much the same point:
     the consequence of this i.e. birth control is that the really
     better-class population are tending to diminish, and more and
     more the unruly element tends to increase ... the unfit, the

unstable, are tending slowly but surely to supplant those on
whom in the past the British nation has largely had to depend.
It is the influence on the general birth rate that which seems of
such importance, because, as Tredgold has pointed out, 'the nation
which advises birth control is soon likely to be overwhelmed by
those other nations who continue to propagate' (Henderson and
Gillespie, 1927).

THE PROBLEM OF ECLECTICISM

An analysis of the contents of Henderson and Gillespie's (1927)
book is revealing since above all it demonstrates the lack of
consistent theory in the psychiatry of this period. There are
detailed discussions of symptomatology and the classification of
illnesses, and yet sections of the book dealing with specific
forms of mental disorder and general discussions of psychopathology
are obviously influenced by psychoanalytic ideas. The book therefore has the appearance of being eclectic, and yet there is an
underlying assumption that mental disorders are in fact forms of
illness.

Henderson and Gillespie's views were very similar to those of
other leading psychiatrists, including J.R. Lord, the editor of
the 'Journal of Mental Science'. In 1926 Lord's presidential
address to the Royal Medico-Psychological Association was considered important enough to be published in book form (Lord, 1926).
In his address he attempted to outline the recent developments
that had occurred in psychiatry and related sciences, such as
psychology and physiology. In the final analysis he too adopts a
reductionist position, as the following quotation demonstrates:
    Though the physiological and psychological viewpoints, however
    much harmonised, will always be necessary to a clinical under-
    standing of mental disorders, they are in a sense only means
    to an end - which is to establish psychiatry if possible on
    the firm basis of pathology, which is fundamental to all medical
    services. Freud recognised this when he stated that 'The
    edifice of psychoanalytic doctrine which we have erected is in
    reality but a superstructure which will have to be set on its
    organic foundation at some time or other.' (Introductory
    Lectures on Psychoanalysis, 1922)
Admittedly, Lord argues that both the 'physiogenic' and the 'psycho-
genic' schools should continue their work independently, but nevertheless he supports the basic assumption that pathological and
organic explanations are of primary importance.

THE PROBLEM OF THE PERSISTENCE OF REDUCTIONIST APPROACHES

The position adopted by Henderson and Gillespie and by Lord was
not as extreme as some other psychiatrists. As Russell Davis
(1970) has pointed out, many of the textbooks published subsequently
in the 1940s and 1950s were far more limited in their conceptualisation than earlier books. For example, Sargant and Slater's
book, 'An Introduction to Physical Methods of Treatment in

Psychiatry' (first published in 1944), reflects the swing towards faulty-machine models that occurred as the physical treatments caught the attention of the psychiatric profession. Significantly, the frontispiece of the book consists of the following quotation from Henry Maudsley:

the observation and classification of mental disorders have been so exclusively psychological that we have not sincerely realized the fact that they illustrate the same pathological principles as other diseases, are produced in the same way, and must be investigated in the same spirit of positive research.

The extreme reductionism of this position is naturally reflected in the book itself. For Sargant, psychiatry is a branch of medicine and its appropriate methods of treatment are physical and bio-chemical ones. It is therefore particularly apt that the publishers of the fifth edition of the textbook should elect to use the one word 'psychiatry' as the summary title that is entered on the book's spine.

Mayer-Gross monolithic tome 'Clinical Psychiatry' (first pub-lished in 1954) is an example of the same genre (Mayer-Gross et al., 1954). This influential book is, in fact, conceptually more limited than Henderson and Gillespie's. It pays less attention to psychological and sociological factors, stressing instead the importance of hereditary, biological and neurophysiological factors in the causation of mental disorders.

The dominating role of this type of approach can also be illus-trated by examining the type of research papers that appeared in the 'Journal of Mental Science' from the 1920s onwards. An approx-imate content analysis of the journal can be established by looking at the cumulative indexes for the journal covering the years 1923-34 and 1935-49. The journal in the first period is dominated by papers concerned with symptomatology, and with the pathological, physiological and biochemical changes occurring in the course of mental illness. One of the largest sections of papers is concerned with the cerebro-spinal fluid, and there is also a large section on the use of chemical treatments, especially for syphilis. In comparison with the wealth of papers on these topics, the sections on the psychological aspects of mental disorders, psychotherapy and psychoanalysis are very weak. Sociological topics receive scant attention, and there is virtually no discussion of important issues as to early treatment of patients or the functioning of outpatient clinics. Interestingly, and as Ewins would predict, there are a comparatively large number of papers concerned with occupational therapy. The later index shows that this trend is continued, with stress being given to medically orientated approaches to mental disorders.

It is important to stress that the psychiatric establishment still adheres to the medical model. In 1973 the newly founded Royal College of Psychiatrists submitted a memorandum to the Department of Health expressing their views on the possible role of the psychological services in the Health Service. The memo-randum contained the following unequivocal statement defending the medical model (Rachman and Philips, 1975):

It is recognised that there is a school of thought which denies the concept of mental illness and considers that the symptoms

hitherto classified as mental illness, mental disorder, tensions,
psychosis, personality disorders etc. should be regarded as
psychological behavioural maladjustments and should be treated
outside the medical ambit. These views are not acceptable to
the College.

The Royal College's statement did produce protests from some
sections of the profession, but the medical model still dominates
the thinking of most psychiatrists. For example the stuffy tones
of the Royal College are strangely echoed in Anthony Clare's
widely publicised book, 'Psychiatry in Dissent' (Clare, 1976).
Clare's argument in favour of the medical model is more sophisticated, but it ends with the same conclusion that only medically
trained practitioners should be responsible for the treatment of
the mentally disordered. In his book Clare is concerned to demolish
other models of mental disorder and he focuses his attention on
what he terms the 'organic orientation', 'the psychotherapeutic
orientation' and 'the sociotherapeutic orientation'. The organic
orientation (Davis's faulty-machine model) has already been discussed by us and Clare attacks it in much the same way, but his
presentation of the psychotherapeutic orientation is decidedly
idiosyncratic. To begin with, it starts with the singular pro-
nouncement that 'it is not entirely accurate to equate the position
adopted by ... Thomas Szasz with the "psychotherapeutic" view of
mental illness'. But having made the statement, he then proceeds
to attack Szazs's position in great detail and avoids discussing
the work of any other major therapist. His presentation of the
sociotherapeutic approach is equally selective as he fails again
to deal with major theorists such as Maxwell Jones.

But the most problematic part of his argument is reserved for
his presentation of the medical model, which is slipped into the
discussion in an almost absentminded way. In his own words (Clare,
1976),

I have made no mention of the so-called 'medical model'. It is
often erroneously believed that this model and the 'organic'
orientation ... are synonymous. The medical model is an evol-
ving one in which scientific methods of observation, description,
and differentiation are employed, in which an illness is concep-
tualized as 'a process that moves from the recognition and
palliation of symptoms to the characterization of a specific
disease in which the etiology and pathogenesis are known and
the treatment is rational and specific'. Such a process may
take years, centuries even, and while many medical conditions
have moved to the final stages of such understanding, others
are still at various points along the way.

This definition is, of course, very traditional and is in no way
distinguishable from Lord's which we have already quoted. But
Clare adds a rider to his definition which serves only to illustrate just how vague the medical model is. His alternative
presentation is as follows:

The medical model does not envisage disease as something which
'happens' to a person independently of any action he may take.
... Medical diseases do not exist independently of the people
who are sick. The medical model, in short, takes into account
not merely the symptom, syndrome, or disease, but the person

who suffers, his personal and social situation, his biological,
psychological, and social status. The medical model, as applied
to psychiatry, embodies the basic principle that every illness
is the product of two factors - of environment working on the
organism.
This portmanteau type of model seeks to embrace all other theoretical positions. Reading between the lines of Clare's argument,
one can see that his model can overarch all other approaches. As
he says himself, 'it can be seen that the variety of ideological
positions within psychiatry, the biological, the dynamic, the
social, the behavioural, represent different emphases.' But Clare
insists that if psychiatry is to progress psychiatrists must continue to be eclectic. They must avoid giving their allegiance to
any one model and avoid being dogmatic.
     At the same time, however, it is clear from Clare's argument
that he feels that only a suitably trained psychiatrist is capable
of taking responsibility for the treatment of the mentally disordered. He never in fact spells this out in so many words, but
when he comes to discuss the anatomy of the ideal psychiatrist he
is really discussing the anatomy of the type of professional who
can be expected to take responsibility for the treatment of the
mentally disordered.
     Clare's ideal psychiatrist is a paragon of virtue and knowledge
since he combines
     scientific attitudes of the sceptic with a powerful impressive
     personality and a profound existential faith sic . He is
     someone with a solid foundation in medicine, the biological and
     behavioural sciences, who is able to cope with the intellectual
     isolation implicit in such a critical eclecticism.
Whether such a paragon could possibly exist is an open question.
What Clare's work represents is yet another attempt to justify
the hegemony of the medical profession. Clare therefore stands
four-square with the psychiatric establishment which insists that
the medical model is the only legitimate model for understanding
and treating the mentally disordered. All other professions are
incapable of working within the model because they lack medical
training - their role must therefore be ancillary.
     Clare's position is strangely confirmed by a singular omission
in his final chapter on the psychiatric services. In reviewing
these he discusses the role of the psychiatric social worker and
the general practitioner, but he fails to pay any attention to the
role of clinical psychologists. And yet elsewhere in his book he
reviewed Eysenck's famous manifesto which insists that psychiatrists should concentrate on treating mental illnesses (i.e. disorders of known organic causation) leaving psychologists free to
treat all other forms of disorder (Eysenck, 1975).
     We would insist, in clear opposition to Clare, that clients
(patients in his terms) should be approached, as a matter of principle, within what we would call a psychotherapeutic mode. No
matter how organically 'damaged' clients may be, they are human
beings first and it is the task of the therapist to relate to
them precisely as human beings. To do otherwise is to relate to
them in other - perhaps inhuman - ways. The doctor-scientist who
relates to his patients as though they were objects or just excuses

for further journal reports is well documented by sociological
research, but such relationships are to be seen as evidence of
the potentially alienating effects of operating the medical model.
The doctor becomes alienated because the model allows him to avoid
examining himself - he remains the scientist, the diagnostician or
the master-detective who finds out what's wrong with the patient,
and then sets about correcting it. The patient's role, needless
to say, is characterised by passivity and dependence.

We would argue that a psychotherapeutic approach can avoid the
pitfalls of the medical approach precisely by insisting that the
therapist must operate within a self-reflexive framework which
enables him to understand the contribution that he makes to the
personal interactions in which he is involved. He must also treat
his client as an equal - as somebody who also strives to make sense
of his own world and his own behaviour. The medical model inevitably carries with it a set of assumptions about patients that is
hostile to psychotherapeutic approaches.

We will return to some of these issues in greater detail in our
final chapter, but it is necessary to return to the main theme of
our argument. This point involves a detailed examination of the
forms of therapy that played a crucial role in expanding and con-
firming the hegemony of the psychiatric profession.

Chapter 3

An evaluation of physical and pharmacological treatments in psychiatry

Several new forms of treatment were introduced in the decade following the 1930 Mental Treatment Act, but it is important to realise that these treatments took place predominantly in the old asylums (now renamed mental hospitals). The conditions within these 'hospitals' gradually improved, but in practice they remained largely custodial in their functioning although there was a tendency to separate acute and chronic patients by building villas in the grounds of the hospitals. Jones (1972) argues that two new hospitals (Runwell and the new Bethlem Hospital at Beckenham) were specifically built to incorporate the ideas embodied in the Act; but in fact several other hospitals (such as Barrow Gurney near Bristol and Cefn Coed near Cardiff) were also built in this period. It remains true, however, that the vast majority of patients received treatment in the older established hospitals, although many of them passed through a system of observation wards which were situated either in the workhouses or in the general hospitals. Such wards generally did not undertake treatment but were more concerned with diagnosis and establishing whether patients required court orders for transfer to the mental hospitals. Outpatient clinics were also developed in this period in an effort to avoid the necessity for hospitalising patients.

LIFE IN THE MENTAL HOSPITALS (1920-40)

Before the introduction of the new methods life in the mental hospitals remained remarkably unchanging. Jones, despite the comprehensiveness of her book, gives her readers little insight into details of everyday life in such settings. Fortunately Clark (1964) in his book on administrative therapy has provided us with a graphic picture of the day-to-day activities of the patients and staff in the ex-asylums. The picture he paints is a complex one, as the following quotation demonstrates.

> These hospitals were not always inefficient or unhappy places; the asylum cricket team was often famous, or the doctors' shooting parties; many of the better patients were well adjusted to a life of contented servitude, working as orderlies, storemen,

or domestic servants in a cosier world than that outside. Among
the younger doctors, too, there were those of energy and endeavour who conducted researches - innumerable post-mortems,
or biochemical assays - or who made massive therapeutic on-
slaughts on the inert mass of misery confronting them, removing
tonsils wholesale, or liberally dispensing thyroid extract ...
there were of course many vigorous, enthusiastic psychiatrists
in the 1920s and 1930s but their energy found its scope outside
the mental hospitals. They left to work in outpatient clinics,
or in private practice, following the exciting new developments
in psychotherapy, in psychoanalysis or the physical treatments,
for it was here that the future seemed to lie.

Needless to say in the mental hospitals the traditional medical
model was accepted. The doctor carried out a 'mental examination'
of the newly admitted patient; he made a diagnosis; he prescribed
treatment; and the nurses and attendants carried it out. The
doctor's attitude towards the hundreds of 'chronic patients' was
one of resignation. They were seen as suffering from incurable
psychoses, mostly hereditary, and it was assumed that there was
little chance of their ever leaving hospital. The duty of the
hospital and the doctor was, therefore, to provide them with humane
custody. However, as Clark (1964) points out, the relationship
between the staff and patients took many varied forms.

Toward some of them, attachment, even friendship, could be
developed; these were the quiet melancholics and paraphrenics
who looked after the doctor's children or cultivated his garden;
a joking relationship was comfortable with some of the deluded
who would report each morning on the state of their influencing
machines; but with many - the 'flexibilitas' cases who stood
statue-like in a puddle of their own urine for days, weeks, and
years on end; the catatonics with their wild outbursts of
dangerous violence; the 'caution' patients who were forever
attempting bizarre self-mutilation - little contact was possible
and the doctor could only attempt to limit the physical damage
to the patient and to those about him. A certain amount of
personal danger and of involvement in degradation and brutality
were accepted as inevitable if regrettable aspects of mental
hospital work.

Clark argues that the doctor who devoted his life to working in a
mental hospital therefore faced a dilemma. Since the majority of
patients were chronic cases with little apparent hope of rehabilitation, he had to accept many features of custodial care - strait-
jackets, padded cells, forced feeding, etc. - and yet these conflicted with his image of himself as benign healer. Given the
entrenched nature of staff attitudes and the dead weight of
tradition, little change could be initiated even when ther was
a will to do so. The most able and sensitive doctors either left
the hospital and went into private practice or became the type of
medical superintendent who interested himself in committee work,
hospital administration or specialist topics such as forensic
psychiatry.

THE IMPACT OF THE NEW TREATMENTS

What then happened to change these backwaters? Clark (1964) makes
no mention of the Mental Health Treatment Act, but he does insist
that:

> the first break into this static world came with the physical
> treatments - insulin coma therapy in the mid 1930s, convulsion
> therapy, first with cardiazol and then with electroshock, in
> the early 1940s. These treatments made a tremendous change in
> the atmosphere of the hospitals. The doctors, the nurses, and
> the attendants could all feel they were really doing something;
> many patients made dramatic recoveries from years of withdrawal.
> A wind of enthusiasm - which at times rose to a tornado of furor
> therapeuticus - swept through the hospitals.

Clark probably overestimates the significance of these new treatments, but nevertheless he is acutely aware of the paradoxical
basis upon which the new treatments actually worked. He pays
special attention to insulin coma therapy, which was introduced
by Sakel in 1935 and which became rapidly adopted as a treatment
for schizophrenics (Clark, 1964):

> Many chronically ill patients, given up as hopeless, made
> dramatic recoveries; many acutely ill patients recovered far
> quicker than was expected. Because it was a dangerous and
> occasionally fatal treatment, a well-organised and highly
> trained staff team was necessary. Many hospitals set up an
> 'insulin unit'; because this was often the most exciting and
> rewarding section of the hospital, it attracted the keen, eager,
> well-qualified young doctors, nurses, and attendants. They
> formed tightly knit teams, working together through crises and
> long dramas of life-saving so that they came to know and trust
> one another as colleagues and comrades. The patients were
> mostly young schizophrenics with changing symptomatology; though
> often very disturbed, they were accessible and emotionally open,
> so that warm relationships sprang up. To a visitor it was
> striking how different the relationships in a good insulin unit
> were from the rest of the hospital. The staff were on easy,
> confident terms with one another, with private jokes and a
> special jargon; the patients were spoken to warmly by their
> Christian names, spoon-fed, and encouraged; all played games
> together in the afternoon, patients, nurses and even doctors.
> But little of this was mentioned in the publications, which
> still discussed varieties of insulin, dosages, potentiators,
> frequency and depth of comas, symptomatic prognosticators, and
> such individual, unemotional 'objective' considerations.

Clark's discussion is particularly important for our argument since
it introduces a dimension that is normally neglected. New treatments are usually examined in very prescribed terms so that there
is no attempt to evaluate the nature of the context or milieu in
which they are utilised. Clark himself is a representative of a
small but influential group of British psychiatrists who attempted
to develop hospitals as carefully structured therapeutic communities. The most famous member of this group is, of course,
Maxwell Jones, whose original work at the Belmont Hospital is
internationally known, but a number of other psychiatrists at

other hospitals such as Claybury (in Essex) and Fulbourn (in
Cambridge) were also pioneers. The development of milieu therapy
in Britain has been very limited, however, because the approach
challenges so many entrenched ideas within the medical profession.
Staff involvement in such settings is far deeper and more complex
than in traditional settings, and several studies have demonstrated
that the staff necessarily have to endure much greater stress as
they can no longer distance themselves from the patients.

It is not our concern to discuss the intricacies of milieu
therapy here, but it is important in terms of our argument to note
that there is a considerable body of research that indicates that
changes in the administration and hence in the day-to-day running
of hospital wards can have profound effects on the behaviour of
patients. This point takes us back to Clark's argument concerning
insulin coma therapy, since it is essential to establish what
features of the therapeutic regime were actually crucial in producing changes in the patients' behaviour.

THE EFFECTIVENESS OF INSULIN COMA THERAPY

In fact, a properly controlled study of the effectiveness of
insulin coma therapy was not undertaken until roughly twenty years
after the treatment was first introduced, when Ackner, Harris and
Oldham (1957) demonstrated that insulin was not the effective agent
in causing therapeutic change. Their study entirely vindicated the
criticism put forward in 1953 by a junior psychiatrist, Bourne
(1953), who had the temerity to question the effectiveness of the
treatment. The psychiatric establishment had duly attacked
Bourne's criticisms only to lose face when the results of Ackner's
study were published four years later.

The history of insulin coma therapy is even more bizarre than
Clark allows. The use of insulin in treating mental disorders is
a classic example of medical pragmatism. Medical practitioners
have always shown a keen interest in applying any newly developed
drug to all types of medical conditions. In 1922 Banting, Best
and MacLeod isolated insulin for the first time. Its successful
use in controlling diabetes made a major impact in medical circles.
Since insulin was known to stimulate appetite (by reducing the
amount of circulating blood sugars), it was often used to stimulate
appetite in patients with chronic physical and mental illnesses.
Several physicians (Steck in Switzerland, Munn in America and
Haack in Germany) noticed that insulin had beneficial effects on
the mood of agitated psychotic patients, but it was Sakel who was
responsible for introducing its systematic use with psychotics.
According to Alexander and Selesnick (1967), Sakel developed his
ideas concerning the importance of insulin as a result of his
experiences with treating morphine addicts in a Berlin hospital.
During their withdrawal from the drug the addicts became highly
excited, so Sakel attempted to counteract this tendency by using
insulin.

Sakel argued that the excitement was due to over-activity of
the adrenal-thyroid endocrine system, which in turn caused increased
activity throughout the sympathetic nervous system. Insulin was

assumed to counteract this process but it took high doses to
produce any effects. Eventually Sakel used such high doses that
his patients became comatose. Undeterred by the life-threatening
aspects of his treatment, Sakel emphasised the beneficial effects
that it produced with schizophrenic patients. His report, which
first appeared in 1933, caused widespread interest in psychiatric
circles, and the treatment became widely established throughout
Europe and America by the end of the 1930s despite adverse criticism from some psychiatrists who attacked the vagueness of his
theoretical rationale for the treatment. Because of its dangers,
unreliable results and high cost (because of the necessity of
providing highly trained staff capable of dealing with the sort
of medical emergencies that the treatment involved), it began to
become unfashionable from the late 1940s onwards. However, it
should be noted that its decline was not because of any definitive
evaluation of its efficacy. In practice, it declined because
another form of shock treatment devised by Meduna began to super-
cede it.

OTHER FORMS OF SHOCK TREATMENT

Meduna was originally interested in epilepsy, but as a result of
carrying out autopsies on the brains of epileptics he believed he
had discovered that they had become abnormally thickened. A comparative study of the brains of deceased schizophrenics revealed
that their glial tissue was atrophied. On the basis of these
findings (which were not confirmed by subsequent more carefully
executed studies) and erroneous epidemiological reports that
schizophrenics rarely, if ever, suffer from epilepsy, Meduna
insisted that schizophrenia and epilepsy must be incompatible
diseases and that a convulsive agent administered to schizophrenics
would therefore be therapeutic. In fact, as Alexander and Selesnick
(1967) point out, he showed no originality in suggesting that convulsive agents should be used in treating mental disorder, and the
particular drug he first used - camphor - had also been used by
doctors in the eighteenth and nineteenth centuries. In 1933 he
began his experiments, first using camphor and then Metrazol
(Cadiazol), a less toxic synthetic camphor preparation. In practice, Metrazol had several shortcomings, among them an unpredictable
time lag between the injection of the drug and the onset of the
convulsion. During this latency period the patient became fearful
and unco-operative, which was scarcely surprising as he probably
knew (and as his therapist certainly knew) that convulsions were
frequently severe enough to cause fractures of the spine, ribs and
limbs.

ELECTRO-CONVULSIVE THERAPY

It was perhaps fortunate for the patients who lived through this
period that another researcher, Cerletti, was also taking an
interest in the possible pathological effects of epileptic seizures.
While undertaking autopsies of epileptics in Genoa he noted a

hardening in a part of the brain known as Ammon's horn. Cerletti's main research interest was to establish whether the hardening was a cause or an effect of epileptic seizures. For theoretical reasons, he was against the use of drugs for inducing shocks so he turned to electrical stimulation instead. But the use of this method was problematic because nobody knew how to establish a correct 'dose'. Amazingly, the correct level of stimulation was roughly established by Cerletti and his co-worker Bini by observing the practices of slaughterhouse men who used electrical stimulation to stupefy and paralyse pigs so that their throats could be cut more easily. In 1938 Cerletti and Bini applied an electric shock to the head of a schizophrenic patient, hence establishing electro-convulsive therapy (ECT) as part of the armamentarium of the modern psychiatrist. ECT replaced other forms of treatment largely because it was more economical and much less life-threatening. For insulin coma therapy to be effective at least thirty to fifty hours of coma had to be produced. Nursing care had to be continuous, and only highly trained doctors skilled in insulin administration were capable of preventing the occurrence of such emergencies as irreversible coma or circulatory or respiratory collapse. The only major hazard of ECT was the production of fractures, but this problem was largely solved in 1941 when Bennet pioneered the intro-duction of curare-like drugs which effectively inhibit the con-traction of the muscles during the administration of the shock. Since ECT is now administered under anaesthetic, the only hazard is the normal one associated with anaesthesia. However, this is not the whole story because it is well known that ECT can cause amnesia in some patients.

It would appear that ECT was a major step forward when compared with the other forms of shock treatment, but as Brewer (1975) has recently pointed out, no definitive, adequately controlled study has been undertaken to prove that ECT is anything other than a powerful placebo. ECT can be effective in alleviating symptoms, but nobody yet knows the basis of this effectiveness. Brewer (1975) has fittingly summarised the position as follows:

For a dramatic description of the placebo effect of ECT, one can hardly improve on Cerletti's account of the very first patient to receive the treatment in 1938. The patient was described as a catatonic schizophrenic, who spoke only gibberish and was unable even to give his name. The first shock was not strong enough to produce a convulsion, though it must have been rather painful in the absence of anaesthesia. Even so he first started to sing, and then, seeing that a further shock was imminent, he sat up and spoke clearly for the first time. What he said deserves to be better known: 'Non una seconda: Mortifera!' (Not another one: It'll kill me!) In the circum-stances, this seems an eminently reasonable comment, and the expression of it alone might have been taken to indicate a worthwhile improvement. Cerletti, however, was clearly anxious to make history, and the second shock was followed by a satis-factory convulsion. The patient was proved wrong, but so, in the event, was Cerletti, for the new treatment made no impact on schizophrenia. Its value in depression remains to be proved, and it is my hope that this article may provoke someone to make

the answer available in time for the 40th anniversary of
Cerletti's bold experiment. No commemoration could be more
fitting: or more belated. And for those who doubt the need,
there can be only one reply: 'Remember insulin'.

PSYCHOSURGERY

The history of lobotomy, the third major form of physical treatment
introduced in the 1930s, also makes dismal reading. As a result
of an extensive study of patients with obsessional symptoms, Moniz,
a clinical professor of neurology at the University of Lisbon,
came to believe that 'morbid' ideas could cause persistent rever-
berations in neuronal circuits in the brain. He focused his
attention on the frontal lobes as the likely locus of these rever-
berating circuits largely because of the prior research at Yale
by Fulton and Jacobsen: they had noted that monkeys whose prefrontal lobe fibres had been severed (in order to destroy the
connection between the prefrontal areas and the main sensory relay
station of the brain, the thalamus) seemed to accept frustration
better and were easier to manage because of diminished emotionality.
Moniz was also aware of a number of clinical cases in which the
removal of a tumour from the frontal lobes resulted in personality
changes which were apparently beneficial since the patients appeared
both less anxious and less inhibited.
   Moniz, in collaboration with the neurosurgeon Lima, performed
the first frontal lobotomy in 1935, but five years elapsed before
the first British operation took place at the Burden Neurological
Institute in Bristol. The ethical objection to the use of such a
technique was circumvented largely on the basis that the patients'
suffering was so great that any treatment that had some possibility
of success was justified.
   The attitudes of advocates of such treatments is well expressed
by the psychiatrist Fleming, who reviewed progress in prefrontal
leucotomy (a modified form of lobotomy involving the cutting of
fibres rather than the excision of parts of the cortex) in 1944
in a special supplement to the 'Journal of Mental Science' (Fleming,
1944):
   there has been some hostile criticism of the operation by medical
   men with no experience of it [sic] and little experience of
   psychiatry. Time alone can tell whether the initial success
   is going to be developed until the operation is accepted as an
   essential part of our therapeutic equipment. It seems a pity
   that such a technical matter as prefrontal leucotomy should be
   discussed in the lay press, and we can only deprecate very
   strongly the action of medical men who have encouraged this.
The arrogance of Fleming's position is all too obvious, but his
attitude to the mortality rate associated with leucotomy is similarly cavalier. Under the heading of mortality he says 'the death
rate is distinctly low' and then quotes figures indicating that
15 deaths had occurred in a group of 517 cases, a mortality rate
of nearly 3.5 per cent. Alexander and Selesnick (1967), reviewing
leucotomy give a lower mortality rate of 1.2 per cent in 1967 but
they point out that the effects of the operation were much more
severe than was allowed by its enthusiastic supporters:

> Patients ... were not really calmer - much of the time they were
> reduced to being placid 'zombies'. Many post-operative patients
> lacked ambition, task orientation and imagination; although the
> patients themselves may have felt more comfortable, their
> families did not. Anxiety was relieved but at the price of a
> loss of self-respect and of empathy with others. Furthermore
> patients with recurrent severely morbid thoughts ... were not
> relieved of their symptoms. A major difficulty was that psycho-
> surgery, which mutilated irrevocably a part of the brain, was
> final.

Leucotomy, admittedly in a highly modified form, still has its
advocates today, but it is alarmingly true that the first randomly
controlled trial of leucotomy in Britain was not initiated until
1972 and is still not complete at the time of writing. Historically, the use of leucotomy and other forms of physical treatments
declined from the early 1950s onwards not because of carefully
controlled clinical trials which demonstrated their ineffectiveness
or otherwise, but because psychiatric practice was changed by the
introduction of new types of psychotropic drugs.

DRUG THERAPIES

Before discussing the importance of what Jones and others have
described as the 'pharmacological revolution', it is worthwhile
reviewing Alexander and Selesnick's (1967) summary of the various
types of pharmacological agents that have been used to treat
mental disorders. Their approach serves to demonstrate that the
idea of a pharmacological revolution is itself not new since
drugs have been widely used in treating mental disorders for over
a century. As they argue,

> Sedatives like chloral hydrate were first synthesized about
> 1870 and were used in psychiatric disorders; bromides were also
> prescribed extensively during the nineteenth century to produce
> heavy sedation, and in the early twentieth century barbiturates
> came into use for the same purpose. As for stimulants, the
> effects of alcoholic beverages and of caffeine have been known
> for centuries. Synthetic drugs used extensively during the
> 1930s to treat depression were the amphetamine derivatives
> (Benzedrine and Dexedrine), but their disagreeable side
> effects - they caused loss of appetite, palpitations, and an
> increase in heart rate and blood pressure - interfered with
> widespread acceptance. Stimulants, like sedatives, act for
> a limited period of time; they do not produce permanent changes
> of mood. In the first years of this century, on the assumption
> that excitement interferes with clear thinking, prolonged
> administration of barbiturates in excited states was proposed.
> In 1922 Jacob Klasi recommended prolonged sedative induced
> sleep, on the basis that excitement was a result of an inflam-
> matory process in the brain that could be relieved through
> rest, as other inflammatory conditions were. Prolonged-sleep
> treatment preceded insulin therapy and may be considered a
> forerunner of the shock treatment.

Alexander and Selesnick add a salutary rider to their review, since an examination of the history of drug treatments of mental illness is in many ways as depressing as an examination of physical treatment:

> In general the pattern of drug therapy for mental illness has been one of great initial enthusiasm followed by disappointment. Twenty years after Balard discovered bromides (1826) they were widely used in psychiatric illnesses. During the latter part of the nineteenth century and in the early years of the twentieth, physicians found that uncontrollable states of excitement could be markedly relieved by the administration of bromides. By the mid-1920s, even some psychiatrists writing in the official journal of the American Psychiatric Association were claiming that finally a drug - bromide - had been discovered that could alleviate serious symptoms of disturbed behaviour. The American public, following the lead of physicians, so desired bromides that by 1928 one out of every five prescriptions was for bromides. As is usual when drugs are hailed as the solution to mental illness, disillusionment gradually set in. Patients had to be continuously maintained on bromides in order to show improvement. Nonetheless, despite the repeated shattering of the drug dream, physicians still hope eventually to alleviate man's inner strife by chemical means.

The use of bromides was never as widespread in Britain as it was in America, but it is significant that it has been estimated that in contemporary Britain one night's sleep in ten is induced by sleeping tablets (hypnotics); i.e., 3.5 million people rely on such tablets to get a night's sleep. However, the most important change in drug usage in relation to psychiatric problems that has occurred since the Second World War relates not to the use of hypnotics but to tranquillisers and anti-depressants since a series of new ranges of drugs has been developed as a result of intensive research. DHSS statistics clearly reflect this trend. In 1961 32 million prescriptions for psychotropic drugs (costing £7 million) were issued in England and Wales, but in 1973 the comparable figure was 45 million (costing £22 million). These general figures obscure the fact that there has been an approximately 50 per cent decline in the prescribing of barbiturate hypnotics and stimulants and appetite suppressants (such as the amphetamines), while in the same period there has been a three-fold rise in the prescription of tranquillisers and non-barbiturate hypnotics. The decline in prescribing barbiturate hypnotics and the amphetamines relates clearly to the dangerous addictive nature of these drugs.

The first major development in the production of effective new drugs occurred in 1952 when two French researchers reported the beneficial effects of Chlorpromazine (a phenothiazine derivative) in treating psychotic patients. This led to the discovery of further drugs, which are commonly called major tranquillisers but should be more accurately called neuroleptics. Various forms of neuroleptics, particularly various alkaloid derivatives of the plant Rauwolfia serpentiqua, had been in use since the 1930s, but they often had severe side-effects, including the induction of severe depression, so the new drugs were welcome as useful alternatives. A series of minor tranquillisers (now more technically

called anxiolytics) were also developed - the most widely used in
this group was Meprobomate, which was developed by Berger in
America, but other types of anxiolytics such as the benzodiazapines
are now preferred as they are much safer drugs to use. In addition
to the new neuroleptics and anxiolytics, a group of anti-depressant
drugs was also introduced. Iproniazid, a drug used in the treatment
of tuberculosis, was known to have a psychotropic effect on many
of the patients who received it, and subsequent research revealed
that its euphoria-inducing properties were related to its abilities
to inhibit the activity of the enzyme monoamine oxidase which normally destroys neuro-transmitters in nerve cells. Iproniazid was
then the first of the new monoamine oxidase inhibitors (MAOIS);
but yet another group of drugs, the tricyclics (including drugs
such as Imipramine), were also shown to have anti-depressant
effects.

But just how effective are drug treatments? This is an enormous
and complex question, but it is important to tackle it from first
principles, without getting bogged down in discussions of the individual efficacy of particular drugs.

Klass (1975), in his recent book 'There's Gold in Them Thar
Pills', takes a highly sanguine view of the significance of drugs:
    For most of my lifetime I have been actively engaged in the
    practice of medicine, particularly in the speciality of surgery,
    I have been involved in the 'care of the ill' on a person-to-
    person basis. I have observed the growing dependence upon drugs
    in all levels of society and in particular the increasing
    reliance upon mood-elevating drugs for the depressed, as well
    as the enormous consumption of sedative drugs for the tense. I
    have witnessed and sometimes I have been a co-operator in the
    efforts of the drug industry to sell more and more of their
    profitable produce. I have seen the industry succeed ...
    because of its special kind of directed research, because of
    its highly efficient method of production but mainly because
    of its sophisticated promotion and marketing. I am convinced
    that its success derives from the fact, not recognised by
    doctors, that the drug industry has made captive my profession,
    the profession of medicine.
Interestingly, he illustrates this captivity by referring (among
other examples) to the over-prescribing of Valium:
    in considering over-prescribing, Valium is a good illustrative
    drug for several reasons. Firstly the enormity of its sales
    is an indication of the amount of psychotropic or mood-altering
    drugs being consumed in our time. Secondly, the mammoth sale
    indicates the success that can be confidently expected from
    skilful promotion of a drug to the profession. The promotion
    includes a constant level of direct mail or medical journal
    advertising, endless supplies of free samples to doctors and
    intensive and repeated detailing on a personal basis to each
    doctor by company representatives. The promotion also includes
    the free provision of Valium in hospital pharmacies, so that
    residents and interns - young doctors at the threshold of their
    prescribing career - become indoctrinated in the use of this
    drug while pursuing the hospital part of their training. The
    young doctor who has never prescribed Valium for his patients

while continuing his training in hospital must be rare.   This
effectively shuts off any knowledge and experience he might
acquire about other drugs that have a similar tranquillizing
effect and have been accepted for many years prior to the
arrival of Valium.   This artificial creation of obsolescence
of other useful drugs having similar physiological effect is
especially important, because the doctor will never know that
in most cases where Valium is prescribed there are other drugs
as effective and less costly.

THALIDOMIDE AND THE QUESTION OF EFFICACY

Klass also refers to the shocking history of thalidomide to illustrate both the profit-seeking motivation of the drug industry
and the confusion created by the industry in marketing its products.
Thalidomide (which, it should be remembered, is classified as a
tranquilliser) was marketed under at least thirty-seven different
names, and the reasons for this are obvious.   It is the glut of
names that ensures a profit for the company holding the patent of
the drug.   A babel of different names is created so that there is
maximum confusion in the doctor's mind as to the active constituent
of a particular preparation.   When the doctor is called upon to
write a prescription, given that he could have many alternative
names to choose from, it is the best promoted and advertised drug
that he is likely to recall.   So it is the drug company with the
greatest 'promotional muscle' that is the one that wins the battle
for the prescription pad, as Klass graphically puts it.
    However, the argument is not just about good or bad drugs or
over-prescribing; it is about the overall efficacy of drugs.
Klass's (1975) comments on the relationship between psychiatry and
drug prescribing are very significant:
    In psychiatry the battle rages regarding possible improvement
    in public health in this area.   It is true that mental hospitals
    are being emptied, and for this all of us should sing praises -
    but not necessarily to the drug industry that has quickly
    claimed the credit.   Part of the outflow from mental hospitals
    is due to a healthier public attitude to those with psychiatric
    handicaps and to more rigid criteria for admitting and retaining
    in hospital individuals who are merely 'peculiar'.   Some part of
    the reduced mental hospital population is due to the near dis-
    appearance of the ravages of syphilis upon the nervous system.
    Syphilis itself, through preventive care and perhaps through
    the natural fluctuation of disease, was diminishing in occur-
    rence, and by no means can all the credit for the reduction of
    the effect of syphilis on the nervous system be credited to
    drug treatment.
    But parallel to this reduction in the population of mental
    hospitals has come a massive increase in the use of so-called
    mood-controlling or psychoactive drugs.   In the United Kingdom
    (1971) prescriptions for barbiturates reached twenty million
    per year; for phenylthiazine tranquillizers, six million; for
    amphetamines, five million; for non-barbiturate hypnotics, five
    million.   Such amounts in the use of any class of drugs might

be expected to show evidence of solid gain in public health.
What is indeed evident is a vast increase in drug dependency,
in adverse drug effects, in hospitalisation for overdosage and
in accidental and suicidal deaths.

And so, overall, where are the gains to justify the enormous
expenditure of time, brains and money in industrial research
and industrially sponsored and promoted mood-altering drugs?
One must conclude that the greatest gain lies in the coffers
of the drug industry.

DRUGS AND DISEASE

Klass's sanguine view of the efficacy of psychoactive drugs is
set against a general evaluation of the efficacy of drugs and
other forms of individual therapy. He argues that the efficacy
of drugs in the treatment of major diseases has been grossly over-
estimated precisely because the social and economic factors contributing to the decline in such diseases have been universally
ignored.

The work of McKeown and Lowe (1960), Cochrane (1972), Powles
(1973) and Illich (1975) has done much to deflate the view that
it was hospital-based medicine that has been largely responsible
for the improvement in health and life expectancy over the last
century. In fact, the most marked improvement in this period has
been the sharp drop in infant mortality (particularly since 1900),
but what caused this? It is customary to cite improvements in
hospital care, better training of medical staff, the development
of preventative treatment of infectious diseases, etc. But it is
equally true that this period was one of important and significant
improvement in environmental factors, better nutrition, improved
sanitation, better control of the purity of water and milk and a
growing public acceptance of birth control measures which resulted
in smaller families.

Which of these factors contributed most significantly to the
decline in mortality? The real value of improved medical care is
illuminated by examining, for example, the decrease in deaths from
scarlet fever, diphtheria, whooping cough and measles between 1950
and 1965. Ninety per cent of the improvement in death rate had
already occurred prior to the introduction of immunisation and the
use of antibiotics. As Klass has recently concluded, 'while not
denying the usefulness of immunization and anti-biotics for a
share of the improvement in child mortality it seems obvious that
other factors were already creating a favourable effect prior to
the introduction of these agents' (Klass, 1975). A similar argument has been advanced by McKeown in relation to tuberculosis,
which was a major cause of death in adults throughout the nineteenth century. The death rate from tuberculosis in fact declined
by nearly 50 per cent between 1860 and 1900, and yet medicine's
contribution to this decline was negligible.

Faced with these approaches to the history of therapeutics,
it becomes increasingly difficult to sustain the argument that
developments in medical care take place simply because of
'scientific' discoveries within the discipline. A number of

researchers (e.g. Powles, 1973, Richards, 1975) have attempted to
explore the social and economic contexts within which innovations
in medical care have occurred. While their findings are illuminating, there is as yet no major authoritative study upon which
to draw. However, the existing research clearly indicates that
there is every justification for challenging the medical profession's explanations of why particular innovations are made. In
this context the introduction of psychiatric drugs is therefore no
exception, but the justification for the wholesale introduction
of such psychotropic drugs raises particular difficulties because
of the underlying problems of the conceptualisation of mental disorders.

This leads us back to a major theme of our argument. Psychiatry,
in adopting a medical view of mental disorders, inevitably tends
to view their causality as a question of individual pathology. Any
drug that can be shown to alleviate symptoms such as anxiety or
depression is therefore viewed as efficacious. Provided the side-
effects of such drugs are not too serious such a drug will then be
added to the armamentarium of the psychiatrist.

Clearly, the notion of a 'cure' is dependent upon the underlying
conceptualisation of mental disorder that is adopted. Therapists
who reject the medical model in favour of psychological explanations
of mental disorder must also reject the use of drugs (except perhaps
during periods of acute crisis) because drug therapies are construed as being merely palliative.

THE PHARMACOLOGICAL REVOLUTION IN PSYCHIATRY

But the dispute between the rival approaches is not just of academic
interest. Many of the recent developments in psychiatry are claimed
as evidence that drug therapies have played a crucial role in
revolutionising patient care, but Klass's (1975) analysis warns us
against accepting any such claims. Indeed, the much proclaimed
'pharmacological' revolution of the mid-1950s requires very detailed
analysis because the exact basis of this 'revolution' has been
largely obscured, even by writers like Kathleen Jones who are aware
of the complexities of the changes in the 1950s.

In her book Jones (1972) presents the problem in the following
way:

In the early 1950's three new movements started: new kinds of
drugs ... were used ... mental hospitals began the 'open-door'
movement ... and the Government ... appointed a Royal Commission
on the law relating to Mental Illness and Mental Deficiency ....
From the point of view of therapy or of public policy the coin-
cidence of these three movements was fortunate, since each reinforced the other. From the point of view of social analysis
it was less so since it made it impossible to trace cause and
effect with any confidence. The three strands of development
crossed and recrossed, becoming so interwoven that it will
probably never be possible to determine what influence each had.
Jones's statements appear to be uncontroversial at first sight,
but in our opinion they serve only to confuse the issue. We would
argue that the changes occurring in the mental health services

during the 1950s could have occurred without the intervention of
new forms of drug treatments. We wish to establish this fundamental point for one obvious reason, i.e. to contradict the simple-
minded claim that drug therapies can legitimately form the basis
for a reconstituted mental health service. Our argument is
difficult to document, largely because of the dead weight of
orthodox opinion which has accepted the validity of the counter-
argument; but fortunately several British psychiatrists have
similarly objected to the accepted view of the changes in the
1950s. However, before examining this work it is essential to
point out that there are examples of rates of hospitalisation
being reduced by administrative procedures.

In 1944, an editorial in the 'Lancet' reviewed a paper by Sommer
and Weinberg (1944) that had originally appeared in the 'American
Journal of Psychiatry'. The paper reported that the State of
Illinois had decided to stop the steady increase of patients
residing in the state mental hospitals. In fifty years the patient
population had multiplied eight times with a sharp increase
occurring from 1937 onwards. Owing to the wartime restrictions on
building it was decided to attempt to freeze the number of available
beds. More active treatment and discharge procedures were introduced together with more extensive rehabilitation programmes once
the patient was returned to the community. Preventive programmes
were also devised, so that less seriously disturbed patients could
be treated in outpatient clinics rather than being hospitalised.
These policies were introduced from May-June 1941 onwards, but it
is noteworthy that the resident population had begun to fall from
March 1941. This was influenced by the fall in admissions which
began in 1939 and continued throughout 1940 with a sharp drop
occurring during the last months of 1941 before a flattening
occurred in 1942. The number of patients receiving treatment in
general hospitals trebled between 1935 and 1942, so it is possible
that this contributed to the decline in admissions to the state
mental hospitals.

The number of discharges from these occurring prior to the introduction of the new policies was unsurprisingly lower than under the
new regime, but it is significant that the number of re-admissions
declined also, indicating that the new policies were not replacing
relatively long-stay patients with ones who merely returned to the
hospital more frequently.

Sommer and Weinberg correctly argue that it is difficult to
attribute the changes in the hospital population directly to the
new programme since social and economic changes were going on con-
currently as the American economy became geared to the war effort.
But nevertheless, their findings do serve to illustrate the point
that we are trying to make - that to attribute the mid-1950s
decline in mental hospital bed residency merely to therapeutic
innovations is obviously simplistic. As Sommer and Weinberg report,
some of the discharges that occurred in the course of their study
were merely the result of the introduction of adequate procedures
for reviewing the reasons for particular patients being in hospital.
In some cases patients could be easily discharged through the
introduction of boarding-out systems or through getting their
families to take an active interest in their welfare.

   The use of industrial therapy as a basis for rehabilitation programmes adds a further dimension to the argument since it becomes
obvious that the retention of mental patients in hospital is often
arbitrary. As Cooper and Early commented in 1961, 'a large proportion of all patients under care in mental hospitals show no
serious disturbance of behaviour and their retention is determined
largely by social factors' (Cooper and Early, 1961). A survey of
chronic patients carried out by Cross in 1957 provides a suitable
illustration of this point. He found that two-thirds of his sample
required only routine care. In practice the degree of supervision
given to patients depended as much on ward tradition and administrative policy as on the degree of the patients' mental disturbance. It is therefore not surprising that the introduction of
more active discharge policies, the development of special
'rehabilitation' units, the systematic use of tranquillisers and
the increased use of day-hospital facilities and outpatient clinics
could decrease the chronic population of mental hospitals. But
as Cooper and Early pointed out, the effects of specific forms of
treatment in contributing to this picture was limited. Quoting
figures from Early's own hospital (Glenside in Bristol), they showed
that the discharge rate for long-stay patients did increase during
1955 and 1956 (following the introduction of new drugs) but declined
again in 1957. The highest-ever discharge rate resulted from the
introduction of a programme of industrial therapy in 1958. Cooper
and Early's work raises the interesting question of whether the
earlier introduction of industrial therapy would have produced the
same results in the long run. Unfortunately they did not debate
this point, but they did make some fundamental points concerning
the general impact of 'social methods on psychiatric practice'
(Cooper and Early, 1961):

   how great a change may ensue from the development of social
   methods is a matter for conjecture. At one extreme of opinion
   it is held that all such measures are of necessity only make-
   shifts of the kind to which resort is always made in medical
   practice until the appearance of a specific therapy. That such
   specific treatment can be found for the major psychoses is by
   no means certain; unless and until it is found the prevention
   of complete social disability, and of loss of normal contacts
   so often arising from psychiatric illness, must be regarded as
   one of the most important goals of treatment. Moreover, in a
   large proportion of the current mental hospitals the major
   problem is one of institutional dependence rather than gross
   mental disorder, and here social measures alone can be effective.
The inadequacies of community care for ex-mental patients remains
a national scandal but it is important to stress that this issue
does not relate only to chronic patients. A recent survey by
McCowen and Wilder (1975) carried out for the Psychiatric Rehabilitation Association highlights the general problems of
isolation that the majority of hospitalised patients suffer from.
The PRA survey investigated the life style of 100 psychiatric
patients residing in a hospital with an East End of London catchment area. The majority of them were diagnosed as suffering from
schizophrenia or depression but a large minority were labelled as
having behavioural problems. Seventy-seven per cent of the patients

had been in mental hospital before (compared with a national figure
of 57 per cent) and there were more men than women in the sample so
that it cannot be taken as representative. However, the findings
of the study demonstrate that the major problems facing patients
coming from urban centres are concerned with social isolation and
the inability to find employment. The latter is a complicated
issue since it in turn encompasses many other issues - such as the
state of the job market, the question of stigma and the lack of
motivation to hold down a job. But, nevertheless, it is clear that
Cooper and Early's points are well supported by the study, since
without effective social rehabilitation the ex-mental patient gains
little from a period in hospital.

THE ROLE OF DRUGS IN THE REHABILITATION OF LONG-STAY PATIENTS

Hordern and Hamilton, in their paper 'Drugs and Moral Treatment'
(1963), have pointed out that the introduction of the new drugs
took place in a specific historical context. The advent of the
National Health Service (NHS) led to improved standards of care
(open-door policies, rehabilitation programmes, vocational training
schemes, etc.) and an improved career structure for psychiatrists,
so that promotion did not necessarily involve transfer to administrative duties. Psychiatry therefore began to recruit more able
and better trained doctors who began to influence the standard of
care. Interestingly, the role of the new drugs in contributing
to the improvement in care was seen to be secondary by many contemporary observers. Aubrey Lewis, for example, speaking at the
First International Congress of Neuropsychopharmacology in 1958,
argued that traditional methods of treatment (such as ward activity
programmes and occupational therapy) could produce results as
satisfactory as those produced by Chlorpromazine.
    But Hordern and Hamilton add an interesting dimension to the
issue by developing an argument about the crucial differences
between British and American experience in relation to the introduction of the neuroleptics. The essence of their argument is
contained in the following quotation (Hordern and Hamilton, 1963):
    It would appear ... that there have been two main patterns of
    response observed and reported with neuroleptics since 1954.
    1 In Britain generally and in the small highly staffed psycho-
       therapeutically orientated psychiatric hospitals of the
       United States some advantages have been noted from their
       use but in the main there has been little enthusiasm for
       these drugs, since they do not appear to have shown any
       striking advantage over established methods of treatment.
    2 In the large state hospitals of North America and in mental
       hospitals in other countries, particularly those with meagre
       programmes of treatment, the efficacy of neuroleptics has
       been reported as being little short of miraculous.
Hordern and Hamilton explore the relationship between the therapeutic status of the hospital and the reported efficacy of neuro-
leptic drugs in some detail. As they pointed out, the most
enthusiastic reports of drug effectiveness tended to come from
the mental hospitals with the most backward therapeutic resources.

These were hospitals in which custodialism still prevailed.   Staff
morale and enthusiasm were low and patients suffered from what
Barton has termed 'institutional neurosis', a condition in which a
patient's behaviour deteriorates precisely because of the imper-
sonal and bureaucratic nature of the hospital setting itself
(Barton, 1959).
The results obtained using neuroleptics and better treatment
programmes were very different, although the number of adequately
designed research studies that sought to demonstrate the factors
influencing therapeutic outcome was surprisingly small.   Meszaros
and Gallagher (1958) demonstrated that a treatment regime involving
the use of drugs and occupational therapy was significantly superior
to a regime involving the use of drugs only, a finding that was
confirmed by Grygier and Waters (1958) and Evangelakis (1961).
However, the most interesting study carried out in this period was
by Hamilton himself.   Using an elaborate statistical design, he
investigated the interactive effects of drugs and occupational
therapy.   Patients who had received drugs or occupational therapy
improved significantly during the period of treatment when compared
with a placebo control group.   But Hamilton reports that the group
of patients receiving both drugs and occupational therapy showed
less improvement than either of the other group; i.e., the drugs
seemed to exert some inhibitor effects on the improvement obtained
with occupational therapy.
Hordern and Hamilton's scepticism about the claims of drug
therapy was confirmed independently by Odegard (1964), who surveyed
the pattern of discharge from Norwegian psychiatric hospitals
before and after the introduction of psychotropic drugs.   Odegard
compared all discharges in a 'control' period, 1948-52.   His most
important finding was that the two periods did not differ significantly as far as the overall discharge pattern was concerned.   In
the drug period there was an increased rate of discharge for short-
stay patients suffering from functional psychoses, but the re-
admission rate also increased.   One striking feature of the results
was the marked variation in individual hospitals discharge rates.
In five of the seventeen hospitals the discharge rate was greater
(in one case by 33 per cent) and in five it was smaller (in one
case by 23 per cent), leaving seven hospitals in which there was
no significant change.   But the most interesting of Odegard's
results from our point of view was his discovery that there was a
marked negative correlation between the pre-drug discharge level
of the hospital and the improvement brought about by the drug
therapy.   In hospitals with a favourable therapeutic situation the
drugs produced little or no improvement or even a decrease in the
rate of discharge.   But in hospitals with a low pre-drug rate of
discharge, the improvement was considerable.   Such results can be
explained in a number of ways, but Odegard (1964) offers an explanation that is similar to Hordern and Hamilton:
It is possible that pre-drug therapeutic efficiency differed
from one hospital to another because modern milieu therapy can
be seriously handicapped by local defects in the structure,
equipment and financing of the hospitals. For such handicapped
hospitals the drugs were a real blessing, because they are
(perhaps) more independent of such milieu factors than were

the earlier methods. In the more privileged institutions the
drugs simply meant that one form of therapy was replaced by
another and equally efficient one.

But Odegard adds another dimension to his argument by making a
further analysis of the discharge rates. This analysis involves
a three-way comparison of the rates for the periods 1936-40,
1948-53 and 1955-9. Such analysis reveals that significant changes
in discharge rate were occurring prior to the introduction of drug
therapies. As Odegard (1964) comments,

> evidently the efficiency of our psychiatric hospitals made
> great strides ahead between 1936 and 1948 and the curve of
> therapeutic improvement shows a much steeper climb than during
> the following period of drug treatment.... In England Norton
> has published similar findings.

But what was responsible for this improved therapeutic climate?
Odegard reports that somatic therapies (ECT, insulin shock therapy,
etc.) may have had an influence from 1939-40 onwards but the most
significant factor was a social one. From 1946 onwards Norway
experienced 'over-employment' rather than the chronic unemployment
of the 1930s. Patients could therefore obtain jobs very easily so
rehabilitation into the community was a real possibility. Odegard
therefore concludes that:

> we do not know what might have happened to the discharge pattern
> between 1948 and 1959 if the psychotropic drugs had not been
> discovered. But it is reasonably certain that some progress
> would have been made even then and so the modest improvement
> which we have been able to show cannot entirely be credited to
> the psychotropic drugs.

Odegard's conclusion is necessarily cautious because of the difficulties of interpreting mass data of the type that he has collated.
But we would argue that his work amplified the independent research
of Hordern and Hamilton in many significant ways. We would therefore conclude that the changes in mental hospitals in the 1950s
that are normally attributed to the drug therapies could have been
achieved by other means. This is not to deny that drugs played
some role in the changes, but we do insist that many other factors
(such as administrative changes, changes in staff attitudes and
changes in rehabilitation policies because of the improved economic
climate) also contributed very significantly. The role of these
types of factors has been underestimated in our opinion - largely
because the psychiatric profession has a vested interest in
stressing the importance of drugs (which, of course, can be prescribed only by members of the profession).

THE IMPACT OF THE 'PHARMACOLOGICAL REVOLUTION' ON POLICY-MAKING

In fairness to psychiatrists, however, it is also necessary to
point out that the profession's attitude to the use of drugs is
very variable. Aubrey Lewis's view was supported by many psychiatrists, based in the larger mental hospitals, who had active rehabilitation policies for their patients. But the dispute over
the efficacy of drugs is no mere debating topic. The assumption
that drugs were the effective agent in decreasing the length of

stay of patients in hospital became enshrined in government policy
from 1960-1 onwards, and the psychiatric unit in the general hospital began to emerge as the new focus of the mental health services. The extent to which the pharmacological revolution dominated psychiatric and lay thinking is well illustrated by the
statement by Sir Keith Joseph in introducing the 1971 White Paper,
'Hospital Services for the Mentally Ill'. He had the following
to say about this issue:

> Psychiatry is to join the rest of medicine ... since the
> treatment of psychosis, neurosis and schizophrenia have been
> entirely changed by the drug revolution. People go into
> hospital with mental disorders and they are cured, and that
> is why we want to bring this branch of medicine into the scope
> of the 230 district general hospitals that are planned for
> England Wales.

Joseph's statement can of course be challenged on a number of
points but it is important to stress that there is indeed a crucial
relationship between the drug revolution and the policy of developing psychiatric units in general hospitals. In essence, the
drug revolution has provided a means of controlling patients'
symptoms so that they can be maintained in the community. During
periods of acute crisis a short stay in hospital is assumed to be
effective in overcoming the patients' difficulties so the patient
can then be returned to the community once more.

THE IMPLICATIONS OF THE WIDER USE OF DRUG THERAPIES

We would argue that the policy changes that have been introduced
are based on the myth of the efficacy of drug treatments. And
the economic reasons for this cannot be overlooked. Drug treatments, in comparison with other forms of treatment, are cheap
because all other forms of treatment require the provision of
costly facilities, large numbers of staff, etc. A well organised
outpatient clinic providing drug treatments can process very large
numbers of patients - and even such minimal psychiatric services
as these can be short-circuited by GPs prescribing the drugs
instead. Recent figures documenting the number of new outpatients
seen show that the number of consultations reached a peak in 1969
and then showed a consistent decline during the period 1970-3.
But the prescribing of psychotropic drugs within the NHS has continued to increase steadily. In 1961 the total volume of prescriptions was 32 million for England and Wales, whereas in 1973
there were 45 million prescriptions in England alone. (During
this same period the prescribing of tranquillisers trebled - OHE,
1975).

  If this trend is maintained it will mean that the psychiatric
services will be progressively short-circuited. The implication
this has for the effective social control of psychiatric problems
is truly alarming. Psychiatrists who adopt the medical model as
their credo will look upon these figures with equanimity, arguing
that psychiatry is successful in preventing hospitalisation and
allowing individuals to cope with their problems in the community
without disrupting their normal functioning in work and family

roles. But critics of contemporary psychiatry, and we include ourselves among them, would argue that drug therapies are nothing more than bromides which enable patients to avoid coming to terms with crises that reflect underlying interpersonal or social or economic problems.

Protagonists of drug therapies tend to overlook the fact that there is currently a serious epidemic of drug overdosing - and the most commonly used drugs are psychotropic drugs prescribed by GPs and psychiatrists (Morgan et al., 1975 a and b). This strange form of iatrogenesis (which Illich strangely overlooks) is a suitable tribute to the inability of drugs to make any basic change in patients' lives. But there is yet another, perhaps more insidious, dimension to the argument over drug therapies.

The use of drugs as forms of behavioural control is an enormous topic which we cannot adequately explore. However, it is essential to mention briefly their use in therapeutic settings such as psychiatric units in general hospitals. A recent paper by two British psychiatrists, Oldham and Bott (1971), provides a striking example of this tendency. An extract from their paper illustrates the peculiarly myopic approach they adopt:

the rapid and effective control of excitement is daily becoming important as the tendency for psychiatric treatment to be given in general hospital departments increases. In the mental hospital setting states of excited behaviour may be tolerated which in a general hospital would cause fear and annoyance to nearby patients, staff, and visitors. The use of tranquillizers for this purpose has probably proved more effective than other forms of treatment, and the main limitations have usually been found in their more severe side-effects such as hypotension. The lack of such dangerous side-effects is a great asset to any major tranquillizer used in the treatment of excitement. Haloperidol, in our experience, possesses this asset.

We view this paper as marking a nadir in British psychiatric thinking. To argue that patients require tranquillising because psychiatric care is now carried out in psychiatric units in general hospitals rather than in mental hospitals is decidedly bizarre, since such units were developed precisely because it was argued that they could cope with all types of patients. In our next chapter we take up this discussion in greater detail when we seek to establish that the psychiatric unit in the general hospital is nothing more than an administrative expression of the medical model. In terms of this model, physical and mental illnesses are to be viewed as essentially similar - it is therefore logical that they should be treated under the same roof.

Part two

The development of general hospital psychiatry

Chapter 4

The origins of psychiatric units in general hospitals

The idea that the mentally ill and the physically ill should be treated under the same roof has a very long history. Medical historians are fond of pointing out that Thomas Guy, in founding his now famous hospital in 1722, insisted that twenty beds should be set aside for lunatics. (This ward was comparatively short-lived but another ward, the York Clinic, was opened much later, in 1861.) Some other London hospitals, such as the Middlesex Hospital, had similar arrangements, but the Manchester Lunatic Hospital, which was opened in 1766 alongside the existing Royal Infirmary, also deserves some mention.

Jones discusses the latter hospital in some detail since she maintains that it played an important role in the history of the treatment of lunatics. According to her (Jones, 1972) the significance of the hospital lay in:

its insistence on the importance of keeping records and case histories which sprang from the close connection with the Infirmary, and the fact of that connection brought a new factor into the treatment of insanity. For the first time treatment was recognised as being allied to the treatment of bodily illness ... the terms 'hospital' and 'patient' were published in the local newspapers. It was the first attempt to treat mental disorder in the way that physical ills were treated - with matter-of-fact compassion untinged by sensation, moral condemnation or concealment.

But Jones fails to establish how effective the hospital was in influencing attitudes towards the treatment of mental illness. This is a difficult question to answer, but it is significant that in Liverpool the Infirmary and Lunatic Hospital originally occupied a site together, while at York, Newcastle and Exeter separate hospitals were provided, but these also had close links with the local general hospitals. It therefore appears that the Manchester Lunatic Hospital was really one example of several similar hospitals built during the hospital-building movement in the second half of the eighteenth century.

The knowledge that such hospitals existed in the eighteenth century is important for the present discussion, since it indicates that the idea of the essential continuity of physical and mental

illness is by no means a new one. It is also significant that in
some cases hospitals for lunatics were actually built immediately
adjacent to a general hospital. Their physical juxtaposition is
an interesting reflection of the notion that physical and mental
illness are to be treated similarly. It is also noteworthy that
these hospitals were situated at the centre of towns, serving the
needs of the surrounding community. The subsequent geographical
isolation of mental patients in asylums in the countryside is a
later development which was determined by the terms of the County
Asylum Act of 1808.

Some of the early asylums (such as Nottingham and Bedford) were
indeed built very near the centre of the cities they served, as it
was hoped that medical men could be encouraged to attend the
asylums on a part-time basis, but from 1815 onwards it became
fashionable to emphasise the importance of healthy, airy sites, a
pure water supply and enough space to permit recreation. The
actual choice of a site for an individual asylum was increasingly
determined by its proximity to county towns, the ease with which
the site could be reached using public transport and the need for
it to be at the centre of the catchment area to be served by the
asylum. Asylums built in the latter part of the century were of
increasingly large size, and it was assumed that they needed substantial estates surrounding them. Since land prices had soared
they were inevitably pushed further into the countryside. Needless
to say, the geographical isolation of the asylums also led to the
isolation of the nursing and psychiatric staff whose lives became
dominated by bureaucratic rules in much the same way as the
patients.

The subsequent development of the asylums cannot be explored in
any detail here, but it is necessary to stress that the movement
towards creating psychiatric units in general hospitals was a
direct response to the increasing custodialism that dogged the
activities of the asylums, especially from the passing of 1890
Lunacy Act onwards. The Act, which was designed to protect the
rights of the individual against wrongful certification and compulsory incarceration in the asylum, effectively converted the
asylums into prisons. At the same time the size of the asylums
increased alarmingly. The average size of the asylum in terms of
beds increased from 116 in 1827, to 542 in 1870, to 961 by 1900.
By 1930 the figure was 1,221.

ALTERNATIVES TO CUSTODIAL CARE

Given the largely custodial nature of the care provided by the
asylums, a number of attempts were made to avoid sending patients
to them. In 1889 the first outpatient clinic was opened at St
Thomas's Hospital by Rayner, and a number of other general hospitals and asylums (such as Wakefield Asylum) followed suit.
However, the most interesting event during this period was the
establishment of a psychiatric unit at Barnhill Hospital in Glasgow.
This development was not surprising since some important innovations
in the treatment of mental patients had already been made in
Scotland.

In the 1870s and 1880s a policy of open doors had been started
first at the Fife and Kinrose Asylum but spreading to other hospitals. In addition, the introduction of hospital-trained nursing
staff and the copying of methods used in general hospitals influenced the life of mental hospitals. The Barnhill Unit was a
very interesting development, since it was a genuine treatment
centre rather than an observation ward. Patients entering the
unit did so only after prior screening undertaken in the course
of a domiciliary visit.

In England the first real impetus to the development of both
inpatient and outpatient centres in general hospitals arose from
the crisis in the asylums caused by the First World War. As a
response to the increasing difficulties resulting from the workings
of the Lunacy Act and shortages of both staff and facilities, the
Board of Control proposed in 1918 that the early treatment of acute
cases could be improved by providing treatment in general hospital
settings. The recommendation fell on stony ground, largely because
inpatient treatment of voluntary patients could not be carried out
without going through a certification procedure. It is salutary
to remember that prior to 1930 the Maudsley Hospital (opened in
1923) was the only public hospital in England in which inpatient
care could be given without certification. In 1929 the Jordanburn
Nerve Hospital and Psychological Institute was opened in Edinburgh
in order to perform a similar function, but it is also true that
a number of the more recently built asylums began to develop a
policy of making better provision for acute patients (Walk,1964).
Hospitals such as Hellingly in east Sussex and Napsbury, near
St Albans, included small self-contained units built in their
grounds. Patients entering these were able to receive a complete
treatment programme without entering the main building.

THE PROBLEM OF UNSATISFACTORY RECOVERY RATES

Part of the impetus for these innovations was the realisation that
recovery rates in the mental hospitals were declining or static.
For example, Lord (1929) drew attention to the fact the recovery
rate calculated on an admissions basis to county and borough hospitals for the period 1871-80 was 40.32 per cent but the comparable
figure for the period 1919-28 was 31.3 per cent. Two years later
another psychiatrist, Leeper (1931), gave a slightly different
version of these figures, indicating that the rate was more or
less static since a 1910-19 recovery rate was recorded as being
32 per cent while the 1920-9 rate was 31 per cent.

Despite these depressing figures, Lord argued that 'scientific
psychiatry ... has enormously reduced the sum total of suffering,
both mental and physical, in mental hospitals' (Lord, 1929). The
only reasons that these successes had not been reflected in
improved rate was the failure to treat patients in the early
stages of their illnesses. But Leeper (1931) gave a far more
critical answer to the question of whether scientific psychiatry
had failed:

  my answer ... is that scientific psychiatry has not failed
  but that many modern developments which we have been inclined

to regard as scientific, are not really scientific at all, and
that until we have radically remodelled or discarded many of
these theories and methods, we cannot expect an improvement in
recovery rate.

In particular, Leeper attacked both the 'mental analysis' of
psychotic patients and treatments designed to eradicate 'toxic
foci' as prime examples of damaging forms of treatment, but he
also criticised the use of ultraviolet light, electrical treatment and the blanket prescriptions of sedatives. It is not clear
from his article what modern forms of treatment survived his
criticisms, but he also concluded that legislation aiding early
treatment would play a part in improving recovery rates.

Such legislation had been enacted the year before, but it is
important to realise that the Mental Treatment Act did not result
in the universal provision of new types of inpatient care. Outpatient clinics attached to teaching hospitals did develop more
widely, but the already existing system of observation wards
attached to general hospitals and workhouses continued to function
in much the same way.

THE ROLE OF OBSERVATION WARDS

There is very little research concerned with the functioning of
observation wards to draw upon, but fortunately Pentreath and Dax
published a detailed account of one in 1937. The unit was run by
the London County Council (LCC) and it contained eighty-two beds.
Its catchment area contained approximately 750,000 people and it
admitted about 1,000 patients per year. The unit was staffed by
two medical officers and a psychiatric social worker, but the
medical superintendent from the Maudsley also acted as a consultant for difficult cases. Patients requiring inpatient or outpatient care were often sent to the Maudsley but there was a
reverse procedure for patients who needed to be sent to a mental
hospital for longer-term treatment. The unit also received some
patients from the special annexe at King's College Hospital which
was staffed by personnel from the Maudsley Hospital.

Mental observation wards of this type can be seen as prototypes
for the psychiatric units in general hospitals that were developed
in the wake of the 1959 Mental Health Act. In some cases observation wards became psychiatric units through a direct process of
evolution in which the changes contained in the Mental Health Act
played a crucial role. The extension of the minimum observation
order from seventeen to twenty-eight days enabled the units to
devote more of their attention to treatment rather than diagnosis
and classification.

As Pentreath and Dax (1937) pointed out, the observation ward
that they directed was responsible for carrying out a multiplicity
of functions. The LCC had a policy of avoiding certifying patients
and removing them from their homes directly to the overcrowded
mental hospitals that were situated many miles away in the countryside. Instead, patients were sent to centralised observation
wards where they could be detained first on a relieving officer's
three-day order and then on a medical officer's fourteen-day order.

During this period they could be assessed so that their needs
could be catered for more realistically. At the end of the
detention period they could be transferred from the ward to a
suitable institution for treatment, or discharged if they showed
improvement.

THE CONTROVERSY OVER THE THERAPEUTIC POTENTIAL OF OBSERVATION WARDS

In practice the functioning of the observation wards was very
dependent on the adequacy of the staff and the resources that were
allocated to them. For example, the Board of Control's report for
1935 contains several highly critical references to the observation
wards in municipal hospitals and institutions. These were so badly
staffed (by largely untrained attendants) that the Board recommended that patients should be immediately transferred to the
appropriate mental hospital which in general was 'the only place
able to provide the specialised experience and therapeutic resources necessary for successful treatment'. The Report also concluded that 'every improvement of the observation wards increases
the temptation to undertake active treatment, a practice quite
inconsistent with the main purpose of such wards which is the
diagnosis of doubtful cases'.
   Since the members of the Board of Control were traditionally
recruited from retired physician-superintendents of mental asylums,
it was to be expected that the Board should make such a recommendation. However, the medical profession's opinion was clearly
divided on the issue. The growth of outpatient clinics and the
provision of better staffed observation wards provided an alternative approach that had many advantages. An editorial in the
'Lancet' in October 1936 provides a classic example of rebuttal
of the Board's recommendations. It argued that the report failed
to consider the problem of the stigma associated with entering a
mental hospital ('Lancet', 1936):

   the public has not yet come to regard the mental hospital in
   the same way as it does the general hospital, the partial sub-
   stitution of voluntary for compulsory treatment has done much
   to counteract the general prejudice, but it is still possible
   to suffer economically and socially because one is known to
   have been in a mental hospital. This injustice and hardship
   may rest as heavily on the patient who was voluntarily in the
   mental hospital as on those under certificate ... the use of
   the observation wards for treatment of the case that will clear
   up within three or four weeks has therefore still much more to
   be said in its favour. The issue must turn on the facilities
   available in the observation ward, and the extent to which the
   public has been or can be brought to an unprejudiced notion of
   mental hospitals. Where the observation ward is improvised,
   staffed by people with no psychiatric experience, or used as
   a common dumping ground for chronic patients, low grade and
   mental defectives as well as the acutely insane, there can be
   no valid argument for its retention; immediate admission to
   the mental hospital is far preferable. But where the observation ward serves its proper purpose in the coordinated

psychiatric services of a district, it is at once the reception
hospital for acute or dangerous mental illness, the distributing
and diagnostic centre, and the place of treatment for very
transient conditions, such as some toxic and symptomatic
psychoses or suicidal attempts of neurotic or reactively
depressed patients who soon become suitable for out-patient
treatment.

The editorial's enthusiasm for well-staffed admission wards contrasted strikingly with the Board of Control's enthusiasm for
admission units in mental hospitals. The report argued that the
admission of uncertified patients to mental hospitals would in
time lead to a modification of the popular dislike of mental hospitals. But the 'Lancet' editorial contradicted this - a better
strategy would be to provide facilities for prompt and early treatment in a setting that would be more acceptable in the first place.

Pentreath and Dax's (1937) review gave some support for the
editorial's standpoint on a number of issues. For example, some
patients were indeed successfully returned home without being sent
on to mental hospitals. However, in assessing the role of their
observation ward they made some interesting points which are still
relevant to the functioning of psychiatric units in general hospitals. They acknowledged that observation wards were still in
their infancy as far as their developmental possibilities were
concerned but they were clear as to their general advantages. One
advantage canvassed by them concerned the wards' ability to provide
patients for teaching purposes. It was becoming increasingly
recognised that medical students needed to be taught psychiatry
and they needed access to acute cases. Observation wards also
provided rich research material and the possibility for gaining
experience in treating patients at an early stage in the onset of
the disease process.

But at a more fundamental level, if observation wards were
properly constituted they could function as follows. They would
dispose of 'justifiably certifiable' patients which Pentreath and
Dax describe as 'patients who should be transferred under the
Lunacy Acts as soon as grounds for certification can be found'.
Voluntary patients and temporary cases could also be rapidly dealt
with since their stay would be very short, coinciding with the
length of time it took to get their papers duly completed. However, the main activities of the ward would be concentrated on a
much larger group of patients who required both investigation and
active treatment. A large percentage of these would in fact make
a rapid recovery so that they would not be sent on to a mental
hospital. Patients would therefore avoid the problem of becoming
stigmatised since the general public viewed entry into the mental
hospital as a major disaster.

The work of observation wards such as the one described by
Pentreath and Dax provided important new experiences in handling
acute patients. The LCC developed a policy of appointing consultant psychiatrists to attend such units on a regular basis, but
despite this the main impetus for developing inpatient care within
general hospitals came from a different quarter. The Mental Treatment Act contributed to the development of psychiatric outpatient
clinics so that by 1936 there were at least 160 such clinics.

However, the provision of inpatient care was still predominantly
confined to the mental hospitals. In 1938 an editorial in the
'Lancet' reviewed the provision of inpatient care in general hospitals, providing the following interesting international comparison ('Lancet', 1938). While the United States had seventy-
eight inpatient units, Canada had four, Germany had seven and
Denmark had two. Britain had no units, but six beds in general
wards were provided both at Guy's and at the Middlesex. (In fact,
the editorial overlooks the annexe at King's College staffed by
personnel from the Maudsley Hospital.)

The editorial argued that it was essential to develop such units
since they avoided the problem of stigma, provided better diagnostic facilities and allowed hospital staff to gain by having
closer contact with psychiatrists. However, the main advantage of
such units was surprisingly that they facilitated the teaching of
medical students. In the words of the editorial,

> it is to students however that such a clinic within their
> medical school offers most. The present system of occasional
> demonstrations at a distant mental hospital gives little en-
> couragement even to those few students who feel naturally
> attracted to psychiatry and leaves the average student ... with
> an impression comparable to that obtained from a series of
> visits to the Zoo.

Some sections of the medical profession saw the educational opportunities that such units provided in training in psychiatry as
being of crucial importance, but an editorial in the 'British
Medical Journal' published in 1936 also stressed their importance
in bringing psychiatry and neurology closer together. It argued
that the voluntary hospitals ought to take on a larger share of
treatment of psychiatric patients because they were potentially
the best centres of treatment for acute cases ('BMJ', 1936):

> Extension in this direction will diminish the discrimination
> between neurology and psychiatry which has been artificially
> exaggerated by the concentration of so much psychiatric material
> in mental hospitals ... the difference in the intramural and
> extramural life and training of the two disciplines is perhaps
> the largest factor in the misunderstandings and difference in
> point of view which exist today.

In practice little was achieved in developing such units in the
1930s. St George's planned a fifty-bedded clinic as part of its
rebuilding programme and Guy's eventually constructed a forty-two-
bedded unit but this did not open until 1944. The war undoubtedly
prevented initiatives being taken but other factors also contributed to the slow development of such units. It is obvious,
for example, that there was a great deal of scepticism about the
efficacy of psychiatry which would have influenced decision-making
by hospital governors. For example, in 1937 the governors of the
Middlesex Hospital finally recognised as autonomous the Department
of Psychological Medicine which had been in existence for fourteen
years.

The reasons for neglecting the importance of psychiatry in this
period were complex but one explanation was put forward by a
'Lancet' editorial ('Lancet', 1937):

> the question may be asked whether the psychiatrist is in fact

sometimes neglected because he does not give much help - whether
his performance in short is as great as his pretensions. It is
true that in the mouths of some enthusiasts the pretensions are
excessive, and non-psychiatric colleagues who take the claims
of ardent psychotherapists over-seriously become disillusioned
and too liberally derisive.

However, the editorial stressed that psychiatry was in 'most part
a sober branch of medicine, not only keenly aware of its limitations ... but capable of giving much practical help in treatment'.

Interestingly, the editorial quoted American evidence to support
this argument since it referred to a review by Billings (1941) of
the experiences of the Colorado General Hospital in treating psychiatric cases.

PSYCHIATRIC SERVICES IN AMERICAN GENERAL HOSPITALS

Billings's work was considered important because it reported that
one in seven new outpatients attending the hospital required psychiatric treatment while one in thirteen patients admitted to the
medical wards 'presented a conspicuous personality disorder that
accounted for their disorder'. Of the total new cases either seen
in the various outpatient departments or admitted to the wards,
nearly 4 per cent were promptly referred for psychiatric treatment.
The 'Lancet' editorial comments that the figures confirmed the
view 'already generally held in principle in English teaching hospitals, that psychiatry is not only one of the essential services
but one of the most likely to develop further'.

Kasanin (1937), who was director of the department of psychiatry
at the Michael Rees Hospital, Chicago, contributed a paper on the
'Function of a Psychiatrist in a General Hospital' to the same
edition of the 'Lancet'. It is equally interesting as it raised
a number of issues concerning the domestication of psychiatry
within a general hospital setting. Kasanin sets out to answer the
crucial question of how the psychiatrist could demonstrate the
effectiveness of his approach to the sceptical medical man and
even more sceptical medical student. He argued that the most
effective method of making psychiatry accessible and understood
by the medical man was by establishing psychiatric clinics with
sufficient personnel to take care of the psychiatric referrals to
such clinics. But it was not enough just to establish such clinics
and wait for referrals to flow:

in the first place there is a definite tendency to refer to the
psychiatric clinic those patients in whom the medical man loses
interest. When a case becomes therapeutically hopeless, when
it becomes a chronic liability, or if the case is poorly understood, it is 'dumped' into the psychiatric clinic. When such
a case is rejected by the psychiatric clinic and sent back to
the referring physician it only arouses his anger, with a
counter attack on psychiatry as being ineffective and useless.

Other difficulties such as problems of communication could also
intervene, so that even when the psychiatrist has been able to
achieve good therapeutic results he may still remain isolated

because his colleagues have lost interest in the case that they
had referred to him weeks or months before. Kasanin argued that
the only solution to such problems was for the psychiatrist to
become a member of any one of the established medical clinics:
   there he becomes a sort of 'floater' accessible to all the
   men in the clinic, a man whom they can consult freely and with
   whom they can discuss their cases without any constraint or
   suspicion ... it is only when the medical man works in close
   contact with the psychiatrist that both develop mutual confidence and faith in each other and begin to appreciate each
   other's point of view.
Kasanin reported that such working relationships had been established in the thyroid clinic, a gastro-intestinal clinic, a general
medical clinic and the general admission clinic at the Michael Rees
Hospital. The main role of the psychiatrist in these settings was
to provide psychotherapy for patients who presented with somatic
complaints that were psychological in origin, but the psychiatrists
also functioned in the outpatient clinics where they received
direct referrals for psychiatric treatment. The predominant method
of treatment was the so-called 'anamnestic-cathartic' method developed by Meyer, but interestingly Kasanin argued that most treatment of 'maladjustments and neuroses' should be carried out by the
'general medical man'. He assumed that, if the psychiatrist could
communicate and teach the medical man some of his techniques and
points of view, he would more than justify his existence in a
general hospital.

   The development of psychiatric units in general hospitals
occurred much earlier and on a broader front in America. From
Haun's review published in 1950 it appears that the first unit
was set up in Christ Hospital, Topeka (Kansas), in the early 1920s.
American psychiatry seems to have been more aware of the commercial
possibilities of treating patients in general hospitals - indeed,
Haun's review itself is concerned almost exclusively with comparing
different architectual plans for such units - a clear indication
that there was a growing market for them (Haun, 1950).

   Six years later Bennett et al. (1956) published a review of
'the practice of psychiatry in general hospitals' which gave a more
comprehensive picture of the growth of the movement in the United
States. The book was in fact specifically designed to act as a
handbook, giving meticulous and detailed advice on all aspects of
the running of such units.

THE ORIGIN OF PSYCHIATRIC UNITS IN BRITISH GENERAL HOSPITALS

The strength of the movement in America in the postwar period
contrasted markedly with the very limited developments in Britain.
However, it is important to stress that the movement towards
psychiatry in general hospitals in Britain developed largely as a
result of the impact that the new physical treatments made from
the early 1940s onwards. An editorial in the 'British Medical
Journal' ('BMJ', 1943 a) confirms this point in an interesting way:
   Whatever may be the ultimate scope of the new physical methods
   in the treatment of mental diseases they have collateral

advantages of no inconsiderable kind. Their tangibility makes
them easily acceptable to the layman, sometimes perhaps dan-
gerously acceptable; and for the same reason they have an appeal
to medical men in general, who, somewhat to their own detriment,
are still apt to regard mental diseases as things apart from
their concern. The actual physical treatment of mental disease
... should have the effect on many people of bringing mental
diseases within the same category of thought as physical ill-
health.

The editorial also explored the impact of the new methods in
raising staff morale but it assumed that the patients would be
most profoundly affected:

about their moral effect on the patients themselves there is
no doubt whatever. They above all people appreciate the reality
of the methods and the amount of attention that they receive
from doctors and nurses in the process - even apart from the
actual results in curtailment of suffering ... early treatment
becomes more possible because both patients and relatives are
willing to accept it and ... a general hospital can become a
suitable place for the treatment of many mental illnesses which
hitherto have had to be sent to special hospitals.

The editorial based its views mainly on some research carried out
at the Sutton Emergency Hospital by Dr Dalton Sands, who claimed
a success rate of 80 per cent in returning patients to the community, following treatment using insulin, electroshock, continuous
narcosis and leucotomy (Sands, 1943). Sands's results led the
editorial to argue that the introduction of psychiatric wards in
general wards was both more practicable and more desirable than
ever. It also argued that the reorganisation of the medical
services which was then being planned by Beveridge should involve
the integration of 'mental medicine' with 'physical medicine'.

MENTAL HOSPITALS VERSUS PSYCHIATRIC UNITS - THE CONTROVERSY BEGINS

The editorial itself provoked a wide-ranging correspondence which
dealt with a number of issues that were to dominate discussions
of the psychiatric services for the next three decades. A letter
from Rees and Shepley (from Warlingham Park Hospital) was particularly significant as it contained a number of classic objections
to developing psychiatric units in general hospitals as advocated
by the editorial. The letter acknowledged that such units had a
place if attached to the 'great teaching hospitals', but it
insisted that the mental health of the community would be best
served if more funds were allocated to the existing mental hospital
system. The justification for this policy was three-fold. First,
Rees and Shepley argued that the better mental hospitals were
capable of producing as good results as Sands's unit. Second,
they argued that it was naive to assume that the question of stigma
was avoided by sending patients to 'neuropsychiatric' wards - in
practice these wards became popularly known as 'mental' wards so
nothing was gained. (As a rider to this point they added that the
stigma of entering a mental hospital had been successfully overcome
at hospitals like Warlingham, since over 80 per cent of the

patients were voluntary ones.) Finally, they argued that the
introduction of the new units would 'relegate the mental hospitals
to their former melancholy role of custodianship largely of the
chronic incurable' (Rees and Shepley, 1943).

Rees and Shepley clearly acted as spokesmen for the psychiatrists
working in the mental hospitals. They felt threatened by the new
proposals because they implied that the mental hospitals would
eventually be run down or indeed pulled down. Interestingly another
contributor to the correspondence - A.M. Spencer (writing from the
Joint Counties Mental Hospital, Carmarthen) - must be credited with
being among the first to suggest that they should indeed be pulled
down. In fact he suggested that they should be replaced by temporary hospitals consisting of isolated single-storey wards each
containing twenty-five patients at the most (Spencer, 1943). But
the correspondence in the 'British Medical Journal' is interesting
from another point of view - it clearly reveals that the profession
of psychiatry was split into different camps.

PSYCHIATRIC UNITS AND THE TEACHING HOSPITALS

This division within psychiatry was commented on in a further
editorial in the 'British Medical Journal' (1943b), which contained
a review of the recommendations of the Langdon-Brown Committee
on Postgraduate Training in Psychological Medicine:
    many psychiatrists ... still suffer from the fact that mental
    hospitals, where most of them live and work, provide a limited
    though valuable and indispensable type of experience, but one
    which fits them in only a one-sided fashion for the great bulk
    of extra-mural psychiatric work ... on the other hand there are
    many psychiatrists who have never held an appointment in a
    mental hospital ... this deficiency in the experience of the
    most serious and profound mental disorders is not by any means
    completely compensated by residence and work in a psychiatric
    clinic or hospital for 'early' or 'recoverable' cases exclu-
    sively.
The editorial partly blames psychiatrists themselves for having
allowed these accidental and unfortunate differences of experience
to create divisions within the profession, but it also points out
('BMJ', 1943b) that psychiatric institutions also contributed
    the cause of these schisms lies largely in the nature of our
    psychiatric institutions ... (examinations as well as hospital
    organization) ... almost alone of Western countries Britain has
    failed to develop in-patient accommodation in special units
    inside general teaching hospitals. The advantages of such
    units ... are many but in general they help to confer not only
    on future psychiatrists but on medical students a comprehensive
    outlook on mental disorder, and a psychological as well as a
    physical orientation towards the problems of everyday practice.
It can be seen from this editorial that there was a growing consensus that psychiatric units needed to be established in teaching
hospitals because of the needs of medical students and trainee
psychiatrists. But at a deeper level there was also a consensus
that psychiatry needed to be fully integrated into medicine. This

viewpoint was clearly expressed in a memorandum on the Future
Organisation of the Psychiatric Services which was put forward
by committees of the Royal College of Physicians, the Royal Medico-
Psychological Association and the British Medical Association
('Lancet', 1945).   The memorandum advocated a more adequate measure
of domiciliary consulting service, outpatient consultant centres
and inpatient accommodation in teaching hospitals and the larger
non-teaching hospitals.   Divisions within the psychiatric profession were to be overcome by instituting a system of rotation
between the mental hospitals, the general hospitals and the outpatient clinics.

The last proposal is in fact the most significant for our purposes, since in practice it would often involve upgrading observation wards so that they became early treatment units which were
departments of, or readily accessible to, general hospitals.   However, despite these far-reaching policy proposals there was little
change in the psychiatric services in the immediate postwar period.
The reasons for this are obviously complicated, but it is important
to stress that there was persistently considerable disagreement
over how the psychiatric services should be organised.   For
instance, the influential Blacker report published in 1946 recommended closer links between general and mental hospitals and the
provision of extended outpatient clinics (Jones, 1972).   But it
also recommended that small independent psychiatric units should
also be developed.   There was no suggestion that psychiatric units
in general hospitals should become an essential part of the
services.

Surprisingly, even the advent of the National Health Service in
1948 did not affect the structure of the services in any far-
reaching way.   Indeed, an editorial in the 'Lancet' in January 1950
pointed out that the bias of the NHS, at least in its initial
phase, was towards the development and improvement of the existing
hospital care.   A letter in response to the editorial bemoaned the
fact that under the NHS the psychiatrist was once more being yoked
to the municipal hospital or the mental wards of the old municipal
hospitals since the mental hospital was to remain the focus of
treatment.   In this climate attempts to develop preventive and
community based services were stymied (Edelston, 1950).

THE SIGNIFICANCE OF THE MANCHESTER REGION

Given the stagnation in the overall reorganisation of the services,
some psychiatrists experimented with admitting suitably selected
patients to medical wards within general hospitals.   In the
Manchester region, as we have already noted, the services began
to be reorganised from 1948 in order to give psychiatric units in
general hospitals greater prominence, but on a national scale no
major changes occurred until the deliberations of the Royal
Commission on the Law Relating to Mental Illness and Mental
Deficiency began to create a new climate of change.   Some isolated
experiments in changing psychiatric care were undertaken.   These
were of two fundamentally different types - one group comprised
those that further improved the existing mental hospitals, creating

firmer links with general hospital outpatient services and in some
cases inviting other departments to move into empty wards or villas
and so turning the mental hospital itself into a general hospital.
The other group consisted of comprehensive psychiatric services
located in and operated from the general hospitals of which they
had come to be an integral part.

In the next chapter we will explore this division of opinion
within the psychiatric profession in greater depth since we seek
to establish the basis upon which government policy changed in
order to give psychiatric units in general hospitals a much enhanced
role within the psychiatric services. The fact that a policy change
of this type occurred is significant to our argument since we would
postulate that the social control function of psychiatry is, in a
peculiar way, embodied in such units. Such units were initially
developed in a piecemeal fashion because of the introduction of new
physical and pharmacological types of treatment. But they are
largely antipathetic to other forms of treatment (psychotherapy
and group therapy) which require very different settings and staff.
The latter forms of treatment are also far more problematic when
viewed from the angle of social control. This is not to deny that
all forms of therapy are potentially controlling but to argue that
the philosophy and approach of many modern forms of psychotherapy
are, in fact, opposed to inducing dependency and passivity in
patients.

We should also hasten to add that we clearly have no brief for
supporting the traditional mental hospitals either. The social
control function of psychiatry can be equally well discharged in
such hospitals, but it is nevertheless true that many important
positive innovations in therapy have been developed in such
settings. This is not surprising, given the much greater flexi-
bility that is possible in mental hospitals because of their often
superior resources.

Chapter 5

The ascendancy of psychiatric units in general hospitals

An American psychologist, Hershenson, donning the mantle of
C. Northcott Parkinson, has wryly proposed a new law of human
behaviour (Hershenson, 1961):

> The amount of research effort expended on a problem by psycho-
> logists is in inverse proportion to its significance for
> humanity. For example, the time and energy expended on sexual
> pursuits is much less than the 40 hours per week most people
> spend working (with the possible exceptions of prostitutes, in
> whose case the two issues are confounded) yet the over-whelming
> bulk of clinical studies are concerned with sexual impulses.

Anybody studying the recent changes in the psychiatric services in
Britain will readily agree that at least in this area Hershenson's
'law' has been richly confirmed. Substantial changes in psychiatric
care have occurred since the Hospital Plan of 1962 and yet the
amount of research devoted to such changes by psychologists or
indeed anyone else is remarkably small. Policy-makers have been
singularly undeterred by the lack of adequate research, although
from time to time the medical profession has sounded the alarm.
For example, in 1962 a leading article in the 'Lancet' contained
the following strange plea: 'From the people who are initiating
and conducting such in-patient units we need to know more of their
plans and problems and of the range of cases they treat and how
they manage them' ('Lancet', 1962). Naively, one might have assumed
that a major change in health policy would have occurred only after
a number of carefully executed research studies had taken place.
But this, of course, is not the way the National Health Service
works. Cochrane (1971) and other critics have eloquently attacked
the endemic lack of research into the effectiveness of treatments
within the NHS, but nevertheless the exact reasons for this neglect
are puzzling given the degree of change involved.

RECENT RESEARCH INTO PSYCHIATRIC UNITS IN GENERAL HOSPITALS

Some clues to the answer can be gleaned from examining the work of
a number of psychiatrists who have been intimately involved in the
development of psychiatric units in general hospitals. Little's

(1974) book 'Psychiatry in a General Hospital' is perhaps the most
fruitful starting point for this discussion. It is primarily concerned with documenting the activities of a psychiatric unit in
St James's Hospital in Leeds; but although the empirical data in
the book were collected between 1964 and 1966, the study was not
fully published until 1974. Little explains the general lack of
research into the functioning of psychiatric units in classical
terms - lack of funds provided by the NHS and lack of time because
the psychiatrists involved in many such units are paid to be
clinicians, not researchers.

Both points are obviously valid and he elaborates his arguments
with some intriguing points which require detailed examination.
Thus he writes (Little, 1974):

> The Department of Health and Social Security launched a massive
> programme to establish psychiatric units in every district
> general hospital in England and Wales ... yet one is aware of
> slender evidence ... demonstrating in any scientific manner
> the effectiveness of such services. This is not to say that
> the Department of Health is misguided; many of the decisions
> involved depend of necessity on value judgements. Methodo-
> logically it is far from easy to assess scientifically the
> psychological advantages to staff and patients of the general
> hospital therapeutic setting.... We had a very strong impression
> in Leeds that patients' relatives and general practitioners
> preferred the general hospital, often for subtle but important
> social reasons if no other.... But it is doubtful now whether
> studies pursued according to accepted standards of scientific
> vigour would stem the surge of 'progressive' opinion in its
> desire for change.... Intuitive human judgement may well prove
> more sound than a pseudoscientism which misses the target
> through failure to take cognizance of what is truly relevant.
> At a similar level, one might have expected before now a greater
> reporting in depth of the activities of general hospital units,
> for lack of which there has been much misinformed speculation
> and criticism.

This passage is quoted (more or less) in full because it illustrates
many of the issues that have preoccupied us in writing this book.
Little's final conclusion is that research money and resources
should be made available to the clinicians actually involved in
running psychiatric units, since most research is undertaken by
university-based departments of psychiatry, which are usually not
involved in the everyday running of comprehensive services. This
plea for more research is, of course, a classic example of closing
the door after the horse has bolted. One can readily agree that
some alternative to the traditional Victorian mental hospital must
be developed, but why should 'progressive' opinion assume that
psychiatric unit in the general hospital is the only alternative?
The quotation marks around the word 'progressive' really give the
game away - indeed, if the term 'progressive' is replaced by the
phrase 'medical and psychiatric', we arrive at the essence of the
matter.

The medical profession, particularly through its psychiatric
wing, has increasingly played the key role in defining the nature
of mental disorders. Mental disorders are seen as 'illnesses'

essentially similar to physical illnesses, so only medically
trained specialists can be legitimately responsible for treating
patients. The patients, since they are suffering from illnesses,
should be placed in a general hospital alongside patients suffering
from physical illnesses. Given this inexorable style of arguing,
it is not at all surprising that psychiatrists who have examined
the work of psychiatric units in general hospitals have failed
to explore the alternatives to such approaches. They unquestionably
adopt a paradigm which insists that mental disorders are illnesses,
and hence they view the development of the psychiatric services in
Britain as a logical progression.

From the turn of the century onwards, the mostly Victorian built
lunatic asylums were increasingly called mental hospitals - a
change reflecting the development of the psychiatric profession
which was increasingly influenced by attitudes concerning mental
disorders. The psychiatric unit in a general hospital eventually
emerged as a replacement for these mental hospitals when more
active medical treatments began to become available. But the idea
that the psychiatric unit in the general hospital is the only
logical setting for treatment can be challenged. It is striking
that in America psychiatric services have developed in a very
different way since the end of the 1960s, and yet in both the
United States and Britain the same challenge had to be met.

AMERICAN AND BRITISH POLICIES COMPARED

In both the United States and Britain the large, mostly Victorian
built mental hospitals, providing largely custodial care, needed
to be replaced by units capable of providing more active and personal treatment programmes. The American solution, incorporated
into the Mental Retardation Act of 1963, was far more radical and
far-reaching than the equivalent British solution contained in
the 1962 Hospital Plan. President Kennedy in his now famous
speech to Congress in 1963 proposed a 'bold new national mental
health program' which had the aim of shifting 'the homes of treatment of the mentally ill from state mental hospitals into community
mental health centers'. Community mental health centres were
essentially conceived as administrative units rather than physical
structures of a particular sort. One might assume that a 'centre'
would be a single building somewhat like a community hospital,
but the regulations issued in conjunction with the Act merely
required that a centre should provide a wide range of services.
It permitted these services to be physically separated as long as
they were administratively integrated. Psychiatric units in
general hospitals, providing inpatient care, could constitute
part of the 'centre' so that they contributed to the overall range
of services rather than being the core of the services.

The British solution, outlined originally in the 1962 Hospital
Plan, places much greater emphasis on the psychiatric unit in the
district general hospital. The latter was conceived as a large
hospital which would cater for all medical specialities and hence
would lead to the phasing out of specialist hospitals, such as
mental hospitals, hospitals for the chronic sick, etc. The

essence of the plan was, therefore to establish the hospital service
as a short-stay service for acute patients only.   Such a system
would, of course, work only in the context of the provision of
adequate, well co-ordinated community services, but it is ironic
and significant that there was a year's gap between the publication
of the 1962 Hospital Plan and the publication of the associated
document, 'Health and Welfare: the Development of Community Care',
which was concerned with the planning of community services.   The
latter document not only lacked the panache and clarity of the
Hospital Plan, but singularly failed to spell out a rationale for
community care.   This abnegation of leadership by the government
was crucial in influencing subsequent developments.   While it was
clearly government policy to reduce the number of beds by half,
the provision of community services was to be left to the discretion
of the local authorities - a strange and almost anarchic policy
since it would inevitably lead to great disparities in the provision
of community services.

This complex issue really requires detailed discussion in its
own right but it is clear that district general hospitals are being
developed irrespective of the adequate development of community
services.   It is also clear that the treatment of the majority of
mentally disordered patients will remain under the effective control
of the psychiatric profession.   The contrast with American practice
is very striking on both these counts.   A crucial feature of the
Community Mental Health Center Act was to establish the principle
that no one profession had the exclusive right to provide therapy
for mentally disordered patients.   Psychologists, psychiatrists
and social workers could contribute equally to treatment programmes,
and the directorship of the community health centre was not to be
the preserve of any one profession.   Equally, there was a concerted
attempt to provide community-based services rather than hospital-
based ones.

The American example, therefore, serves to illustrate a crucial
point in our argument - that the policy of replacing mental hospitals with psychiatric units in general hospitals reflects both
the power of the medical profession and the weakness of other
professionals (such as social workers and psychologists) in
influencing policy-making.

Until very recently clinical psychologists as a body have never
effectively challenged the supremacy of the psychiatric profession
in deciding what sort of therapies should be administered to
patients in mental hospitals.   Admittedly, Eysenck's manifesto,
'The Future of Psychiatry', does represent an effective challenge
to psychiatry, but it is remarkable that this challenge should be
made so recently (Eysenck, 1975).   Similar challenges occurred
much earlier in America - indicating the much greater strength
and maturity of psychology, both as a discipline and a profession.

THE SIGNIFICANCE OF THE POLICY OF DESEGREGATING THE MENTALLY ILL

But to return to the main line of our argument, it is our contention that the 'desegregation' of the mentally ill, which involves
the eventual replacement of large geographically isolated mental

hospitals by psychiatric units in (the now renamed district)
general hospitals, has both a manifest and a latent function.
Ostensibly the change in policy was for the benefit of patients,
but certain sections of the profession of psychiatry clearly had
a vested interest in achieving such a change in a field which, in
medical terms, has traditionally been out in the cold, and which
finally achieved the status of respectability when it took its
rightful place alongside other specialities in the hospital. It
is therefore entirely just that the Royal College of Psychiatrists
should be founded at a time when the DHSS pressed forward with
plans for the large-scale development of psychiatric units in
general hospitals. The psychiatric profession has achieved its
own desegregation in a formal sense at least, but what price, if
any, have patients paid in the process?

It is no surprise that there is virtually no published research
that can answer this question. The psychiatrists who have been
intimately involved in establishing and running psychiatric units
in general hospitals have been preoccupied with answering one
question and one question only - can the new units provide a comprehensive form of care which caters for the psychiatric needs of
a local community? This question is, of course, important to
answer, but it is entirely secondary to the more fundamental
questions that must be answered first - where and why did the idea
of psychiatric units originate?

Again, these apparently simple questions are difficult to answer
satisfactorily. Amazingly, Little (1974) fails even to mention
these issues in his book. If one turns to Hoenig and Hamilton's
much quoted book, 'The Desegregation of the Mentally Ill' (1969)
there is at least some attempt to explain the origin of psychiatric
units in general hospitals, although the authors' interest is
largely in the Manchester area. However, their brief account draws
very heavily on Jones's book, 'Mental Health and Social Policy'
(1960), and this book has many weaknesses, as we have already
pointed out. To take one example which is particularly relevant
to the present discussion - one section of her book is devoted to
exploring the changes in the mental asylums that occurred as a
result of the First World War. Hoenig and Hamilton refer approvingly to her 'very vivid' description of this period, but in
fact her account subtly obscures the depth of the crisis (Treacher,
in preparation). Surprisingly, Jones also fails to bring out the
significance of one of the key documents of the period in sufficient
detail - she refers in passing to Dr Lomax's book, 'The Experience
of an Asylum Doctor' (Lomax, 1921), but fails to include it in her
bibliography, and yet this book was the centre of controversy at
the time. Lomax was a GP who became an assistant asylum superintendent in a mental hospital in Prestwich during the closing stages
of the war. Since his was only a temporary appointment (replacing
medical staff away at the war) he was fully prepared to publicise
his experiences without fear of dismissal. The dismal and fright-
ening picture of asylum life that he portrays in his book was
probably typical of the asylums during this period, but Jones
fails to grasp the extent of the crisis at this time and also
fails to deal adequately with the protest movement that developed
in response to it.

LOMAX AND THE DEVELOPMENTS IN THE MANCHESTER AREA

Lomax himself was instrumental in getting an ex-patient's account of asylum life published. This book, 'Experiences of an Asylum Patient' (Grant-Smith, 1922), related the experiences of a female patient who was certified insane during a period of depression following the death of her husband. Over a period of twelve years she was an involuntary patient in five different hospitals and was exposed to many forms of ill-treatment. Several similar accounts from patients, amplified by anonymous accounts from asylum attendants, also received wide publicity during the same period. Jones only documents the official reaction to such events, although she does mention that there was a popular outcry at the time.

Surprisingly, Hoenig and Hamilton also pay little specific attention to Lomax despite his involvement in the Manchester area - they argue that the outcry following the inquiry into Lomax's book 'prefaced the way for subsequent developments leading to the return of psychiatry to the medical field'. This may well be true, but it remains a puzzle as to why Manchester became the centre of the new developments in psychiatric care.

Hoenig and Hamilton hint that it was precisely because the Manchester region had got such a bad reputation as a centre of custodial care that active attempts were made to correct the balance by first of all introducing outpatient care and then in- corporating psychiatric units in general hospitals. The Manchester region's development of outpatient clinics dates from 1918 when the Board of Control (responsible for monitoring the operation of the 1890 Lunacy Act) made its first recommendation in favour of voluntary and early treatment in outpatient clinics. When the NHS came into being in 1948, Manchester took the opportunity to re- organise psychiatric care, introducing psychiatric units in general hospitals. These units were, therefore, well established before the Mental Health Act of 1959 finally removed the legal distinction between general and mental hospitals, so that every hospital was now given the legal right to treat compulsorily detained patients. Eventually units similar to the Manchester one were developed in some shape or form throughout England and Wales.

Hoenig and Hamilton fail to explain why psychiatric units in general hospitals developed so much earlier in the Manchester region, and yet their explanation of natural developments are equally unsatisfactory. Jones's account is also strangely un- illuminating, largely because she does not set herself the specific task of exploring why such a policy emerged.

DEVELOPMENTS IN THE 1950S

On a national scale the mid- and late 1950s was a period of con- siderable social change and innovation as far as mental hospitals were concerned but it is a striking fact (as we have already noted) that remarkably little innovation was taking place at the other end of the psychiatric spectrum. Indeed, one can justifiably argue that psychiatric units in general hospitals were in the doldrums apart from developments in the Manchester area. In fact, prior to

1961 it is impossible to assemble more than a handful of research reports dealing with their activities.

In 1955 Dr J.T.C. Keddie, the medical officer of health in Oldham, reported on the activities of the psychiatric unit in the general hospital in his borough at a meeting of the Royal Society of Medicine (Keddie, 1955). The unit was a very large one containing 228 beds and was supervised by Dr Arthur Pool who had taken up his appointment in 1950. In fact Keddie's report was remarkably lacking in detail. It is clear that the necessity for the unit arose largely for administrative reasons. For historical reasons Oldham seems to have been poorly provided for in terms of hospital beds so the provision of a unit (in reality a small hospital) was sufficient to solve the problem. Interestingly Keddie's report is prefaced by a comment on the chronic shortage of nursing staff at the time as it would appear that economic and staffing difficulties also contributed to the experiment of locating a psychiatric unit within a general hospital complex.

Significantly, Keddie's discussion of the Oldham services was presented to the Royal Society at a meeting at which another speaker (Professor A. Querido) talked about the psychiatric services in Amsterdam. Amsterdam like Oldham did not have its own city mental hospital; instead it was provided with a series of psychiatric settings (including a 200-bedded university hospital with associated outpatient clinics, twenty polyclinics, two psychotherapy clinics and three child guidance clinics). The Amsterdam system placed a great premium on treating patients in their own homes in order to avoid hospitalisation so that in many ways it conformed to the community mental hospital model put forward by the World Health Organisation (WHO) in 1953 (Querido, 1955).

It was not until 1960 that the full details of the Oldham scheme received wide publicity when Freeman (1960) published a short paper in the 'Lancet' summarising its details. Freeman's report agreed in general with the earlier findings of Leyberg, who in 1959 had discussed the activities of similarly organised services in Bolton (Leyberg, 1959). The general conclusion of both reports was that psychiatric units could cope with the full range of patients and therefore operate completely independently provided some provision could be made for psychogeriatric cases. Freeman stressed the importance of the adequate provision of community services as being crucial for the successes of the scheme, but interestingly pointed out that elsewhere in the country mental hospitals had been equally adventurous in developing them. He therefore cited the famous Worthing service (which involved a mental hospital developing extensive community services independently of local authority services) and a similar system developed in Nottingham.

Other research of relevance to the policy change in 1961 was a statistical survey of London mental hospitals and observation wards which appeared in 1959. This meticulous study, carried out by Vera Norris, contained some interesting documentation of the functioning of the observation wards in London. Norris (1959) is at pains to argue that the wards freed approximately thirty-five hospital beds each year from being occupied, since in the period 1947-9 patients spent a total of 34,000 days in such units. Since no less than 15 per cent of all patients died within three days of

admission, the wards also prevented dying patients from being
inappropriately sent to mental hospitals. But perhaps the strongest
argument in their favour was that nearly a quarter of the patients
were discharged home or to general hospitals because they needed
no further psychiatric treatment. (On a national scale this would
mean that about 7,000 patients would not have to be sent to mental
hospitals.)

THE BASIS OF THE POLICY REVISION (1961-2)

The striking lack of concrete research into the functioning of
psychiatric units in general hospitals leads inevitably to the
conclusion that the policy change in 1961 was taken on a political
and social basis which had little or nothing to do with the proven
efficacy of one form of psychiatric system as opposed to another.
It can be argued that the decision was based upon experiences in
the United States where psychiatric units in general hospitals had
been developed on a broad basis, but this argument is difficult to
sustain. As we have pointed already, in 1963 (the year after the
Hospital Plan) the US Government put forward its major proposals
for community mental health centres which did not involve using
psychiatric units in general hospitals as the key element in a
spectrum of services. But nevertheless, it is possible to demonstrate the influence of American experience on British policy-
making. The British psychiatric profession was affected by the
movement in the United States, but it is peculiarly paradoxical
and ironic that British policy change influenced by American experience occurred precisely at a time when a major American policy
change was taking place in order to negate that experience.
American policy-makers were clearly influenced by psychologists,
social workers and community psychiatrists who did not accept the
traditional medical model as the only framework within which
psychiatric care could be provided. In Britain policy-making was
dominated by the sections of the psychiatric profession who accepted
the medical model and who accepted that general hospitals were the
natural and logical settings for psychiatric treatment to take
place; the comparative weakness of the professions of social work
and psychology meant that the psychiatrists' position could not be
effectively challenged.
   As Jones (1972) amply demonstrates, Powell's announcement of the
new policy in 1961 did provoke a mixed response, both from the
psychiatric profession and more generally, but it is important to
establish which sections of the profession supported and which
sections opposed the new proposals. Jones argues, from examining
the correspondence in the medical journals at the time, that the
group that supported Powell's policy was mostly 'optimistic,
politically right-wing and inclined to the organic school of
psychiatry, which most easily assimilated with the general ethos
of medicine' (Jones, 1972). The group that opposed Powell tended
to be 'pessimistic, politically left-wing, and with a stronger
interest in psychotherapy and the contribution of the social
sciences'.
   We would certainly agree with this analysis but we would add

one important rider. It is essential to acknowledge that Powell's
proposal occurred at a specific time when there was an emerging
disenchantment with mental hospitals as therapeutic centres. In
the late 1950s the effects of institutional life upon the behaviour
of long-stay patients was beginning to be explored in detail.

Russell Barton's book 'Institutional Neurosis' (Barton, 1960),
which contained the controversial hypothesis that institutions
actually induced a specific style of neurotic responding, was the
first major publication in this field. Goffman's much more famous
book, 'Asylums' (Goffman, 1961), appeared one year later in 1961,
although his work had been circulating in the United States from
the mid-1950s, but it is again intriguing that his research became
widely known only after the major policy change in 1961. 'Asylums'
was followed by a whole series of books and articles attacking
mental hospitals and other forms of total institutions. With the
benefit of hindsight it is possible therefore to see why so little
attention was paid to researching psychiatric units in general
hospitals and other forms of services that were being put forward
as alternatives. The reaction against the mental hospitals seems
to have been so powerful that little attention was paid to planning
and developing alternative systems. And yet during the 1950s a
number of energetic physician-superintendents were busily restruc-
turing the hospitals they directed. Perhaps the most radical of
these was A.A. Baker, whose famous paper 'Pulling down the old
mental hospital' (Baker, 1961) received wide publicity when it was
published in the wake of Powell's speech. In fact, Baker had published a precursor to this paper in 1958 under the less radical
title of 'Breaking up the mental hospital'. Baker proposed to
adopt the WHO approach and attempted to split the massive hospital
in which he worked into a series of semi-autonomous sub-units
which would function in parallel (Baker, 1958).

There is also another element involved in the argument.
Powell's hospital plan was linked to proposals for developing
community services as partial alternatives to hospital care. These
proposals served to unite many behind the proposals so that there
was a peculiar alliance between radicals, who saw the proposals as
providing a viable alternative to mental hospitals, and the psychiatric right-wing, who saw the psychiatric units as a perfect
expression of psychiatry's manifest and justifiable claim to be
the dominant profession in the treatment of the mentally ill. The
sections of the psychiatric profession who sought to defend the
status quo remained isolated in this situation, particularly in
a period when a growing series of publications attacked mental
hospitals as being counter-therapeutic. Many hospitals rightly
deserved such reputations, but it was equally true that some hospitals had been remarkably innovative and flexible in their provision of care.

DIVISIONS WITHIN THE PSYCHIATRIC PROFESSION

In practice Powell's proposals served to uncover a historic split
within the psychiatric profession itself. But this split is not a
trivial matter - indeed, exploring its historical origins in some

depth will return us once more to the issue of conceptual frameworks in medicine and to certain aspects of Ewins's analysis of
the rise of psychiatry as a dominant profession within the mental
health services. We touched on this issue in the last chapter,
but it is essential to reiterate that many influential policy-
makers remained firmly opposed to such units. For example, the
World Health Organisation's Expert Committee on Mental Health
(whose British representative was Dr T.P. Rees) published a report
in 1953 which categorically opposed developing psychiatric units
as the central element in a psychiatric service. The report is
worth quoting at length since it once again spells out the classic
objection to such units (WHO, 1953).

> In much modern writing on the subject it is taken as axiomatic
> that psychiatric wards in general hospitals are the most desir-
> able form of provision for psychiatric medical care. The
> committee cannot accept this view as axiomatic. It is true
> that in a teaching hospital this may be considered the most
> convenient method of making clinical material available to
> students; but, as the committee has emphasized, the psychiatric
> hospital does not do its job best by imitating the general hos-
> pital. Too often the psychiatric wards of a general hospital
> are forced by the expectations of the hospital authorities to
> conform to a pattern which is harmful to their purpose. Patients
> are expected to be in bed and nurses are expected to be engaged
> in activities which resemble general nursing. The satisfactions
> of neurological diagnosis are enhanced by the prestige in the
> general hospital of clear-cut physical pathology, to the detri-
> ment of interest in the average psychiatric patient whose case
> does not exhibit such features; and it is difficult to obtain
> recognition of the overwhelming importance in psychiatry of
> the factors (which can only be described as the atmosphere of
> the hospital).

Elsewhere in the report the Committee had attempted to define what
it meant by this 'atmosphere':

> the most important single factor in the efficacy of the treatment
> given in a mental hospital appears to the committee to be an
> intangible element which can only be described as its atmosphere;
> and in attempting to describe some of the influences which go
> to the creation of this atmosphere, it must be said at the out-
> set that the more the psychiatric hospital imitates the general
> hospital ... the less successful it will be in creating the
> atmosphere it needs. Too many psychiatric hospitals give the
> impression of being an uneasy compromise between a general hos-
> pital and a prison. Whereas, in fact, the role they have to
> play ... is that of a therapeutic community.

It is obvious from this presentation that the Committee felt that
psychiatric wards were incapable of creating and sustaining such
a therapeutic atmosphere, but this also raised another objection -
that mental hospitals would become the dumping ground for chronic
cases with bad prognoses. They would therefore be turned once
more into 'madhouses', and would not be able to carry out their
role as therapeutic communities. In effect, the Committee did not
assume that these difficulties were insurmountable but in order
for them to be avoided they had to be recognised in the first place.

At a practical level the Committee felt that the problems could
be avoided by making the staff of the mental hospital also responsible for the psychiatric wards in any general hospital. Such a
policy would ensure that the two activities would be run in close
association so that neither would function to the detriment of the
other.

The Committee itself was in favour of developing a new model
for providing mental health services. They placed great stress
on the necessity to provide a variety of services - inpatient, outpatient, domiciliary care, day care, hostels and so on. These
would be operated as 'tools' in the hands of the community, but
the mental hospital would become one of a wide range of tools
rather than the only one. As Jones (1972) has commented, this
concept of a community mental health service was still far from
reality in the England of that time, but it formed part of the
thinking of the Royal Commission on Mental Illness (1954-7).

The Expert Committee's report is also important because it contained specific recommendations about the building of mental hospitals and also about ways of reducing the size of existing ones.
In practice it insisted that no mental hospital should have over
a 1000 beds - indeed, the Committee felt that the ideal might be
nearer 300, given sufficient funds. But it also recommended that
any new hospital built should consist of groups of small buildings
capable of easy conversion and modification. The Committee
correctly sensed that any proposals they put forward would be
subject to considerable modification within a few years.

THE BRITISH RESPONSE TO THE WHO REPORT

It is possible to detect the influence of the WHO Expert Committee's report on some of the changes that subsequently occurred
in the British mental health services, but it is interesting to
note that its major recommendation, that mental hospitals should
become community mental hospitals, was never taken seriously. The
reasons for this are complicated and difficult to document, but it
is obvious that there was a fatal flaw in the Committee's plans
anyway. A community mental hospital can, of course, become a
reality only if it is suitably located at the centre of the community it serves. Since most British mental hospitals are located
miles away from the communities they serve it was not conceivable
that they could play the role advocated by the Committee. New,
smaller hospitals built at the right locations would have been the
only solution, but the older hospitals with their immense resources
and capital investment would have to be phased out at the same
time. It is therefore not surprising that successive ministers of
health looked for other less costly and less radical solutions.

According to Jones (1972), the prophet that was turned to was
McKeown who was Professor of Social Medicine at the University of
Birmingham. In practice McKeown's views (McKeown, 1958; Garrat et
al. 1958) supported those of the right wing within psychiatry although much of his own research work is famous for its explicit
critique of the medical establishment (as we demonstrated in
Chapter 3). McKeown was fully aware that the whole of the hospital

system was outdated. Hospitals were on the wrong sites, were
often of the wrong size and were concentrating on the wrong forms
of treatment, forms that were out of step with the needs of the
majority of patients. The solution to these multiple problems lay
in developing 'a balanced hospital community' where a common staff,
on a common campus, could organise the treatment of patients in a
far more comprehensive and rational way. Such a hospital could
have less complicated and hence better relationships with general
practitioners and with the social services. McKeown's plan
naturally assumed that psychiatric services would form an integral
part of the new hospital complex (or district hospital, as it was
to be called).

   McKeown's proposals for the provision of psychiatric services
were based on a large survey of the needs of patients in Birmingham
mental hospitals. This survey reported that 13 per cent of the
patients actually needed full hospital services while 12 per cent
needed none at all. The remaining 75 per cent needed either supervision (because of their mental state) or 'simple attentions
referred to as basic nursing'. Given such patient needs McKeown
proposed that three types of accommodation were required. Patients
in the first group would require both traditional ward accommodation
and hostel-type accommodation (with or without supervision), while
the second group would require just hostel accommodation without
supervision. The third group would require the same facilities as
the first group but the accent would be on hostel accommodation
with relatively little provision of ward facilities. In practice,
when McKeown was faced with making concrete proposals for reor-
ganising Birmingham's hospitals he suggested that four types of
facility should be set up. The first would effectively be a general
hospital providing full services for acute, chronic and mentally
disordered patients. The second would cater for chronically sick
and mentally disordered patients who required hospital facilities
of a limited type but no mental supervision. The third type would
cater for similar patients who actually needed mental supervision,
and the fourth type was merely hostel accommodation for patients
with very limited needs. Needless to say, McKeown insisted that
all these facilities needed to be grouped together on a common site.

   Elements of McKeown's proposals have clearly been absorbed into
government policy in relation to the development of district
general hospitals, but it is clear that the impact of inflation
has prevented any full-scale attempts to reorganise the hospital
services in the radical way that McKeown proposed. But it is not
our purpose to explore that issue or to evaluate possible criticisms of his proposals. It is more important for our argument to
point out that McKeown's work contributed to the growing consensus
that the distinction between mentally and physically ill patients
should be no longer recognised as being of fundamental importance
in deciding the provision of facilities. The 1959 Mental Health
Act contained a crucial clause which allowed any hospital to admit
mentally disordered patients so the special designation of mental
hospitals was ended. The way was now clear for a basic policy
change - psychiatric units in general hospitals rather than mental
hospitals were to be the main centres for treating the mentally
disordered.

THE UNDERLYING REASONS FOR POWELL'S POLICY CHANGE

But the policy change occurred for other reasons as well. It
should be remembered that it was a Conservative government that
introduced the hospital plan. Indeed it was entirely fitting that
Enoch Powell should be minister of health at the time - his hos-
tility to increasing public expenditure undoubtedly influenced the
policy decision, as the running down of the mental hospitals would
eventually lead to cost-cutting. However, the successful adoption
of the new policy also depended on another factor.

Powell made his famous speech announcing the new policy in March
1961, at a time when it was becoming clear that the size of the
resident population in mental hospitals was beginning to fall.
Opinion differed as to the size of the fall. A ministry circular
estimated that there would be a fall from 150,000 to 80,000 over
a sixteen-year period. This projection was based on the work of
two statisticians, Tooth and Brooke, who had reported that the
number of occupied psychiatric beds had declined by 8,000 between
1954 and 1959. Tooth and Brooke cautioned against drawing any firm
conclusions from their data but the circular was far less cautious.
In practice, the projection has proved to be fairly accurate since
the 1973 figure for beds occupied is 99,800 and the figure is still
declining.

The factors that had contributed to these declining figures are
complicated and we have explored some of them already, but it is
obvious that three factors (changes in treatment methods, changes
in hospital administration and changes in the legal system) had
contributed the main sources of change.

In Chapter 3 we argued that changes in hospital administration,
in rehabilitation programmes and in admission policies could play
a significant role in reducing admissions and speeding recovery.
But it is clear that elements within the psychiatric profession
were able successfully to establish the myth that changes in forms
of treatment (especially the introduction of psychotropic drugs)
were primarily responsible for the gains that had been made. Since
the new forms of treatment could be administered only by the medically trained, the policy change clearly had the latent function
of reasserting the hegemony of the psychiatric profession.

PSYCHIATRIC UNITS AND THE PROBLEM OF THE MEDICALISATION OF LIFE

At a deeper level it is also possible to argue that the provision
of therapy within the general hospital setting represents the
culmination of the general process of 'medicalising' mental health
problems. We have attempted to demonstrate that the real impetus
to developing psychiatric units in general hospitals was derived
from the introduction of physical methods of treatment and then
from the introduction of psychotropic drugs. These means of treatment significantly regard the patient as mere object - they are
essentially manipulative and have a latent ideological content
which conspires to amplify the passivity that is inherent in the
sick role. Or to put this more bluntly, the sick role absolves
the patient from responsibility for his condition - the use of

drugs strangely confirms this passivity. The patient not only becomes dependent upon the doctor for his 'cure' (because the doctor alone can be responsible for prescribing the drugs), but he also runs the risk of becoming physically dependent on the drugs. The current drug overdosing epidemic adds another dimension to the argument since it is a peculiar irony that the much acclaimed psychotropic drugs are being increasingly used in suicide attempts. Admittedly, the majority of these attempts are not seriously designed to result in suicide, but nevertheless they clearly indicate the palliative nature of drug therapies (as we pointed out in Chapter 3). The political content of therapies based upon drugs also becomes clear in this context since the manipulation of the psychological state of a patient cannot be equated with forms of therapy that attempt to deal with the social, inter-personal and economic factors that influence patients who seek help.

Our argument may once again appear dogmatic at this point, but it is important to establish that there is significant evidence for this view. For example, a number of studies of British psychiatrists (by Kreitman, 1962, and also by Walton and Drewery, 1966) have shown that psychiatrists who are interested in the sig- nificance of psychological processes in influencing mental dis- orders tend to be reflective, self-analytical and interested in abstract ideas; whereas those interested in physical treatments tend to have the obverse characteristics. Later work by Pallis and Stoffelmayer (1973) has intriguingly shown that a pro- Conservative political attitude is also associated with a pre- dilection for physical methods of treatment.

Since our argument has been a long and involved one it is now time to summarise it. At a policy level psychiatric units in general hospitals are ordained to become the key element in the psychiatric services for the following reasons.

1 Physical and pharmacological forms of treatment have a degree of effectiveness in alleviating symptoms so their extensive intro- duction enabled the mainly right-wing, organically orientated, psychiatrists to establish the claim that there is an essential continuity between physical and mental illness. Having established this continuity to their own satisfaction, they then argue that the psychiatric unit in the general hospital is a logical setting for forms of treatment which do not differ in principle from other forms of treatment carried out in such hospitals.

2 At a political level such forms of treatment have a political content that is congenial to those who seek to deny that mental disorders are significantly influenced by social, political and economic factors.

3 At an economic level, psychiatric units with their policy of short-stay treatment held out the attractive prospect of cost- cutting.

4 With hindsight it is clear that the attacks on the mental hospitals mounted by sociologists and indeed by some psychiatrists created a climate of opinion that sought alternatives to tra- ditional hospital settings. The prospect of the provision of community services allied to the psychiatric unit in the general hospital served to confuse the issue and conceal the fact that the psychiatric profession was able to retain its control over salient

features of the services.   (In America a similar reorganisation
had a far different result.)

5 Given the weaknesses of social work and psychology as professions, and the manifest strength of the medical profession,
no effective challenge to the new policy was mounted. Eysenck's
famous and sustained attacks on psychoanalysis served to strengthen
the claims of the psychiatrists using physical methods of treatment. The subsequent flowering of behaviour therapy and other
forms of psychological treatment not based on psychoanalysis cannot
conceal the fact that there was no coherent and substantive body
of evidence that could demonstrate that psychological methods were
more effective.

MORE RECENT STUDIES OF PSYCHIATRIC UNITS IN GENERAL HOSPITALS

Ironically, once the policy decision had been taken there was a
minor flurry of papers dealing with newly established psychiatric
units in general hospitals. Many of these originated from the
Manchester region but two studies dealt with the evolution of
observation wards into properly constituted treatment units. Thus
Benady and Denham (1963) reported on the activities of the unit
at St Clement's Hospital in London. They showed that the unit
became more effective as a treatment centre following the passing
of the 1959 Mental Health Act. Patients stayed an average of five
days longer in the unit but twice as many were able to be discharged to their own homes. In the same year, Dunkley and Lewis
(1963) provided a report dealing with 'North Wing', the former
observation ward of St Pancras Hospital which was converted into
a psychiatric unit, but they fail adequately to document the
changes that occurred. Two years later Snaith and Jacobson (1965)
described the conversion of a Brighton observation ward into an
emergency treatment unit. This unit did not function in quite the
same way as the London units as it apparently sent a larger proportion of its cases on to a mental hospital. As its name implies,
it did receive a large number of emergency referrals from GPs and
from its parent hospital but its treatment policy was obviously
less comprehensive than for comparable units.

Interestingly, Snaith and Jacobson's approach (which saw the
psychiatric unit more as a screening device than as a treatment
centre) received subsequent support from a study of the admission
unit at the Royal Edinburgh Hospital. In her review of the unit,
Woodside (1968) argued that there was a necessity for providing
a short-stay unit where 'psychopaths, chronic alcoholics and
others unamenable to in-patient treatment could be screened out;
and where ... community support could be mobilised for those in
social difficulties'. This alternative approach clearly reflects
Scottish thinking on the issue since it is significant that the
Scottish section of the Royal College of Psychiatrists has been
noticeable for its criticisms of the new policy of introducing
psychiatric units in general hospitals (Royal College of Psychiatrists, Scottish Division, 1973).

In areas such as Manchester, where new units were set up in
order to cope with crucial deficiencies in the already existing

services, it is noticeable that there was more concern with the crucial question of whether such units could deal with the full spectrum of possible patients.

Early reports by Leyberg (1959) and Freeman (1960) had revealed a disagreement on this point since Freeman felt that the units had the potential to do so while Leyberg felt that they were incapable of offering the best conditions for the rehabilitation of chronic patients. A later study by Hoenig and Hamilton (1966) claimed that only a tiny percentage of patients (1.3 per cent) in their sample became long-stay but this rather ignores the point that 7.4 per cent of their sample was admitted to the mental hospital directly.

A later study by Hoenig (1968) serves to illuminate some of the complexities of this question, however, since she compared a mental hospital with a psychiatric unit. Unfortunately the patients they dealt with came from different communities, so there are intrinsic methodological difficulties, but it is clear that there were interesting differences in the functioning of the two systems. The unit used day care more frequently, outpatient services less and domiciliary visiting equally. Contacts between the mental hospital and GPs were weaker than for the unit, but this was partially counterbalanced by the fact that the hospital used social workers more extensively. Admission policies differed in that the hospital admitted patients only after a long contact period but once the patients had been admitted they stayed longer.

Owing to methodological problems concerning the failure to match samples, these results can only be treated as suggestive. However, a much more careful prospective study by Copas, Fryer and Robin (1974), once again comparing a unit with a hospital, indicates that it is possible for a unit to avoid admission by using community contacts. The unit they studied was superior on many counts, but in fairness to the hospital they point out that it had a singular disadvantage when compared with the unit - namely that it was twelve miles from Southend, deep in the countryside and very inaccessible from the point of view of transport. As Copas comments, if the tables had been turned and the hospital had been located in the centre of the city, then the results of the study might have been strikingly different. Clearly, the question of crucial differences in geographical location brings a confounding factor into the research into the superiority of one system over the other. The WHO community hospital, custom-built with extensive facilities intra- and extra-murally and correctly related to the community it serves, would of course be an interesting alternative to either system.

PATIENTS' VIEWS OF PSYCHIATRIC UNITS IN GENERAL HOSPITALS

In concluding our review of studies of psychiatric units, we need to refer to the most recent and perhaps the most interesting study of all. This survey of patients' opinions of psychiatric units in general hospitals was carried out for the King Edward's Hospital Fund (Raphael, 1974). Patients and staff from fourteen different

units were interviewed, so the study is particularly useful in
providing comparative data. However, in practice it is extremely
difficult to summarise the report. As Raphael herself comments,
   there were striking variations in policy and practice between
   the units visited. Some of these were due to physical factors
   such as location of unit, size, whether purpose-built or adapted,
   and proximity to the main hospital. Others were the result of
   policy on such matters as the method of allocating patients to
   wards, whether the patients' life was ward-centred or unit-
   centred, and provisions for treatment, occupations and social
   activities. Views were sometimes diametrically opposed not
   only between units but between individuals in the same unit.
   Often one doctor would have quite different views from another,
   and it would be grossly inaccurate to speak of views of 'the
   patients' as if they were a generic group.
Raphael insists that it is not her purpose to evaluate these con-
trasting views, although she does allow herself to comment that
perhaps it is because they are so comparatively new that they are
diverse and that nobody can count themselves an expert on them anyway. But we would see her findings in a much different light.
   The 'striking variations' to which she refers we would see as
very concrete proof of the under-researched basis upon which they
were set up. At a deeper level the variations also underline a
crucial aspect of the functioning of the NHS and the lack of
accountability within the service. As we have demonstrated, the
research carried out on such units is utterly haphazard and unco-
ordinated, with the DHSS utterly failing to initiate any evalua-
tive research on a national scale. It is therefore not surprising
that the units differed markedly on a whole series of dimensions.
For example, the units differed in size from 30 to 101 beds; some
were an integral part of the hospital, some formed wings of the
hospital and yet others were in entirely separate buildings. One
unit was remarkable in being three miles from the town it served
while another unit was separated into sub-units several miles
apart. Overall the nurse-patient ratio ranged from 1:1 to 1:4;
patient allocation in some units involved progressive care, with
patients moving from an admission ward to other parts of the unit,
while other units allocated patients to one ward throughout their
stay. In yet other units patients were categorised in groups
according to their age and illness. Irrespective of these differences, some units chose to centre the daily life of patients
around their ward while other units used the unit and all its
different types of accommodation more flexibly. One could go on
endlessly but these examples should be sufficient to make the
point.
   It will be argued by supporters of the present system that such
diversity is healthy and allows for innovation, but we would take
a more sanguine view. Given the lack of research and evaluation
that would justify experimentation, one can only conclude that the
present system is an acute example of the British art of compromise
at its rottenest. Other more sophisticated supporters of the
status quo might argue that the differences that Raphael documents
are superficial ones and that the units will run more or less
along the same lines irrespective of the differences. Again, this

argument is difficult to sustain since there are in fact no data
to base it on, but research derived from more traditional mental
hospital settings indicates that there is no reason to support this
contention.

But to return to Raphael's study. It is important to acknowledge that her findings do reveal some important agreements among
patient and staff concerning many aspects of their functioning.
More crucially for our purposes, she presents findings that
indicate why staff (and a minority of patients who had been both
to mental hospitals and to the unit) preferred the units. These
findings are listed below.

Reasons for preferring psychiatric unit

Better treatment (higher staff-patient ratio, closer and more
friendly contact).
Less stigma.
Building often more modern (units allow more privacy as dormitories
are smaller and there are many single rooms).
Smaller community (enabling more friendliness).
In own area (allowing better contact with relatives, social workers,
ease of visiting).
Shorter stay (stimulating atmosphere and intensive treatment means
rehabilitation is easier).
Liaison with other departments in the hospital.
Food better.

Advantages of large psychiatric hospitals

Better facilities for long-term patients.
Better classification and grouping of patients with different
needs and problems.
Large grounds.
Wider choice of social activities.
Industrial therapy programmes.
Professional advantages due to concentration of staff (enabling
better training, better career opportunities, etc.).
Better staff conditions (more clubs etc.).
Better rehabilitation possibilities because there is less pressure
to vacate space for further patients.

These 'findings' are, of course, based on the opinions of staff
and patients on these issues. As we have already seen, some
psychiatric units may in fact have better rehabilitation programmes
than mental hospitals so it is important not to accept any simple-
minded division on these issues. Until adequately controlled
studies are carried out one has to accept that these findings are
merely indicative.

But this brings us to the starting point of the next stage in
our argument. We now turn from the historical part of our analysis
to our attempt to examine the working of a psychiatric unit in a
general hospital. As we have already noted, no previous attempt

has been made to study the day-to-day activities of such a unit
as it functions. We therefore seek to break new ground - given
the historical and sociological perspective we have developed we
have attempted to understand the functioning of the unit not in
the traditional sense of examining its efficacy but as a unit
that embodies and reflects the historical processes that we have
reviewed in the first five chapters of our book.

Part three

Porchester General Hospital psychiatric unit observed

Chapter 6

The psychiatric unit at
Porchester General Hospital

The empirical part of our work consists of a study of the psychiatric unit at a general hospital which we have chosen to call
Porchester Hospital. The study was, in fact, carried out by one
of us (GB), although we both share responsibility for the methodology of the study and the interpretation of the results. The
study was essentially concerned with documenting the 'careers' of
patients who entered the unit during a nine-month period in 1973
and 1974. At the beginning of November 1973, the researcher began
to visit the unit in what amounted to the role of a medical
student. Medical students from the local university attended an
eight-week course in psychiatry but one or two students taking
postgraduate courses in psychology or sociology were also able
to participate in the course if their research interests were concerned with psychiatry or psychotherapy. After participating in
the course for eight weeks, the researcher was then able to begin
the research phase of the study without causing any disturbance in
the running of the unit. During the eight-week period the researcher was able to acquaint himself with the unit and its staff
in a unique way, and the change to full-time researcher was made
with a minimum of friction. The staff were informed of the researcher's role from the beginning but the researcher's initial
contact with the unit undoubtedly helped the unit to become ac-
climatised to his presence. Throughout the two-month course field
notes were kept in order to provide documentation of the way the
unit functioned, but the observations presented in this and the
following three chapters are based mostly on field notes and interviews recorded between January and October 1974.

METHODOLOGY

The study was designed to document the careers of patients from the
time they were first interviewed by a psychiatrist in the outpatients' clinic until the time when they were discharged to their
own homes after a period of hospitalisation. There were therefore
three stages in the patient's career: (i) an initial pre-hospital-
isation phase, (ii) the hospitalisation phase, (iii) the post-
hospitalisation phase.

93

Interviews

During the period between the patient's outpatient consultation
and admission into the unit, taped interviews were conducted with
the patient and close relatives in order to establish the patient's
personal history and the nature of the presenting problem. In all
the cases that were researched, interviews were carried out during
this stage of the patient's career either in the patient's home or
in the home of a relative. The patient's adjustment to the unit
was explored, in a series of taped interviews with both the patient
and close relatives, while the patient was in hospital and after
the patient had been discharged and was undergoing outpatient
treatment.

Although the interviews were designed to elicit information concerning various aspects of the patient's situation, a rigid pre-
determined set of questions was not adhered to. There were two
reasons for using such semi-structured interviews. First, they
had to be flexible in order to cope with different patients presenting very different histories and problems. Second, much of
the information to be gained was likely to be of an intimate
nature. This meant that the interviewer had to gain the confidence
of the patient and close relatives.

Diaries

Patients were asked by the researcher to keep a daily record of
their experiences while in the unit. Thus, in some cases, it was
possible to have continuous documentation of how the patient was
adjusting to the unit. Some patients were unable to keep a record
of this nature because they felt too unwell.

Observational data

The researcher attended all ward rounds, team meetings and any
other decision-making meetings that were concerned with the staff's
assessment of the patient's problem, their decisions about treatment of the patient and their evaluation of the patient's progress.
Notes of decisions were made either during the meetings or immediately after they had terminated.

Also, whenever possible the researcher observed (and participated
in) some of the activities that formed part of the patient's daily
routine in hospital, e.g. occupational therapy.

Case notes

Throughout the patient's period of treatment the researcher kept
a record of the patient's case notes as written up on a day-to-day
basis by the medical staff, psychiatric social work staff and
nursing staff.

Selection of cases

In selecting cases for study the researcher adopted the procedure
of accepting every case that was offered by the consultants. In
practice, owing to organisational difficulties it proved problematic
to make contact with patients during the preliminary phase between
seeing the consultant in the outpatient clinic and actually being
hospitalised. Since the unit had three treatment teams it was
originally hoped to monitor patients cared for by all three teams,
but in the event only patients from two of the teams were studied
in a comprehensive way. From an original group of eight patients
we have decided to present the full case material for three cases.
These were the most fully documented and one of the cases is a
classic re-admission case which can be considered to be an acid
test of the decision-making processes of the unit.

THE UNIT AND ITS SETTING

Although the unit at Porchester Hospital was situated in the heart
of a large provincial city, its links with the community it served
were extremely weak. This was partly because of geographical
difficulties, since it was located at the extreme northern edge
of the area it serves, and partly because the staff of the unit
made little effort to establish community-based ties with patients
and their families. Domiciliary visits were rarely made and a
valuable opportunity to establish a deeper understanding of
patients' ways of life was thereby lost. The social workers in
the unit saw their role primarily as psychotherapeutic, and domiciliary visits did not fit into this conception of their role.
    Until recently a commonly held stereotype of hospitals for the
mentally ill was that of a large, foreboding Victorian building.
It was hoped that by geographically desegregating the mentally
ill and treating them within general hospitals that this image
would disappear. Unfortunately the architecture of Porchester
Hospital, far from dissipating this negative stereotype, perpetuated
it. The outside of this nineteenth-century building was austere and
was covered with grime as a result of the polluted atmosphere of its
surroundings. The immediate environment in which the hospital was
situated did little to enhance its depressing image. On two sides
of the hospital there were roads which were unusually heavily congested with traffic. There were also empty warehouses in the
immediate vicinity and waterways which were murky from industrial
waste. In fact, the area has been neglected and allowed to run
down for some time. It is an area that the city has scheduled
for redevelopment.
    The hospital itself has virtually no grounds as it was built
on a congested site hemmed in by commercial and other buildings.
The unit, originally a nurses' home, was added on to the hospital
before the Second World War. It too has a hemmed-in feeling, as
it is surrounded on two sides by the main hospital buildings and
on one side is adjacent to a high-rise block of flats. Patients
have access to a small cramped garden next to the unit and there
is also a tennis court, but this is disused. During the period of

the study some of the younger patients, who were seeking somewhere
to play football, embarked on clearing away the rubble and the
remains of the wire netting that were lying all over the court but
their attempts to restore it to a fit condition petered out. In
practice, the lack of facilities meant that patients had no suitable place to relax unless they left the vicinity of the hospital.

The interior of the hospital was as gloomy as its exterior. In
order to enter the unit the visitor had to walk through the gloomy
corridors of the main hospital and then cross an unenclosed bridge
to reach the unit itself. The unit was more brightly decorated
and was adequately furnished in a modern fashion, but since it
was separated from the rest of the hospital it formed an entity.
Its most striking feature, however, was its narrow and congested
nature. It was primarily built to provide sleeping facilities
for off-duty nurses but because it was built on a confined site
it was built as a tall, narrow building consisting of four floors
connected by two stairways and a lift. In practice, most of the
patients' activities were confined to three floors since the ground
floor contained a series of utility rooms and a large seminar room
for teaching purposes, conferences and ward rounds.

The bridge from the main building connected with the first floor
corridor which ran the length of the building. However, owing to
the peculiarities of the building the only really large rooms were
to be found on the top floor. This floor was referred to as the
day centre, since patients spent most of their time during the day
in this area. Patients dined, and participated in occupational
therapy in a room specifically designed for this purpose, on this
floor. There were two other rooms on this floor which were multi-
functional. One, which was large, was used for patient-staff
meetings, teaching, ward rounds and occupational therapy activities
that involved the patients participating in groups. The other,
smaller, room was also used for ward rounds and teaching but contained a record player which patients could make use of in their
free time. The floor below the day centre was referred to as the
hostel floor. This floor was made up of offices for the psychiatric social workers and interviewing rooms. A hallway separated
these rooms from several others, which were originally for the
use of patients who went out to work during the day but slept in
the unit. During the period of study these rooms were used as
dormitories by inpatients. They accommodated either three or four
patients. The first floor contained a ward consisting of approximately twelve beds for female patients, a number of smaller rooms
which contained three to four beds each, and a patients' lounge.
The remainder of the rooms on this floor included the nurses'
station, the sisters' office, a small kitchen, a treatment room,
a bathroom and a washroom.

Since this building was designed as a nurses' home it displayed
certain features that obviously did not lend themselves to a
psychiatric unit. In particular, the fact that it contained four
floors made the task of monitoring patients a difficult one.
Patients in fact could easily 'disappear' within the unit, and
thus there were genuine difficulties in actually locating them - a
state of affairs that was aggravated by the fact that each floor
could be entered by one of three different entrances.

THE STAFF

On entering the unit the researcher was struck by the complexity
of the therapeutic setting, especially in relation to the numbers
and different groups of staff involved. During the period of study
there were approximately thirty-two members of staff who were
attached to the unit in various capacities. They were involved in
the care of a maximum of twenty-nine inpatients, a smaller group
of day patients and a large number of outpatients.

Three members of the medical staff, the consultants, were drawn
from the local university. For historical reasons one of the consultants tended to play a more leading role in the affairs of the
unit than the others. One medical assistant, a registrar and
three senior house officers (SHOs), whose term of employment was
either six months or a year, were employed by the National Health
Service. There was an active psychiatric social work department,
which was part of a larger combined medical and psychiatric social
work department within the Porchester hospital system. For most
of the period of study there were four psychiatric social workers
working within the unit. Although there was a high rate of turnover amongst the nursing staff, the average number of personnel
during 1974 was approximately seventeen. The nursing staff was
composed of three sisters, eleven staff nurses, two state-enrolled
nurses and an auxiliary nurse. The unit also had the services of
two full-time occupational therapists.

All the senior members of staff in each profession were involved
in teaching programmes as well as the diagnosis and treatment of
patients. Thus there were always approximately nine medical students, a smaller number of trainee social workers, student nurses
and occupational therapy students attached to the unit at any one
time. During the period of study all the consultants were male,
there was a predominance of female senior house officers and
nurses, and all the psychiatric social workers and occupational
therapists were female. This distribution was significant in
relation to the treatment of patients, especially when marital
therapy was carried out, as the later case history chapters will
demonstrate.

THE PHILOSOPHY OF THE UNIT

Given the large number of personnel and their diverse social and
professional backgrounds, it is not surprising that staff often
could not agree about basic diagnostic and therapeutic issues.
However, rather than confronting and trying to cope with this
problem there was a distinct antipathy on the part of the senior
medical staff towards discussion aimed at articulating a coherent
unit philosophy.

For example, towards the end of 1973 formal discussions were
initiated among the members of staff with the intention of re-
arranging the structure of the unit, and the functions of members
of staff in relation to patient care. The psychiatric social
workers and junior medical staff argued convincingly that such
changes were dependent on the 'philosophy' of the unit. The senior

house officers were of the opinion that, if treatment of patients was going to be psychotherapeutically orientated, then the psychiatric social workers ought to be allocated more responsibility for individual therapy since they had more training in dealing with psychological problems than the average senior house officer. However, the senior medical staff were unwilling to participate in discussions that involved matters directly to do with the unit's 'philosophy'.

In the absence of a clearly defined position in relation to diagnostic and therapeutic issues, the researcher was forced to rely on observational material for this account. The senior members of staff of the unit had gained a widespread reputation for the teaching and practice of psychotherapy. They considered that the unit's philosophy had progressed from a 'medical model' approach towards mental disorder to a psycho-social one. However, it is fair to say that in practice, in terms of its diagnostic and therapeutic outlook, the unit was eclectic. Nevertheless, there was a bias towards formulating patients' problems in interpersonal terms and applying psychological methods of treatment.

Although the senior medical staff and the social work staff would be considered to have received training in psychotherapy, it is extremely difficult to define precisely the school of thought to which they belonged and to assess the quality of their training. This is hardly surprising when one considers the more general issue of the training and practice of psychotherapy within and outside the NHS. We briefly discussed this in Chapter 1. At the time of writing there are no statutory arrangements within the UK which define the length and type of training an individual is obliged to undergo in order to qualify as a psychotherapist. This state of affairs has allowed the proliferation of a number of bodies with very different therapeutic outlooks which claim to offer training in psychotherapy. Even if an individual does not participate in one of these schemes he may still practice as a psychotherapist if he so wishes, since he is not bound to any kind of formal registration. We will not pursue this issue at greater length. Suffice to say it is in need of urgent resolution especially when one considers the increasing use of psychological methods of treatment within psychiatric settings.

To return to the treatment offered within the unit, it is true to say that when patients were treated with any one of the vast array of physical treatments that are now available to psychiatry, this was typically as an adjunct to psychotherapy.

THE STRUCTURE OF THE UNIT

As a result of the discussions held among the members of staff in 1973 the unit was restructured. Each member of staff was placed into one of three therapeutic teams. Each team, typically, consisted of a consultant, a senior house officer, a psychiatric social worker, an occupational therapist and one or more staff nurses. The teams functioned independently of each other and were responsible for a quota of outpatients, day patients and inpatients. Each team met twice a week in ward rounds and team

meetings in order to assess inpatients' problems and progress and to
make therapeutic decisions. In practice, there was little difference between a ward round and team meeting except that the latter
was of a shorter duration. The only occasion when the teams participated together as one body was at the weekly case conferences,
where the cases of selected patients would be examined. Members of
staff from one team would present the life history and problems of
one of their patients to the rest of their colleagues from the other
two teams. Everyone would then proceed to discuss the case.

As regards the diagnosis and treatment of inpatients, the most
crucial members of each team were the consultant, the senior house
officer and the psychiatric social worker. The extent of involvement of these members of staff in the treatment of inpatients was
inversely proportional to their expertise and training. In other
words, the consultant, theoretically the most experienced and extensively trained member of the team, had little or no contact with
inpatients. The senior house officer, who, typically, would arrive
at the unit with no more training in psychiatry than he had received
as a medical student, was in practice responsible on a day-to-day
basis for the treatment of his team's quota of inpatients. The
psychiatric social worker, who was often better equipped than the
senior house officer to carry out treatment in those cases that
required psychotherapy, usually played a secondary role to the
senior house officer in the case of inpatients. The expertise of
the psychiatric social worker would be used only in a situation
that demanded that a patient's spouse become involved in the treatment programme.

DECISION-MAKING AND THE 'CAREER' OF THE INPATIENT

While the actual practicalities of treatment were carried out by
those members of staff with the least experience, assessments and
treatment decisions were heavily biased in favour of those who knew
the inpatients least of all - the consultants. Thus a new patient
entering the unit via outpatients would be initially interviewed
by the consultant. Having been admitted, the patient's care would
be passed on to the senior house officer (and the psychiatric
social worker if a member of the patient's family became involved
in the treatment programme). The consultant's involvement in the
case would then be limited to participating in ward rounds and
team meetings. His role, typically, would consist of taking the
initiative in assessing the patient's problem and in deciding the
treatment programme, of advising the therapists (on the basis of
their reports about the patient's progress), and of generally
monitoring the progress of the case. After the patient had been
discharged from the unit the consultant would play no further part
in the case. In outpatients the senior house officer would continue to treat the patient. He would have the freedom to pursue
any course of treatment that he favoured, since, in practice, the
care of outpatients was a matter for individual therapists rather
than the team as a whole.

STAFF RELATIONS

A lack of agreement about fundamental diagnostic and therapeutic
issues, the structure of the unit and the method of decision-making
had a divisive effect among the members of staff. Relations
between the junior members of staff and their senior colleagues
were often covertly characterised by resentment and acrimony.
There was little effort consciously to cope with the difficulties
that the unit experienced. Even when staff meetinss did take place
in order to discuss the way the unit was operating, they were not
very productive. For example, a number of meetings were held
during the summer of 1974. A female inpatient had committed
suicide and the senior house officer and psychiatric social worker,
who were responsible for her care, arranged a meeting for the
patients in order to explain to them the circumstances surrounding
the suicide. The nursing staff objected to such a meeting, since
in their view the patients would be unnecessarily distressed and
this would result in more work for individual nurses. The senior
house officer and the psychiatric social worker were incensed by
this reaction. They felt that implicit in the nursing staff's view
over this matter was the notion that patients were not responsible,
adult human beings who could not be trusted with their own feelings.
Furthermore, they felt that something very basic was at issue here,
i.e. the 'philosophy' according to which the unit was going to
operate.

The disagreement between the nursing staff and the senior house
officer and the psychiatric social worker sparked off a number of
staff meetings which were centred around the issue of the 'philosophy' of the unit. However, little progress was made. Certain
matters which ought to have been open to discussion in any meeting
to do with the unit's 'philosophy' were not. For example, during
one meeting a medical student pointed out that, although the unit
by and large opposed the use of the 'medical model', staff inevitably classified the people who were in their care as 'patients'
and their problems as 'illnesses'. Some members of the senior
medical staff rejected this criticism on the grounds that their
usage of these terms was metaphorical. Other members of the senior
medical staff claimed that use of the 'medical model' was entirely
justified since many patients were clearly ill, required active
treatments such as electro-convulsive therapy, and recovered well
as a result of these treatments.

A combination of these views espoused by the senior medical
staff had the effect of stifling the opinions of their junior colleagues. The latter felt that these kinds of assumptions about the
'philosophy' of the unit made meetings arranged in order to discuss
this issue irrelevant. As a result of past experience the junior
members of staff were of the opinion that their senior colleagues
were not well disposed towards frank discussions about the way the
unit operated. This opinion was confirmed by views such as those
expressed by the senior medical staff on the issue of the unit's
use of the medical model. Ultimately these staff meetings, which
were designed to decrease the divisions that existed in the unit
over fundamental diagnostic and therapeutic issues, had the reverse
effect.

THE NURSING STAFF

So far in this account, little attention has been paid to the
activities of the nursing staff. As regards the diagnosis and
treatment of patients, they tended for the most part to play an
ancillary role to the medical and psychiatric social work staff,
although they had more daily contact with inpatients than any
other members of staff.
   The activities of the nursing staff included monitoring the
conduct of patients, talking to them about their problems and lives,
joining in activities with patients such as card games and going
for walks, participating in ward rounds and other decision-making
meetings, and generally nursing the patients, including providing
them with medication.
   Although the scope of the study did not extend to actually
measuring the attitudes of the nursing staff towards patients, some
assessment of their position can be gained from a document provided
by the senior members of the nursing staff for the guidance of
student nurses during their period of training at the unit. This
document was entitled 'General principles in the nursing of the
mentally sick'. On the whole, the principles contained in it imply
that patients were literally sick or ill and were thus unable to
help the way they behaved. The document emphasised that the nurse
should relate to the patient more in terms of her role as a nurse
than as an individual. The following quotations from the document
convey its flavour and also indirectly the attitudes of the senior
members of the nursing staff towards patients:
   'Try to forget some of your own feelings so that they do not
   influence your attitude and feeling towards the patient.'
   'Don't get into discussions over delusions however amiable or
   apparently sensible they may be. Listen politely for a while
   then get the patient off his twisted track by giving him something to do or by turning the conversation to something else.'
   'Mentally sick people tend to become easily dependent, so do
   not neglect or ill treat a patient.'
   'Look at any unpleasant symptom as part of the patient's condition.'
In practice, some nurses tended to relate to patients on a more
personal level. Indeed during the period of study the younger
nurses sought a more active therapeutic role in the treatment of
patients. Unfortunately they were frustrated in this respect by
the senior members of the nursing staff and the nursing officers
of Porchester Hospital. A measure of the latter's intransigence
over this issue was their reaction to the request of the younger
nurses not to wear uniforms. The younger nurses made this request
because they felt that wearing uniforms formalised their relationships with patients and thus prohibited them from forming close
bonds of a therapeutic nature. However, the senior members of the
nursing staff did not appreciate this point and denied their junior
colleagues' request.
   Occasionally some of the junior doctors and psychiatric social
work staff cynically remarked to the researcher that the only
situation that the nurses appeared to be comfortable in were those
in which they were carrying out activities that conformed to the

more traditional aspects of nursing. This remark was often made
in reference to the nursing involved in treating patients with
electro-convulsive therapy. The efficiency and certainty that the
nurses were observed displaying in this situation belied the uncer-
tainty and discomfort that some of them presented in situations
that demanded dealing with patients on a more personal and subjective basis.

The conduct of the nursing staff in these very different situations was not unexpected, since their training did not provide them
with adequate experience of relating to patients on a psychotherapeutic level. However, it did equip them to discharge the
more technical aspects of psychiatric nursing. This bias can be
considered especially ironic when one considers that nurses had
more daily contact with inpatients than any other members of staff.

TEACHING

The psychiatric unit was committed to teaching students and trainees
of the various professions and was one of the centres in the area
for the training programme for doctors taking the examination for
membership of the Royal College of Psychiatrists.

This commitment to education and training had its implications
for the care of patients. During the period of study it was noticeable that a certain amount of tension existed between the unit's
teaching commitment and the treatment of patients.

Students and trainees were attached to one of the three therapeutic teams. A large part of the teaching process was centred
around their gaining clinical experience, either directly or indirectly. For example, medical students during their psychiatric
firm were instructed to elicit life histories from at least three
inpatients and to conduct further interviews at a greater depth
with the latter. Also some psychology students, taking the course
in psychopathology at the local university, and theology students
came into contact with inpatients on one afternoon a week. Inevitably this meant that some patients were saturated with interviewing
and this had its effect on the course of their treatment programmes.
Patients who had undergone this plethora of interviewing sometimes
could not be bothered to impart important information to their
therapists, having already discussed it on a number of other occasions with different people. Another occasional consequence of
teaching students through the medium of clinical experience was
that interviewers would be played off against one another by
patients. The research necessarily involved becoming acquainted
with inpatients and their families at a fairly intimate level.
One of the patients whose career was followed became quite practiced
at disclosing personal information to the researcher and refusing
to disclose it to her therapist. There is no doubt that some
patients genuinely found informal relationships with students or
researchers more rewarding than formal ones with doctors. On the
other hand there were patients who objected to being interviewed
by students or researchers because they did not wish to disclose
intimate information about themselves to persons who had no clinical
responsibility. Another source of objection was the way in which

students conducted themselves towards patients. For example, one
patient whose career was followed told the researcher that a
medical student had upset her by questioning her about her problems
in an insensitive manner.

Problems of a different nature arose in relation to those
students and trainees who were directly involved in the treatment
of individuals. For example, senior house officers came to the
unit to gain some training and experience of psychiatry. Those of
them who did not intend to specialise in psychiatry typically spent
six months working in the unit. The ephemeral nature of their term
of employment, and the fact that they were responsible for the
treatment of inpatients and a quota of outpatients, created problems for those patients who were being treated by senior house
officers who were about to leave the unit. Although the consultants
tried to cater for this situation, inevitably it meant that some
patients were left without a therapist or had to recommence their
treatment with a new and inexperienced senior house officer. The
latter state of affairs occurred particularly when a patient's
treatment programme involved psychotherapy. The new senior house
officer needed time to become acquainted with the patient's problem
and case history and also to develop a close relationship with the
patient. The situations that have been described here were also
evident when trainee social workers were given clinical responsibility for patients.

Obviously, the problems the unit experienced regarding its
teaching function were not unique. They are inevitable in any hospital that combines teaching with the treatment of patients. But
it can be argued legitimately that the problems of the psychiatric
unit were accentuated because too many students were accommodated
for a place of its size.

OCCUPATIONAL THERAPY

As in any other mental hospital or psychiatric unit, occupational
therapy was an integral part of the unit's work. The principal
occupational therapist construed the objective of the occupational
therapy department in two ways. First, it aimed to assess the
behaviour of individual patients in a number of respects; for
example the way patients related to staff and to one another, and
the ability of patients to work, to carry out domestic functions
and to cope with the outside world. The second objective of the
department was based on the assessments made of individual patients.
On the basis of these assessments the occupational therapists
arranged activities and tasks for patients within the scope of the
department's facilities.

The department divided occupational therapy into tasks and
activities for individuals, which took place in the morning, and
group activities and tasks, which occurred in the afternoon. The
former consisted of cooking, carpentry, sewing, pottery, metal-
work, typing, making jigsaw puzzles, etc. Group activities usually
consisted either of team games, such as table tennis, darts and
card games, or of dancing, play-reading, walks, attending lunchtime concerts, etc.

The perennial problem of the occupational therapy department was to do with the fact that all patients were obligated to attend occupational therapy regardless of their needs. This meant that some patients were merely 'occupied' rather than performing activities which were of benefit to them. The psychiatrists only occasionally liaised with the occupational therapy staff over arranging 'custom-built' programmes for individual patients. The occupational therapy staff would have preferred a more flexible arrangement for patients regarding occupational therapy. For example, they recognised that, whereas it was beneficial for some patients to participate in group activities, for others it was not necessary. Unfortunately, the demands of the occupational therapy department for a more flexible approach were not met during the period of study.

THE PATIENTS

Initially, patients were unsettled by the unfamiliar environment of the unit. Nevertheless they soon settled into a prescribed routine.

The patients' day began at 7 a.m. when they were presented with a cup of tea by the nursing staff while they were still in bed. By 8 a.m. they were expected to attend breakfast which was served in the dining room on the top floor of the unit. Occupational therapy commenced at 9.30 a.m. and lasted until midday when lunch was served. From midday until 2 p.m. patients were free. During this period they rested, read, listened to records, chatted or played cards among themselves and with the nursing staff. It was during this part of the day, and on any other occasion when patients were free to pursue activities of their choice, that the division between the nursing staff and patients was most blurred. For example, when they played cards together at lunchtime it was noticeable how informal and amicable the relationships between the nurses and patients were. Of course the division between the two groups was re-established when the nursing staff instructed patients to return to occupational therapy at 2 p.m. From 4 p.m., when they had their tea, until lights out at 10.30 p.m. patients were again free, although they ate supper at 6 p.m. For many patients this was the most eagerly awaited part of the day since friends and family often visited them after 4 p.m. During the evening patients spent their time either watching television or participating in recreational activities similar to those pursued during the lunch break.

There were a number of exceptions to this daily routine. For example, those patients who were involved in either psychotherapy or marital therapy did this when it was convenient for their therapist. Thus a patient might miss part of occupational therapy or part of his lunch break. Patients who had been prescribed electro-convulsive therapy were treated on Monday and Thursday mornings. On those days, owing to the nature of the treatment, they missed breakfast and occupational therapy in the morning. On Wednesdays patients attended the weekly staff-patient meeting between 9.30 and 10.30 a.m. This was the only opportunity for staff and patients to meet as a group in order to discuss issues raised by patients. Although all the patients were obligated to attend the meeting, this obligation did not extend to the members of staff. It is a measure of the 'distance' of the consultants from the patients and the day-to-day affairs of the unit that they never attended any meetings that took place during the period of study. Also the junior members of staff of one of the therapeutic teams were unable to attend this meeting because they were involved in outpatients on Wednesday mornings. Given this state of affairs the importance of the patient-staff meeting was somewhat diminished.

There were other grounds for scepticism over the efficacy of these meetings, particularly in relation to the way they were conducted. Theoretically the patient-staff meeting was meant to be run in a democratic fashion. Issues raised by individuals were meant to be discussed and solved by both staff and patients. On a number of occasions some members of staff were observed taking the initiative over a particular issue and using their power and status in such a way that the democratic nature of the meeting was totally undermined. For example, during one meeting one of the patients wondered whether it was not possible to stay up later than midnight because he was used to going to bed at 1 a.m. and found it difficult to go to sleep any earlier. One of the members of the medical staff duly rounded on this patient and asserted that if he wished to go to bed after midnight he could not be ill and thus should not be in hospital. As a result of this interaction the patient's involvement during the rest of this meeting was virtually non-existent.

Weekends in the unit were by far the most relaxed days of the week. There were no prescribed activities so many patients spent the weekend at home with their families. The remainder of patients often had visitors who frequently took them out. Others not in such a fortunate position were taken out by members of the nursing staff.

One of the main problems confronting any inpatient in a mental hospital or a psychiatric unit is boredom. Although some of the patients found the unit a source of relief and enjoyed being there, others found the daily routine monotonous. The problem was that as a result of the diversity of age groups in the unit, the staff were not able to cater for all the patients all of the time. For example, during the period of study it was observed that some of the younger male patients preferred to play table tennis rather than attend morning occupational therapy, which they found boring. Yet on the occasions when table tennis competitions were arranged as part of the occupational therapy programme these were not suitable for the older patients.

CONCLUSION

In this chapter we have briefly outlined the salient features of the unit, but it should be added that the unit was in fact originally developed to provide a suitable teaching milieu for medical students attending courses at the local university. It did of course develop a crucial role in providing beds for short-stay patients drawn from a large catchment area in the southern sector of the city in which it is located, but nevertheless its development is comparable to many of the psychiatric units in London teaching hospitals. Whether the unit is typical of psychiatric units is an open question. Raphael's survey, which we reviewed in Chapter 5, indicates that it is impossible to talk of a 'typical' unit, as the development of such units seems idiosyncratic in terms of so many dimensions (physical structure, staffing, teaching or non-teaching functions, etc.). However, we would nevertheless argue that some of the problems of the unit are probably endemic to all such units. This is a statement that has to be taken more or less on trust since there is so little comparable research, but our knowledge of other units indicates that there is no reason to assume that the unit is unique.

In order to document the functioning of the unit we have elected to present three case histories of patients who went through the unit during our period of study. The detailed documentation of these patients' 'careers' is presented in the next three chapters.

Chapter 7

The case of Mrs Smith

When Mrs Smith was admitted into the unit she was fifty-five years old and her husband was fifty-nine years old.

Her case is that of a classic 'revolving door' patient. That is to say, she is the type of patient who experiences admissions at recurring intervals. This type of patient typically receives pharmacological treatment or electro-convulsive therapy. The effect of these kinds of treatment is often merely palliative.

THE PROBLEM

The following material is to do with the way the Smiths and Mrs Mary Jones, the patient's sister, construed Mrs Smith's problem. The material is extracted from a number of interviews held with them by one of the authors.

Mrs June Smith

MRS J. SMITH: I seemed to have sort of given in, stopped trying, I think.
INTERVIEWER: Do you find it hard to express what you are feeling at the moment?
MRS J. SMITH: Yes I think so.
INTERVIEWER: Is it because you feel that you have let other people down?
MRS J. SMITH: I do feel a little that I've let my husband down, because he's so good and works so hard and I've probably made him feel worried and he's got enough worries at work anyway without me piling on the agony.
INTERVIEWER: While you were in hospital did you see your problem any differently from the way you saw it before you came in?
MRS J. SMITH: No, because I don't really know what my problem is. It seemed as though I gradually sort of got weak-willed. Could you put it that way? I could see things that wanted doing and I knew I should have done them and I could leave it, you know, which is not my natural way at all generally - if there's something to do I would normally want to get on with it.

I only think it was probably trying to fit too much into a week if you know what I mean. I was doing the housework, rushing to do the shopping, and hurrying up to get ready to go to work in the afternoon, and hurrying up to get the tea, and perhaps we would go out two or three times during the week and it seemed as though I didn't have a minute to breathe, and I wondered if that had not got me down. There seemed to be no breathing space between. Maybe I had done a little too much for somebody of my age, I don't know....

The nerve trouble, or whatever it was, seemed to make me feel ill in myself....

I want my life to be normal again, straight away, as though nothing had happened; to alter things like putting back the clock, as though it had never happened. I want to be a normal housewife again, happy to get ready to go out.

Mr Reg Smith

MR R. SMITH: I've realised with hindsight that certain features have happened in spotted positions in time but they've gradually closed up in time and she's got to the state she's in now. So with hindsight I can see all this happening for the past nine years....

To me there's a will link missing, an impetus link. She can think, she knows she has to go from A to B, but the little link between the think and the action is missing and she knows this quite clearly. She can even relate quite clearly conversations a week ago and I feel that there is some deterioration somehow somewhere that you are going to have a terrific difficulty building up.

You people will manage to charge her batteries up but they will fail on her again. This is going to be the pattern. I've tried to explain it but no one has said to me, 'Yes that's the layman's term for what's happening.' And I feel physically there's a link missing, there's a nerve gone down somewhere. My car wouldn't start the other day, it was a piece of very small wire. All right by the time I finished I realised there was a contact gone, and this is what I feel physically has happened to her, there's something gone. Now whilst you can regenerate that for a while, you can't clean the contact enough to make it permanent. That's my interpretation of what's happened and between the one blob here, i.e. the impetus, the clarity of thought to do something, that little link to start the motor up to do it, to get to these things just ain't there. And that's my version and nobody's saying, 'Yes, you're not far out', or, 'You're talking a load of codswallop'. But this is what I feel....

It's like driving a car across the Sahara and sooner or later you know it's going to break in and you're going to get crunched.
INTERVIEWER: While your wife was in hospital did you change the way you saw her problem?
MR R. SMITH: No because I'm pretty convinced I know what's wrong with her. As I've said all along, she's emotionally short-changed and her courage has oozed out.
INTERVIEWER: What do you mean by emotionally short-changed?

MR R. SMITH: I can take her down the garden, which she is familiar
with, and she'll suddenly be overcome by crying. She's got a
perverse way of crying now at every little thing that means a
decision. What I find now she cries easily, she's trying to fight
it, she's probably over-fighting it. Sunday dinner she was desperately trying to fight it and I tried to make her sit down to a
degree of a little bit of hardness, not force but hardness. I
then realised she was so determined I backed off. So I think she's
fighting to a degree in vain where she can't let go. And as I say,
courage she's short on, which I call emotion, comes out. She isn't
hard enough.

I found out now, she's even ... she's got big feet, eights, but
I know she tried desperately hard, woman's vanity, to get smaller
shoes than she should have. Now I can tell her from St John's
Ambulance days that the mechanics of the foot don't allow you to
do this. And I know now, since she's been out this last month
she's even bought two pairs of size sevens.

Being my wife I like her to walk upright; she's an upright
person, always faced the world. She doesn't, she hasn't, she
hasn't for a long time and still doesn't face the world. She's
certainly lost her courage and hospital hasn't given it her back,
in whichever respect that courage is applied; i.e., you need courage
to make decisions, though we don't realise it; you need courage to
go into shops, though we don't realise it. People that don't behave
in this pattern don't realise that courage is necessary to go into
a shop for some people. And she's in that particular environment
at the moment, that mental sphere of don't want to go.

Mrs Mary Jones (57 years old)

MRS M. JONES: It's only been since eighteen months she's been like
she is now.
[Before quoting Mrs Jones's 'theory' of how June became 'ill'
eighteen months before her admission into the unit, a description
of Mr Smith's background before his marriage to June is necessary
in order to make what Mrs Jones says more understandable to the
reader. This historical information has been extracted from an
interview one of the authors conducted with Mrs Jones during her
sister's first admission.
Mr Smith had already been married before his marriage to June.
After he left his first wife he went to live with June and her
ailing mother in the house the Smiths now occupy in their own right.
At that time he had not yet divorced his first wife, and only did
so after she had given birth to a child by a man who was co-
habitating with her. She and Reg already had two children.
After Mr Smith divorced his first wife and married June he still
retained ownership of the house he had shared with his first wife.
'Anyway the wife took ill two years ago and died' (Mrs M. Jones),
and Mr Smith decided to sell the house and share the money between
the three children and himself. 'The house was still in Reg's name
all the years, he did nothing to change it' (Mrs M. Jones).]
INTERVIEWER: He was sharing it between the children and himself.
MRS M. JONES: Yes, Joan (Mr Smith's daughter) said he altered his

tune when he had the actual cheque in his hand, because I suspect
that house fetched at least six thousand if not more. He gave his
two children so much and put the rest in the bank for himself, and
this is when June started getting agitated.
INTERVIEWER: How long ago was this?
MRS M. JONES: About eighteen months ago. It was just before she
took rough the first time. She came up, she said, 'John (Mr Smith's
son) came to see his dad to ask for more money. He is going in for
another house at Bedmoore and thought he was entitled to have more,'
and she said, 'Our Joan, she wants some more money, she doesn't
think it's fair Reg should have the bulk of it when he never paid
a penny towards that house.' Anyway June was very agitated because
she said she didn't want any of the money, it's nothing to do with
her she's got her own bit of money, and there was a hell of a row
down there and John hasn't spoken to his father since. Reg put
the money in the bank and said, 'It's bloody staying there, none
of you are having it.' So that made a rift between father and son.
Anyway June's very fond of John. She says she couldn't interfere
because it was between father and children. She got all agitated
as I just said. She was doing the housework, going to work, having
to chase about. She just got run down in the beginning, I think,
really run down. Anyway she had an awful row with him one Sunday,
this was the first time she was ill. She must have spoken back
to him and he went beserk because nobody speaks back to Reg. He
called the doctor, he must have been frightened, but the GP didn't
call, it was an emergency doctor and he stayed there a couple of
hours talking to her and next day she started getting ready to go
on holiday quite happily, so she was perfectly OK again.
    [Here Mrs Jones discusses the occasion when her sister began
to feel unwell again. It was during this period that June was
admitted into the unit.]
MRS M. JONES: She was not very well for those three weeks.
INTERVIEWER: Which three weeks?
MRS M. JONES: In March when she took poorly again. She said she
felt poorly and I went down and I said, 'What's up June?' She
said, 'I was in the car going to work and I was going down through
the Ridgeway, and at a red light the brakes failed, that's never
happened before.' And she was too shaken even to get the car over
to a parking lot. So a fellah in the garage on the left-hand side
of the Ridgeway said, 'I'll do it for you,' so she left the car
there. I think Reg fetched it. Then she said, 'Reg's car has gone
wrong. He's had to take it to the garage but he's doing my car
himself. He's done my brakes, but,' she said, 'before I drove it
to work I thought I'd go round the block to see if it's OK.' But
she said she only put her foot down on the brake and it stopped
dead, locked. So she said she was scared to drive it like that, so
she walked to work, went to Redbank where her place was to get to
work and she was crying. She said, 'I was walking along the road
crying, wondering to myself, whatever am I doing wandering along
this road? There's no need for me to go to work.' Anyway she
said Reg came home, he said, 'How's the car?' [Assume that June
shakes her head in a negative fashion.] 'No, why bloody not?'
She said, 'I didn't like the brakes Reg, they were locked, they
were too quick, so I walked.' 'Bloody fool,' he said, 'The car's

all right.' A couple of nights after Caroline, my daughter, and
I went over there and he had to move June's car for Caroline to
get in by the front door, and he came upstairs because June was
in bed, and he said, 'You were right about that car June, the
brakes do lock. I just tried it!'

MRS M. JONES: Anyway this is what June's told me since she's been
in hospital. She said to me when I first went there, 'You did me
good when you spoke to me last time.' I said, 'In what way June?'
She said, 'You've described to me that you and Bob don't have
sexual relations now.' And I said, 'No, we don't.' I was forty-
five at the time, young isn't it really? But my husband, it was
on holiday, and he picked up a germ, one of his testicles dis-
appeared in the end, you know he was really ill and if he was a
young man we wouldn't be able to have any children, you know,
because all that life has gone from him. I was only forty-five
and he was fifty. I said to June, 'As you get older, perhaps some
go on longer, I don't know.' I mean I love my husband and I never
thought him less of a man because he couldn't have sexual relations,
I mean I still love him. But June said, 'That's very good,' and I
said, 'Why?' She said, 'Because Reg is not sleeping with me,' and
I said, 'Why not?' She said, 'Because he says, "You bloody cough
all night, you're bloody twittering, you're jumping and I've got
to get some sleep. I've got to go to work. I'm going in the other
room", and he's never come back.'

INTERVIEWER: How long ago was this?

MRS M. JONES: Over a year ago, she told me. They were making love
as you call it and she fell asleep and he ranted and raved and he
said, 'I'm not bloody bothering with you any more,' and he hasn't
been back in the room any more to put his arms around her once
since.

MRS M. JONES: I kept her in bed for a couple of days, because she
was exhausted, terrible she was, I couldn't make her eat. I don't
think she's ate properly for a couple of months. I said to my
husband, 'What do you think of her, Bob?' He said, 'June looks
bad, she looks worse than our Dave ever did.' [Dave is a deceased
brother of Mrs Jones and June who was cared for at the Jones's
home while he was suffering from terminal cancer.] She just sat
there and she cried. It was something different every few minutes.
So I said, 'What is it now June?' And she was crying, 'Reg said
I've got big feet, bloody feet, and I can't get any shoes to fit
my feet.' He said that to her. There's two pairs of new shoes,
size sevens, that he's been trying to push her feet into and she
takes size eights. And then she said, 'I mustn't eat any potatoes
or I'll get fat.' And I said, 'You won't get fat at all, you're
too thin.'

INTERVIEWER: Why is she afraid of getting fat?

MRS M. JONES: Because of her appearance I suppose. But she kept
on and on about her feet and Reg came in one afternoon and he was
sat with her for three or four hours, and she never moved. She
was sat there with her legs and feet bent under the chair. She
just sat there like that. So when he'd gone I tried to get her
to go to bed and I felt her legs and they were frozen to the core.
I got a hot water bottle. She said, 'What's wrong with my legs
and my feet? I can't feel them.' So I got her a hot water bottle.

Anything I would start speaking to her about she would start
worrying about and forget everything else. So I got her a hot
water bottle and after a couple of hours she couldn't feel that,
so after a couple of hours I began to think there was something
physically wrong with her.

Well she's got this friend Hazel. Hazel came into the hospital
last week while I was there. Reg walked towards the ward where
June is. So I'd never spoken to Hazel, only a couple of times in
June's house, I don't know her, but Hazel seemed very fond of June
and the other way around too. She said to me, 'I wish Reg wouldn't
shout at her, he's always shouting at her.' But then Reg came back
and nothing else was said. I mean you can't get to the bottom of
it all really.

INTERVIEWER: While she was in hospital did you change the way you
saw her problem?

MRS M. JONES: No. I've always known from the start it's Reg, Reg's
attitudes.

INTERVIEWER: And you've held to that throughout this last admission?

MRS M. JONES: Yeah, yeah.

SOCIAL LIFE

Mrs June Smith

INTERVIEWER: Mrs Smith, is it that life has just become very difficult for you?

MRS J. SMITH: Not really, because I've always enjoyed our pleasures.
We go old-time dancing, we always go out at the weekends. I've
always enjoyed that.

INTERVIEWER: Is it difficult to enjoy that now?

MRS J. SMITH: Yes.

INTERVIEWER: What is yourself normally, someone that's active,
someone that does things?

MRS J. SMITH: And very bright and witty and I'd always enjoy a
joke and didn't mind telling one and I used to keep other people
around me quite jolly and laughing.

INTERVIEWER: What are the sort of things you like doing apart from
dancing?

MRS J. SMITH: Going to friends' houses.

INTERVIEWER: Do you like being with people?

MRS J. SMITH: Yes.

Mr Reg Smith

MR R. SMITH: She is more male company than female company. There
is no two ways about this. She is not, although in all respects
she is feminine, she is not a feminine woman. I don't know whether
you have come across that phrase before. But that's my feeling,
she is not a feminine woman. Put her with blokes and she can hold
her own.

INTERVIEWER: How did you see your wife before you married her?

MR R. SMITH: At that period ... I was never a drunkard, but I

always enjoyed a pint and she was of that type, socialising, there
were lots of us going around at that time.
INTERVIEWER: This was when?
MR R. SMITH: 1946, '47, '48, '49, and my pal at that time, we would
get four of us in the car and go out for a pint - my wife in those
days drank a pint, and you'll find if you watch her now, she is
afraid to put a cup to her lips of anything. That's how I met her,
socialising as much as anything, the average social evening, going
out, and probably having a bite of bread and cheese which we still
enjoy.
INTERVIEWER: Are you saying that she was in some way like you at
that time in terms of activity?
MR R. SMITH: Oh yes, for that particular activity that was in vogue
at that time after the war, I would say yes, we fitted.

But as you know we've started going out the last six to eight
years and I'm pretty sure what's failing her now is her ability to
keep up with other females. Inadequacy. She's got no bottom to
her domestic chores. When I say domestic chores, I don't mean
dusting and cleaning, this comes easy, but the hostess side to it.
She's just inadequate.

Another thing she has done, even though we go out a lot, has
never asked anybody to the house. Now she used to work at Michael's
Motors up at the back here, and there's a rather pleasant woman
there I knew other than coming here. Now when June was ill with
the flu this woman would bring her money down. She would never
ask her in and I would say to her, 'Why didn't you ask her in?'
'Didn't want her in here.' I took no notice, she didn't want her
in here, all right, doesn't worry me, it isn't my friend. But I
realise now there's a rejection.

We've never had a party in the house. Now a while ago I was
yearning to have a party. So I said to her, 'It's about time I had
a party.' Because of my long family I've got nieces of our own age
group. I said, 'I'll get eight people in and we'll have a party.'
'I don't know what to do.' Now I feel that she feels she is
feminine-hostess-deficient, short on her standards, and she hates
to be exposed. So I said, 'OK, we'll have a party. We'll get Joe
to do a bit of cooking, now Tina'll do the sausage rolls and all
the other things,' and I said, 'We'll get the table out and have a
few card games,' and I said, 'At nine o'clock we'll have all the
grub laid out in the other room as a buffet and we'll just say,
"Go in there and eat."' 'But there isn't enough chairs for people
to sit on.' I said, 'They'll sit on the floor.' Now I've said
several times since then, 'It's about time we had another party,'
but there's never any agreement to cotton on to this. There's a
rejection of having people for some reason or another.
MR R. SMITH: My wife never asks anybody to the house. She never
says, 'Let's ask so and so to the house, let's get some sandwiches
going.' This type of hostessing, this type of welcoming people.
OK, if people come to the house she'll go and get them a cup of tea
but you never have the effusive enthusiasms.
INTERVIEWER: Does this disappoint you in some way?
MR R. SMITH: Not disappoint, a bit of a hard word ... I notice it.
OK, this is her. I can't change you, I can't change her. This is
something I have to live with. If I want somebody in, I say,

'It's about time we asked so and so here and we'll do it Sunday
night.' And the next thing is, 'What do we do about it?' I say,
'I'll get some beer in, you do some chips or something,' but I do
the cooking usually then. This is the sort of inadequacy I mean.

Well if I say, 'We'll go to a dance,' she says 'yes,' but if
she ever said to me, 'I'd rather not go tonight, I'd rather go
somewhere else,' I'd say, 'OK.' But she's never made a decision
to alter anything.

Now you haven't got rid of this reluctance to do things and you
never will. We went to a dance Saturday night and I think, as I
have explained, it's still there in her, she has a negative attitude. Now I'm the sort I'll get up for a dance, whether I know it
or not because by now I've acquired a fair expertise. I haven't
got three legs any longer, but her attitude is not, 'Shall we
try?' But, 'We don't know that do we?' Negative, so what do I
do? I don't say anything, she knows how I feel about dancing, well
if that is her attitude do I try to convert her to a more positive
attitude? You see what I mean, it's negative....

Mrs Mary Jones

MRS M. JONES: Well my elder sister and her husband went for tea one
Saturday or Sunday a few months ago. Reg never encourages any
family there at all, he don't want to know, he just wants friends
there he can talk cheers and a pint of beer, nothing serious talk
at all, he don't want anything like that all. My sister went for
tea, June made it in the front room nicely, whereas usually they
sit in the kitchen, she made the tea and Reg walked in, 'What the
bloody hell's going on, what's this, having a bloody party?' And
my sister said our June curled up. And Reg said, 'What the bloody
hell's going on?' And if you went there it would be, 'How do,'
he would be down the garage. You can't get through to him.

He just ignores her, and she said he don't tell her anything.
She said that Esther, Reg's niece, and her husband, Roy, kept
coming into the hospital to see June. So June said to Reg, 'Why
don't you ring up Esther and Roy, because we haven't met them at
the club to see how she is because she's had ill health?' He said,
'No can't be bothered, I've got other things to do.' So she said,
'You ought to Reg.' Anyway they went out to Roxham and Ilkton is
on the way out to Roxham so she said to Reg, 'Let's call in to
Esther and Roy because they came in to see me and we can see how
they are.' He said, 'I rang her this morning.' She said, 'You
never told me,' he said, 'Oh I forgot.'

Andrew, I don't know him. And June said, 'Andrew put himself
out for Reg, bought him something to do with the car that Reg
wanted.' She said, 'I felt so unhappy, Reg never even asked him
in, kept him out by the door and gruffly took it from him.' She
said, 'That man was putting himself out for Reg,' and she said,
'Why don't you ask Andrew in?' And he said, 'Oh I can't bloody
be bothered asking people in.'

And it worries June, I don't think there's actually anything
in it, but one of their friends, Vera, who he wants to bring into
the psychiatric unit to see June, she's very attractive, and Joan

said at Christmas she was sat with Reg in his house and she was
kissing Reg in front of June, but our June really loves him with
all her heart. She don't have sexual relations and sees friends
of theirs making a fuss of him, she gets all shattered inside, I
think she does.
INTERVIEWER: You've mentioned something to me about some friends
Reg wanted to bring in to see June at the hospital but she didn't
want them to visit.
MRS M. JONES: To be truthful June said herself, this isn't the
place to bring friends because it's not a very happy, is it there?
She don't mind the family, but she said she don't want friends
coming in until she's better.
INTERVIEWER: But she doesn't mind Hazel coming in.
MRS M. JONES: That's true, well she doesn't in fact want Vera,
this attractive woman I mentioned earlier, and her husband coming
in.
INTERVIEWER: Why?
MRS M. JONES: Well it was them ... well when June's out with Reg,
say you are courting with someone and out with them, and my husband
and I are with you, June might go to the toilet on her own and on
her way back her friend Vera will call out, 'All right for next
Saturday. It's all arranged, cheerio.' So she says to Reg,
'What's arranged?' 'We're going out for a meal.' So she says,
'I wish you'd ask me sometimes Reg if I would like to go - you make
all the arrangements with everybody and I've just got to fall in
line and go with you.' And while she was ill there was a commotion
at a dance one night and Reg didn't speak to her for a whole week,
not one word.
INTERVIEWER: Why was that?
MRS M. JONES: While Vera and her was out to the toilet, they moved
the table somewhere and their bags were there. Reg bent over back-
wards looking for Vera's, and June said, 'I can't find mine,' and
Reg said, 'Well bloody look for it.' And she rounded on him that
night. She said she told him, and because she told him off in
front of company he didn't speak to her for a whole week. I
couldn't live like that, not speaking.
INTERVIEWER: Will you tell me what June's relationship to Reg's
children has been?
MRS M. JONES: Well she's got this friend Hazel ... Oh yes, well
they were out an evening. It came up about the war and June was
in the WRAFs and she said to Reg, 'Can I tell Hazel you were married
before because when I'm talking I've got to pick my words because
you want me to say the children are mine and I don't like doing
that?' You see, Reg has told her not to tell anyone that he had
been married before. 'It's nobody's business,' he says. You can't
pretend all your life those children are yours when they're not.
June had to pretend that the children were hers and Reg's. Reg
said, 'You're not to tell anyone they're children of a previous
marriage; you're not to tell people of our business.' Anyway a
niece of mine met Hazel and said, 'June's not been very well,' she
said, 'I can't understand our June being as poorly as this because
our mum', that's mine and June's other sister, 'said what a fine
girl she is; in the WRAF she was a smart girl and what's she got to
pretend about Joan and John?' And Hazel said, 'What do you mean

pretend?' 'Those aren't June's children.' 'Oh, we've always understood that they were, but we couldn't understand where the children
could have been when June was in the WRAF.' So they must have been
talking among themselves about it, June must know that as well. He
just won't let her do anything.

   She says she hasn't got any clothes but she has, she takes great
care of them, but with the places Reg wants to go all the time, she
can't wear a dress with these kind of people too often because
they've all got different clothes, all of them.

   So I said to June, 'What's wrong June?' She said, 'I feel
alright but....'. Joan and her husband - these are the things
that worry June. Joan lives a stone's throw from where they live;
now Joan and Jim go into hospital to see June, she's discharged.
Reg didn't even tell his daughter. June said Joan had done a lot
for Reg while she was in hospital, 'Not a thank you will Reg give
you or Joan or anyone.' He works at the LAT with his son and his
son didn't know what June had been discharged and was home. He
didn't tell anybody anything.

DOMESTIC LIFE

Mrs June Smith

INTERVIEWER: Do you like doing domestic things normally?
MRS J. SMITH: Yes.
INTERVIEWER: These things, you find them difficult to do now.
MRS J. SMITH: Yes, it would seem I've lost interest.

Mr Reg Smith

MR R. SMITH: I realise I've done more domestic work as regards
cooking and cleaning than possibly the average bloke ever does.
   One thing she wouldn't do is ever buy a dress for herself. She
would never go and shop.
   Well as I say afraid to go shopping, which I never took much
interest in before. I'd say, 'OK you want a dress, let's go and
find one.' Now we'll stand outside a shop window and she'll say,
'Come on away, there isn't one there.' 'How do you know there
isn't one in the shop? Come on in.' So I simply say to the first
person that comes up, usually a young girl, 'The manageress if
she's in I'd like to talk to her, if she isn't I'd like to talk
to you.' I explain what we want and I simply say point blank,
'If you have it we're interested, if you haven't got it don't waste
my time or your time.' My wife is astounded at this.
   Since Christmas 1973 my wife has been totally lethargic, the
will to get up and do anything, the will to shop. I've never been
able to, as other blokes say to their wives, 'Go and get so and so
for me.' I've got a hardware bloke for stones and gravel, I ring
him up, he's a good lad. I know him quite well and I say, 'Paul
will you send me down so and so?' 'Yeah,' and I say sometimes to
the wife, I have said, 'I haven't paid Paul, will you go up and
pay?' So I write out a cheque, she doesn't want to go up Queen's
Street, a ten-minute walk and pay Paul.

I took her to Jones's Supermarket, I won't give her any money
at the moment (not that I won't give her any money, I won't let
her bother to handle it), take her into Jones's Supermarket and
immediately she reacts to that and cries.

I took her around Jones's Supermarket. Unfortunately I whizz
around there because I'm the sort, I'll get a pile of grub in,
bring it home and say, 'Now we know what we are going to have for
dinner.' We don't go out thinking of programming lunch or programming tea and then buy accordingly. I'll buy a load of it, if
it so happens it's all beans then we'll have beans, that's how easy
it is, as far as I'm concerned, to shop. But she was mesmerised,
stood up in the shop and grabbed me and said, 'I can't stand much
more of this.' So I had to shop off, that was it.

We're regimented to, although I would never say it to her,
sausage and mash on Saturdays. Nothing free and easy you see,
meticulous about the house. OK. I don't mind so long as I can sit
on a chair occasionally, 'cos I usually say if I damage the chair
I'll buy another.

And I've had to educate her the way to make modern mashed potatoes. She measures it out and says, 'I hope I'm doing it right.'
So I say, 'Don't worry, don't worry whatsoever, there's three
saucepans, if there ain't enough in that one, we'll boil some more.'
But no, fuss, because the instructions say, a cup of water, so much
milk and you get so much mash. And then she's worried if you don't
get so much mash. And she fidgets over things like this. In the
past she's been so meticulous to a fault.

INTERVIEWER: What has she been crying about, as you see it?

MR R. SMITH: That she can't cope, that she can't make decisions,
that things get on top of her, that's the only way I can describe
it. Things ... having to make decisions even to get meals. Sunday
tea she says, 'What can we have for tea?' 'Well,' I said, 'What
do you want?' Leaving it to her to make the decision. 'All right,'
I said, 'We'll have three eggs and we'll do poached eggs on toast,
is that all right with you?' She said, 'Yeah.' 'That's all right
then I'll poach them.' Normally we've got the little poacher.
'I'll poach them,' I said, 'We'll poach them in some water with
some vinegar, like you like them.' 'Ah well,' she says, 'I don't
like them in there because they're runny.' She likes her eggs hard.
I said, 'It don't make any difference, I can boil an egg til it's
hard in water, all you do is leave it a bit longer.' And she was
going to make a point of that, so I just shifted her out the way
and gave her a shout. So it's fidgety things, things that I
wouldn't dream of making an issue of, that if I don't watch out
can become an issue.

INTERVIEWER: You said you were trying to help her in the last
months. You said something like, 'I tried to get her back on her
feet.' How did you try to help her?

MR R. SMITH: Well her constant theme of being ill was, 'We're in
a frightful muddle, there's a frightful mess downstairs.' I said,
'OK, have a cup of tea, sit quiet for a while and we'll walk around
the house and I'll shift the muddles, I'll shift it.' And I walked
her around the house as I've said, I pointed to that chair, and
I'd say, 'What's wrong with the chair, what do you want done?'
'Well nothing it's all right,' and I'd say 'Yes, do you want me to

move it out to look behind it?' I had to do this in minute detail,
walk around the house, and the one thing she had was the stove.
So Easter Sunday I dressed her and I pulled the stove out myself
and I meticulously cleaned the back, put it back again. I got her
into bed and she said, 'Aren't we in a muddle?' I didn't say anything to her, I realise she's ill. All right, I've done all I
could. I've even stood over her and said, 'Grow up for G....,'
but nothing's been of any avail until we knew; we tried the extreme,
which we knew was going to be a difficult passage for us, i.e.
hospitalisation.

My underclothes she's valiantly washed. I would normally wash
them myself under these circumstances. 'No,' she said, 'Let me try
it.' I said, 'OK, but there's one thing you don't do and that's
iron it.' 'Ah,' she said, 'I like to see nice ironed vests.'
'Look,' I said, 'As far as I'm concerned nobody sees my vest
except you and provided they're dry I'm not interested in them
being ironed.' I said, 'The hankerchiefs, the ones I use day by
day, just fold them up and smooth them with your hands.' I like
to see a nice white hankerchief ironed, but if I'm going to use
hankerchiefs, half a dozen not being ironed saves a chore. But she
practically insists, so I had to say, 'No you do not iron my vests,
I don't want 'em ironed, doesn't matter what you want, I don't want
my clothes ironed, my underclothes.' I had to bang my fist on the
table.

She has a particular trend at the moment, a particular illness
that she don't want to make decisions. That's why I had to do the
hoovering on Sunday - she wouldn't touch that hoover. Not that it
bothers me. I'm only telling you this.

It's probably a bit pointed, but I don't think you people
appreciate, and as I've said before, I've seen people enough in my
life now.... OK, I'm pretty sure she's been living with a facade
of some sort. OK, she's a hard worker, always been a hard worker,
always been meticulously clean which is a fault. All right, you
can be clean, but not meticulously clean which is a fault to me;
but I would never say this, not to her anyway. I would never say
this, OK, I might think there's no need to do that, but if she
wants to, OK, this is up to her. But as you know we've started
going out this last six to eight years and I'm pretty sure what's
failing her now is her ability to keep up with other females.
Inadequacy, she's got no bottom to her domestic chores. I don't
mean dusting and cleaning, this comes easy, but the hostess side
of it. She's just inadequate.

Mrs Mary Jones

INTERVIEWER: June must have been very capable at one time, as you
said she looked after your ill mother before she died.
MRS M. JONES: Yes she's more capable than me or you. It's only been
since eighteen months she's been like how she is now. June was
educated, she's got her name on the Honours board at school. She
taught Reg what French she knows to try and help him in his job at
work.
INTERVIEWER: Does he always go shopping with her?

MRS M. JONES: Yes, Reg does, and she's got to have what he wants.
He told Joan, Easter, to buy June a brown jumper and a black one,
but June wants bright things not dark. He dominates everything
she does.
MRS M. JONES: I said to June, 'Why don't you go out?' She said,
'Because I'm dirty.' I said, 'Who said you were dirty? Reg?'
And she said, 'No, the house is dirty, everything is dirty.' And
she said, 'Look at my sink Mary, isn't it dirty?' I said, 'It's
whiter than I've ever seen a sink.' Everything she looks at she
says is dirty.
INTERVIEWER: Do you think that's what Reg says to her?
MRS M. JONES: Well this is another day I went down there, that
Monday I went down there, she says, 'I can't do his washing, I
can't do it.' So I said, 'Come on, find it out and I'll do it for
you.' Then it starts, 'Oh I've only got one of those rotary things.
I haven't got a line and all the peg marks will be on it and it will
all be dirty again.' I said, 'It won't be dirty, it doesn't matter
if you get a peg mark, it's the wash, if it smells clean and fresh.'
So I washed it, she hovered over me the whole time so I would do it
properly. And I said, 'June I've been washing for forty years and
I can wash better than you so don't hover over me.' So I did her
washing and pegged it out, and she said, 'How do you know when it's
dry, how do you know when it will be aired?'
MRS M. JONES: Apparently now he's doing the front bedroom out. She
said, 'Do you know what he done yesterday, Mary?' I said, 'No.'
She doesn't mention him very often. I said, 'What did Reg do?'
She said that he said the bedspread on the bed was dirty, so he
brought it down, and she said he washed it in the sink. I said,
'What on a Sunday?' She said, 'Yes he did, it was filthy dirty.'
I said, 'I saw the bedspread June, it didn't look dirty to me.'
There's no dirty marks on none of her stuff, but it might have
needed a wash. She said, 'Life is a vicious circle,' and I said,
'In what way?' She said, 'You have things clean, you wear it, it
gets dirty, then you've got to wash it, then you've got to iron it.'
I said, 'June, everybody's got that, all of us, all women have got
washing, ironing, cooking and cleaning to do, that's life.' Then
I said, 'Where's the bedspread, because you haven't got it hung up?'
Because I thought she might have been imagining it. So she said,
'I think he's got it in the garage.' So I said, 'What, the bedspread in the garage?' So I went down the garage, looked in the
doors and there's no bedspread there. So I went back and said,
'There's no bedspread down there June.' And I began to think she
made it up or something. Anyway she said the only place it could
be is in the greenhouse. I said, 'Surely he didn't wash a bedspread
and put it in a greenhouse.' I went down the garden to the greenhouse and it was hung up there to dry. He'd washed it, said it was
dirty.
INTERVIEWER: How did she feel about that?
MRS M. JONES: She felt she was dirty because the bedspread was
there. She thinks everything is dirty, she's looking for every
mark everywhere, she's doubled up.
MRS M. JONES: I wonder about the hoover, she won't use it because
he fixed it up.
INTERVIEWER: I gather Reg bought her a second-hand hoover while June
was in hospital. Why won't she use it?

MRS M. JONES: She said it might explode. And it might be something
to do with that car because he did her brakes on the car and they
failed and he did them again and they locked on her. Whether she's
so poorly that she imagines he's trying to get rid of her that way,
I don't know.

     She likes to have ordinary conversation, like women do, about
the price of food. 'I don't want to bloody hear that rubbish,
shut up.' That's how Reg is. She says to me she's got no conversation anymore, that's because he won't listen anyway. She
won't ask him for any money, he's got loads of money, I know for
a fact he keeps her at a bare minimum. She goes to work herself
and that's what runs the house.

ACTIVITIES

Mr Reg Smith

MR R. SMITH: And as from the time I was fifteen years, I always
had some interest. I took up St John's Ambulance work, I've always
been a basic engineer. I then took up motorbikes, when the time
came around I took up rough riding until I had three accidents,
then it was time to pack in....

     And in between all this [Mr Smith is referring to the numerous
positions he has held during his working life], I've been interested
enough to take cars to pieces, motorbokes to pieces, only about two
years ago I replaced an engine in a car. So all in all I would
say I am very, very active.

     She just got very tired last year, mostly tired. There was no
other noticeable effects other than very tired and taking Yeast
Vite tablets, because I suppose she sees me, I'm the opposite of
her, I can wake up at 4 o'clock in the morning and start reading
and I'm awake. I can wake up at 7.00 a.m. and I can start singing.
She takes two hours to come around, she can't understand this. Now,
I am one of those people, I've analysed myself a little bit, and
I'm one of those persons, I went to bed last night 11.30 p.m., I
was awake at 4.00 a.m., picked up a book about Russia, just simply
started to read it, half an hour later put the book down, went to
sleep again till 7 o'clock. Doesn't worry me. Now she gets
bothered about that and I think she rejects the fortunate vitality
I have.
INTERVIEWER: How else has she been? Has she been weepy?
MR R. SMITH: Oh yes she weeps all right. She begged me not to go
down in the garden on Sunday, and Saturday I was down there all
day. You probably know I'm very energetic, I didn't think anything
Sunday night of putting a new exhaust pipe on my car at 6 o'clock,
and I already had changed, washed and sat down for the evening and
I thought I may as well do that little job. So all right, put a
new exhaust pipe on. I had it in the garage so I thought if I
don't do it tonight, I shall have it tomorrow night to do. So I
think my image tends to upset her a little bit because she knows
I'm so active and she begged me not to go down the garden on Saturday and Sunday and I was down there all Sunday afternoon and
evening during that showery weather.

OUTPATIENTS

A summary follows of the general practitioner's letter written on
19 April 1974 to the consultant psychiatrist in charge of Mrs
Smith's initial outpatient interview.

The GP wrote that Mrs Smith was suffering from severe depression.
He said the first episode was a mild one six years previously but
she had become more severely depressed in January 1973. Apparently
she had responded after some time to Caps. Surmontil, having been
prescribed initially one at night but later the prescription being
increased to two. He claimed that Mrs Smith did not really improve
until July and that by September 1973 she was able to do all her
housework, gardening, decorating and odd jobs that she had been
unable to do for years. He went on to say that in spite of still
taking the treatment, e.g. Surmontil 50mg, two at night and Valium
2mg, r.d.s., Mrs Smith's depression worsened during March 1974. As
a result of Mrs Smith getting slightly obsessional the GP wrote
that he changed the treatment to Anafranil 25mg t.d.s. This did
not seem to help her particularly and she had become very tense.
A fortnight before recommending to Mrs Smith that she should consult a psychiatrist he prescribed Serenacel Caps. b.d., but he
added finally that her depression seemed to be deepening and that
he would be glad of the consultant's advice.

A summary of the consultant psychiatrist's reply to the general
practitioner written on 24 April 1974 after his initial outpatient
appointment with Mrs Smith.

The consultant thanked the GP for asking him to see Mrs Smith,
whom he described as moderately depressed and needing urgent admission.

The consultant wrote that she had been depressed mildly on and
off for several years but more noticeably over the past year. She
had not responded to various anti-depressant medication and was
now functioning at a pretty poor level, unable to live independently
and to do the shopping and the housework. Apparently Mr Smith was
out of the house for a long day and Mrs Smith had no children of
her own. Mr Smith had children from another marriage who lived in
the vicinity. Mrs Smith's attitude towards lack of children was
that she did not want them particularly, and that she had been
looking after her elderly mother for many years.

The consultant was of the opinion that there was considerable
tension in the marital relationship. He described Mrs Smith as
cowed and retarded but Mr Smith as brisk and asserting his reason-
ableness. He had the impression that Mrs Smith was very much dominated by Mr Smith and that he had little insight into what she was
feeling.

The consultant wrote that he had decided to admit Mrs Smith in
view of her long-standing depression and also in view of the fact
that she had not responded to anti-depressant medication. He
assessed the outlook as being very good from a symptomatic point
of view but felt that the marital relationship was unsatisfactory
and would be difficult to influence in a constructive manner. He
said he would let the GP know how the unit got on.

Mr and Mrs Smith and Mrs Jones were interviewed in the time between Mrs Smith's outpatient appointment and her admission into the unit by one of the authors.

Mrs June Smith

INTERVIEWER: What made you come to Outpatients yesterday?
MRS J. SMITH: Well I think my husband was worried because I wasn't making such a good recovery as he hoped and I think he arranged with my doctor I should see someone else.
INTERVIEWER: Did you want to go yourself?
MRS J. SMITH: I don't like hospitals.
INTERVIEWER: In what way did the consultant say he could help you?
MRS J. SMITH: He didn't really say.
INTERVIEWER: If you were offered the following three treatments, ECT, drugs, or talking with someone who understands you, which do you feel would be the most valuable?
MRS J. SMITH: Well I'm hoping against hope all the time there isn't anything wrong with me, that I don't need drugs and things, that I should be able to get better on my own. I don't really want to come into hospital at all.

Mr Reg Smith

INTERVIEWER: In your opinion how does your wife see hospitals?
MR R. SMITH: I'm pretty sure my wife's got a horror of tablets, and I'm pretty sure she's got a total horror of hospitals.
INTERVIEWER: Your wife stayed with her sister, Mary, over Easter. Why was that?
MR R. SMITH: Because I had to go to work. I just didn't dare leave her because over Easter she was talking about wanting to go into a corner and go to sleep and not wake up anymore. When Mary came home from a holiday after Easter I nipped up there. She said bring her straight up and said, 'We'll see if we can't feed her up to get her on her feet again.'
INTERVIEWER: Did Mary agree with the decision for June to seek psychiatric help?
MR R. SMITH: Oh yes, she and I decided. She persuaded me. Mary couldn't get June back on her feet. So the next thing was, 'You ought to get her some treatment.' I said, 'OK.'
INTERVIEWER: Did you attend the Outpatient consultation with your wife?
MR R. SMITH: Yes.
INTERVIEWER: Did the consultant say to you or your wife how he could help June?
MR R. SMITH: Not at all.
INTERVIEWER: If your wife was offered the following three treatments, ECT, drugs, or talking with someone who understands her, which do you feel would be the most valuable?
MR R. SMITH: She's had drugs, she's had sympathy, now the only other thing must be something else and it happens to be electrical treatment.

INTERVIEWER: For how long do you expect your wife to be in hospital?
MR R. SMITH: I would be surprised if two months pulled her round.
I feel there is some deterioration somehow somewhere that the hos-
pital is going to have a terrific difficulty building up.

Mrs M. Jones

INTERVIEWER: Do you know why June is afraid of hospitals?
MRS M. JONES: She's afraid Reg is going to leave her in hospital
and desert her like he deserted his first wife.
INTERVIEWER: What happened before Easter?
MRS M. JONES: 'Oh,' she said, 'the GP's coming and I've got to
tell him I'm better.' This was a couple of days before Easter.
'But June, you're not better.' She said, 'I've got to tell, Reg
said I've got to tell him I'm better.' So the GP came to the door,
she made me stay in the kitchen and said, 'Don't you do anything.'
So I said, 'No it's nothing to do with me June.' So the GP said,
'Hallo Mrs Smith.' She said, 'Hallo,' and he started admiring all
Reg's paintings on the wall. So he said, 'How are you Mrs Smith?'
She said, 'Better thank you.' So he said, 'That's good,' and was
gone.
INTERVIEWER: What happened after you returned from your Easter
holiday?
MRS M. JONES: Before I went away I had told June I would take her
home and care for her when I returned. So on the Tuesday after
Easter Monday Reg really dumped her here, and then didn't come for
two days to see her. The week I cared for her was the hardest week
I've ever had in my life. I couldn't make her eat. She just sat
there and cried. About four days after she got here I said to Reg,
'My husband said he's never seen a girl look so ill,' and he said,
'What do you think?' I said, 'I think she should see a specialist.'
I said specialist because our June was terrified of the word
'psychiatrist'. So Reg said, 'I'll go along with that then.'

THE PSYCHIATRIC UNIT

Mrs Smith was admitted into the unit on the 26 April 1974. She
was immediately placed on Chlorpromazine medication, 100mg three
times per day, in order to combat her tenseness. On the fifth day
of her admission the consultant increased the dosage to 150mg per
day since he felt that June was still tense. This assessment of
tenseness and the consequent increase of dosage was made during a
ward round in the following extraordinary manner. A staff nurse,
when asked by the consultant how effectively Mrs Smith was being
helped by the medication, replied that she did not know since she
had been on weekend leave. The consultant became angry and wondered what was the point of her attending the meeting if she knew
nothing. At this juncture she left the ward round, returned a
minute later and asserted that Mrs Smith was joining the other
patients in occupational therapy. It was on this basis that the
consultant decided to increase the dosage.
  During the first week of her admission the consultant said he

would pursue a treatment policy that was aimed at solving, as he saw it, the apparent incompatibility of the Smiths' marriage. But he was pessimistic as regards a successful outcome to this plan because, in his opinion, there was a lack of contact between husband and wife. He instructed his psychiatric social worker (PSW) to interview, individually, Mr Smith and Mrs Jones.

Part of this plan was carried out. Mr Smith was interviewed by the social worker at the end of the first week of June's admission. The consultant had stated that an interview with Mrs Jones was important as it might shed more light on the nature of the Smiths' marriage. However, even though Mrs Jones visited the hospital every day, she was not interviewed until the day before June was discharged. By this time a different form of treatment had been decided upon and carried out. It is possible that the delay in seeing Mrs Jones had considerable bearing on the management of the case.

It is pertinent to note that a life history was not taken from Mrs Smith until the sixth day of her admission. The policy of the unit was that life histories should be taken as soon as possible after the patient had been admitted.

Mr and Mrs Smith, and Mrs Jones were interviewed towards the end of June's first week in hospital by one of the authors.

Mrs June Smith

INTERVIEWER: Have you been able to strike up acquaintances while you've been in the unit?
MRS J. SMITH: Well only surface-wise you know. You listen when they talk about their troubles. I feel sorry for them as much as I do for myself.
INTERVIEWER: You said to me the other day that you had this feeling that the day was all the same, it's too long. Is that right?
MRS J. SMITH: Yes it is a long day.
INTERVIEWER: Have you still got this feeling?
MRS J. SMITH: Well I think it's really because in the time we've got off around mealtimes I can't get really interested in a book as I'd like to. You know I keep reading bits and trying but I don't seem to remember it after I've read it.
INTERVIEWER: How do you feel about occupational therapy?
MRS J. SMITH: There's not a great deal up there to do. I've been trying to play the games with the other patients but half the people don't think anybody really knows how to organise the people in it.
INTERVIEWER: How different do you feel from when you first came in?
MRS J. SMITH: Well I don't suppose I feel a lot different. I feel I am a different person from what I was a few months ago.
INTERVIEWER: Do you feel tense at all?
MRS J. SMITH: Not in the sense that I'm strung up. I've a fear, I seem to be afraid of something.
INTERVIEWER: Did you have this feeling before you came into hospital?
MRS J. SMITH: Well I got it as soon as I knew I had to come into hospital.

INTERVIEWER: Have the pills you've been having affected you?
MRS J. SMITH: I don't feel that much better with it yet, whether
it's not got through my system yet. No I don't feel suddenly
cheerful, or suddenly myself now.

Mr Reg Smith

INTERVIEWER: Have you been visiting your wife since she's been in
the unit?
MR R. SMITH: Yes I've visited her quite regularly.
INTERVIEWER: Do you feel her state of health has improved?
MR R. SMITH: I don't think her condition has altered much. She's
still scared of hospitals and, in my opinion, is a bad patient.
She constantly asks me not to leave her in here. I always reply:
'How could I, would our friends and family let me?'
INTERVIEWER: How did you see the purpose of your interview with
the social worker?
MR R. SMITH: I don't know where she fits in. I was only hoping
what I said to her was helpful, and if so I can put up with an hour
of my time for helping anybody's case. If what I say from what I
consider to be a fairly lucid explanation helps at all then OK,
because these cases are pitiful. That in fact is the only contact
I've had with the staff. No one's told me what diagnosis my wife's
been given, nor what treatment she's been receiving and what her
chances of recovering are.

Mrs Mary Jones

INTERVIEWER: Have you been visiting your sister since she's been
in the unit?
MRS M. JONES: Yes, every day.
INTERVIEWER: How do you think she's been since she's been in hospital?
MRS M. JONES: The first few days she was terribly upset because
she was in there. She said, 'I can't wash a cup. They expect me
to lay the table one day and wash up. You know I've got to get
somebody to tell me to wash. I don't know what's gone wrong with
me.' 'All I can say June is those tablets must be very strong
that they've deadened your concentration.' She's a beautiful
writer, she's excellent at figures. She can't write, she can't
read, she can't concentrate on the television. I think her concentration has got worse since she's had these tablets.

June's treatment was crucially affected by a ward round that took
place during the second week of her admission. The PSW, on the
basis of one interview with Mr Smith, assessed that June needed to
be dependent on Reg and that he needed to dominate her. Thus she
felt that therapy aimed at altering the Smiths' relationship would
be inadvisable.
    The consultant agreed with this and decided to treat June symp-
tomatically with ECT. He explained to her that Chlorpromazine had
not helped her as he had hoped it would. Nevertheless, June

continued to receive Chlorpromazine as well as ECT throughout
the remainder of her stay in the unit.

Thus the consultant and his team had confirmed Reg's view that
his wife was ill and needed ECT. It is reasonable to suppose that
in doing this they further jeopardised any possibility of Reg's
co-operating in marital therapy (treatment for both husband and
wife), which might be necessary in the future.

Mr and Mrs Smith and Mrs Jones were interviewed at the end of the
second week of June's admission by one of the authors.

Mrs June Smith

INTERVIEWER: Would you describe how you felt after ECT had been
recommended?
MRS J. SMITH: I was very worried. It was because I didn't know
what the treatment was all about. I know that once you are in
here you have to accept treatment but I wanted Reg to know I was
having it and the doctor talked to him about it.
INTERVIEWER: What were your worries about?
MRS J. SMITH: I didn't know what the treatment was and what I was
afraid of was people talking about it in the ward, and when they
said it was electrical treatment and it was something to do with
my head I was afraid it might change my normal character. I might
get spiteful, aggressive, something that I'm not normally.
INTERVIEWER: What made you decide to have it in the end?
MRS J. SMITH: Well I think the doctor told Reg there was nothing
to worry about and Reg convinced me there was nothing to worry
about, and I thought well, if this is going to do me some good I
best have it.

Mr Reg Smith

INTERVIEWER: How did you feel about June being recommended ECT?
MR R. SMITH: Well I was surprised that the staff didn't inform me
before her. They know of her fear of hospitals and it would have
been better if I had broken the news to her. Anyway I arranged
an appointment with the SHO who told me why she was getting it
and what it consisted of. I then explained to her what it was
all about.
INTERVIEWER: What did you say to her?
MR R. SMITH: I told her she would have an anaesthetic and not know
anything about what was taking place. She would have a fifteen-
minute sleep and then wake up. I said she would feel a little
funny in the morning until the ashes had dropped to rest. I told
her that the doctors would not advise her to have it unless it was
in her best interests, and that ECT had been used with considerable
success. I made her understand that the doctors had informed me
that the tablets weren't working. I explained to her that she had
two choices, either she could stay in the unit for a long period
of time until the tablets had cured her, but, I said, this would
be unfair to other potential patients, or she could have a quicker,

well accepted form of treatment. I also said that the doctors
knew what was wrong with her, and their view was the same as
mine, a missing link had gone from that thing called 'will power'.
I told her she had to face up to life and believe in the ECT.

Mrs Mary Jones

INTERVIEWER: As you saw it how did June react to being advised
to have ECT?
MRS M. JONES: Oh she was terrified of it. So she said, 'What can
we do Mary?' I said, 'I haven't seen anyone to ask, I would like
to see the doctor. You're not bound to have it surely.' 'Oh
Reg will say I've got to have it. It's up to Reg, if Reg says
I've got to have it, I've got to have it.'
INTERVIEWER: What did she say to the doctor who recommended that
she have the treatment?
MRS M. JONES: Oh she told him she didn't want it. The tablets
haven't apparently worked. When I was there that day I went up
to the diningroom with her, they were just having their cup of tea.
It was 4 o'clock and I fancied a cup. There was a woman there
called Gladys who comes in every so often for electrical treatment.
Our June said to me, 'Look Mary, that lady there, Liz told me, has
had treatment eight times and look at her, she's no better, she's
worse. And Liz has just had another lot, she's had four lots, but
I don't want to look like them.'
INTERVIEWER: Do they say they are better from it?
MRS M. JONES: They say they are. Liz has no conversation at all,
says June. All she says is, 'You'll be all right June, don't
worry, injection in the arm and then the nurse takes you a cup of
tea, nothing to it, like having a tooth out.' But June says,
'That's all she says from morning till night, she's got no conversation, so how could she be better?' That's all she says all
day long to June.
INTERVIEWER: What about Gladys?
MRS M. JONES: Oh Gladys looks terrible. June's never seen her
before. So Liz said, 'You're better, aren't you Gladys through
having this treatment?' 'Not really,' she said. And she turned
to Liz and said, 'You'll be back again.' [She was, two weeks after
June had been discharged.] Liz said, 'I won't, I've had it four
times.' She said, 'You'll be back again, don't worry.' And June
sat there listening to all that conversation. She was terrified
of it.

June was prescribed three ECTs during the last ten days of her
admission. The consultant's team was of the opinion that as a
result of this treatment June's mood had considerably brightened.
    Two themes emerged from ward rounds during this period. First,
there was the consultant's assessment that ECT had succeeded where
Chlorpromazine had failed. As has been noted before, the latter
continued to be prescribed to June throughout her stay in the unit.
Second, there was the consultant's desire to hold marital therapy
even though he had previously agreed with his PSW that this was
inadvisable. Indeed, on the last day of June's admission he put

forward this plan once again after his SHO had reported to him
on his interview with Mrs Jones. She had confirmed the staff's
view that Mr Smith mistreated June. The plan was dropped when
the PSW reiterated her view that more harm than good might be
done to the marriage.

   The junior staff were pessimistic about June's future. The
SHO felt sure that she would be re-admitted into the unit in the
future. Unlike his colleagues the consultant was more optimistic.
'After all,' he said, 'Mr Smith's behaviour might change for the
better.'

   June was discharged on the 17 May 1974 and responsibility for
her outpatient care was given to the SHO.

Mr and Mrs Smith and Mrs M. Jones were interviewed at the end of
June's admission by one of the authors.

Mrs June Smith

INTERVIEWER: How did you feel after you had ECT?
MRS J. SMITH: I felt much better but I didn't know if it was the
treatment or if it was a feeling of relief that it was over, and
that it hadn't changed my normal character. The first one made
me think of doing something which I hadn't done in a long time
which was to ring up Reg at work. I remembered his number without
having to refer to any paper or anything. One thing that did
bother me was why I continued to take the pills, because the consultant had said to me, when he told me I was going to have ECT,
that they hadn't been working.
INTERVIEWER: Did you have more desire to join in and do things?
MRS J. SMITH: Oh yes I did. Yes, I think I got the feeling that I
probably could help other people a little bit more, you know,
people who appeared to me to be worse than I was. Because I had
a numb feeling when I first went in there, because everything was
so strange and I didn't like the thought of hospitals right from
the start really.

Mr Reg Smith

INTERVIEWER: How did you see your wife's condition after she had
ECT?
MR R. SMITH: She was certainly better. One of the things I did
notice was that she was walking upright which she hadn't been up
to that point in time, and the very first day after the very first
application of this ECT, she certainly was on top of the world
that day because she rang me in the morning at eleven or half past
and I was shattered at the tone of her voice. If I hadn't known
I would have thought it was normal.
INTERVIEWER: You mean it was like before.
MR R. SMITH: Yeah, but obviously the next day she reacted and she
was very, very dull. Now from that time on she became scared,
though she had gone up a couple of notches, each time she had
dropped back one.

INTERVIEWER: Does what you've said apply to the second and third ECT?
MR R. SMITH: Yes, second and third were very much the same.

Mrs Mary Jones

INTERVIEWER: How did you see June's condition after she had ECT?
MRS M. JONES: I thought she was better only after the first one.
You saw Reg and I in the passageway, and June was laughing and
smiling. Oh I was happy, I thought that's our old June, how she
was before.
INTERVIEWER: What about after the other two?
MRS M. JONES: I didn't see any improvement at all. I thought she
was how she was before her first ECT.
INTERVIEWER: In what way?
MRS M. JONES: Not a smile on her face for a start. I said, 'Do
you feel better?' I don't think she did really, but the first day
I saw a marked improvement. I thought she was very happy but when
I asked her about it she said she thought she was so relieved at
getting that first treatment over. It wasn't as bad as what she
thought because she was very worried about it.
INTERVIEWER: What about after that?
MRS M. JONES: The third one she was real worried because the night
before she had that third one she'd moved upstairs to another bed.
When she had the third one, this is what she told me afterwards,
all the three persons that had it were all the same, they couldn't
remember where they were for the time being and nor could June.
She looked across at her bed, knew that she had been sleeping over
there previously, but knew she wasn't there now. But she couldn't
remember about being moved upstairs. Her and another patient had
been moved upstairs the night before. For the time being they
couldn't remember that they'd moved and then they sort of talked
it over together and remembered and then they went upstairs. June
said, 'Oh yes, I had a bath up there last night, our room is upstairs.'

OUTPATIENTS

From the time of her discharge June was in outpatient care for
two and a half months. For the first month she was seen once a
week, and subsequently once a fortnight, by the SHO.
    The consultant had made the decisions as regards June's treat-
ment while she was an inpatient. Once discharged he placed her
under the care of his SHO. Thus, in effect, the latter had the
freedom to choose whatever treatment he felt was necessary, even
though the consultant maintained ultimate responsibility for June's
welfare. The SHO embarked on a policy of paving the way for June
to speak frankly about her marriage, although the team decision
had been not to do this.
    As time went on the consultant became increasingly detached
from the case. There was evidence of this in a letter he sent to
June's GP on 24 May 1974. He wrote that he had seen Mrs Smith at

the outpatient department on 24 April and that she had been admitted two days later on the account of agitated depression which
had not responded to medication and which had been present in
some degree for about six years.

He said that she had remained in this state despite Chlorpromazine 100mg q.d.s. so she was given a short course of ECT following which she made considerable improvement. The consultant felt
that the domestic situation seemed to be at the root of the
trouble. From what he could ascertain there was considerable
tension between Mrs Smith and her husband and that he tended to be
a domineering person who gave Mrs Smith little hope to express her
point of view. ·He said his team were informed by Mrs Smith's
sister that Mr Smith's sons both shared this view about him.

The consultant claimed that he and his team would have liked
to have worked in joint therapy with the Smiths but they felt that
in this instance they were unlikely to be successful and ·that the
best they could do would be to support Mrs Smith on her own. He
said she left hospital on 17 May much improved and that she would
be followed up as an outpatient. He claimed that she was on no
medication. He felt that if there was a recurrance of the tension
that it would respond to moderate doses of Valium if necessary.

The facts were that Mr Smith had a son and a daughter, and not two
sons, that June was receiving medication - Chlorpromazine and
Valium - and that the SHO was doing more than just support June.

During the first three weeks of outpatient care the SHO noted,
in a letter to June's GP on 29 May 1974, that June 'was still
moderately agitated and depressed', and had been staying with her
sister for support on weekdays. Furthermore he was making little
headway in his discussions with June about her marriage. In the
same letter to the GP he wrote:

There is certainly a lot of conflict between her and her
husband. He is being very domineering and overpowering to her
and she cannot bring herself to discuss this with me and I feel
that this is because she cannot bring herself to accept how bad
things really are between them.

Mr and Mrs Smith and Mrs M. Jones were interviewed three weeks
after June had been discharged from the unit by one of the authors.

Mrs June Smith

INTERVIEWER: How have you felt since you left hospital?
MRS J. SMITH: I can't do as much as I'd hoped. But the thing is
I think I hoped for a lot more than some people. Some people don't
care whether they've done this today or they can leave things until
tomorrow, but I'm the type who wants to do everything and do it
properly and feel satisfied with it. I don't feel I'm quite up to
that standard yet. I'm certainly feeling better. I don't want to
lie in bed all the time or anything like that. I feel stronger
bodily and I'd like to do jobs around the house again that I didn't
before. I'd gone right off it. But I still feel that I need some
help, support, I do.

INTERVIEWER: I gather you've been staying with Mary.
MRS J. SMITH: A few of the days during the week, you know.   I'm
all right at home when Reg is there. Of course he works out at
Shipton so he can pick me up from here all right and I've been
going home with him at the end of the week and staying all the
weekend and then have been staying with Mary for a few days during
the week you know.
INTERVIEWER: Why is that?
MRS J. SMITH: I've tried staying at home on my own but I don't
like being totally on my own. I don't know what I'm afraid of.
I'm not afraid of anything in the house but I just feel the need
for company. I think Mary does me good and I'm all right at home
with Reg for support, but I feel I need that little bit of support.
I don't feel wholly independent if you know what I mean.
INTERVIEWER: How do you feel about the sessions you're having with
the SHO?
MRS J. SMITH: I dread the thought of going in, but I feel you just
can't make these appointments with people who are specialists at
their job and not go, because you are preventing somebody else
from going, and their time is valuable. I hope it will help me
because presumably that's what it is intended to do, but what
worried me is the fact that I can't think of anything to tell the
SHO to help him. He's trying to help me by asking questions but
if I haven't got ... if I could say my husband hits me about the
head or anything like that, that's something positive, but I don't
feel I've got anything positive for getting the depression I've
had.

Mr Reg Smith

INTERVIEWER: How, in your opinion, has your wife been since she
was discharged?
MR R. SMITH: All I'm saying is the improvement now we've got her
home is the fact that she is lucid in conversation. She still has
no energy and she is starting to go over again. She's weepy. She
cries about the fact that she can't cope, that she can't make
decisions, that things get on top of her, that's the only way I
can describe it. Things ... having to make decisions even to get
meals.
INTERVIEWER: Why has she been staying at her sister's?
MR R. SMITH: I don't think for one minute she would be happier on
her own until six every night, her courage isn't there. If I was
home all the time she wouldn't go, no problem, frightened to be
on her own. Mary is a motherly sort. I feel, mentally, if somebody feels sheltered their brain or head has got a chance of
healing. I can't imagine she can heal over here on her own. She's
totally worried about things. I know she wouldn't eat during the
day.
INTERVIEWER: Do you think she will have to go back into hospital?
MR R. SMITH: I wouldn't be surprised. I think we've got to get
round it, she's got to come in again for a while for no other
reason that she is not strong in herself yet.
INTERVIEWER: What kind of treatment do you think it would be valuable for her to have?

MR R. SMITH: More ECT. I don't know what ECT does but I would
say whatever it had done it hadn't notched her up notches enough.
But she still has a total horror and I can't tell you how intense
that horror is because she cried here Sunday and said, 'I only
hope I'm not going to be worse because I could not go back into
hospital.' She has a total horror of hospitals, and this is part
of it. It's like driving a car across the Sahara and sooner or
later you know it's going to break in and you're going to get
crunched. She's completely terrified of hospitals, there's no
two ways about it.

Mrs Mary Jones

INTERVIEWER: Do you think June's any better compared with before
she went into hospital?
MRS M. JONES: No, not really, I don't think.
INTERVIEWER: Is there no improvement?
MRS M. JONES: She's not so agitated I don't think. I expect you
saw June at the beginning, she was very agitated, trembling and
that. All that's gone, she's very calm in her actions like, but
there's no excitement, no enjoyment, no laughing at all. But she's
not agitated like she was before. I think it's done her good that
way, but if you saw her yesterday you wouldn't have thought she
was any better.
INTERVIEWER: What happened?
MRS M. JONES: As you probably know she's been staying here during
the week. Well we thought she might have a long weekend at home
rather than coming here on Sunday night. I suggested that she
should stay at home on Monday morning when Reg had gone off to
work and that I'd pop over at lunch time to see how she was. If
she was all right I'd come back on my own and she could come over
Tuesday and stay the night so we could go to the hospital together
on the Wednesday. The idea was that each week she could go home
earlier and come back here later in the week, you know, gradually
ease off. Any way I got to her on the Monday and I knocked on the
door and she came out crying her eyes out. She said, 'Mary I'm so
pleased you've come, I didn't think you were coming.' The tears,
I had a job to console her for a couple of hours.
INTERVIEWER: How does June feel about going to see the SHO?
MRS M. JONES: It worries her. She said she don't know how to
answer him because, she says, there's no trouble between her and
Reg. She said that that's what the SHO is looking for, one spe-
cific thing, but she says it's a lot of things, though she never
says what.
INTERVIEWER: Would you think if June didn't get better it might
be an idea for her to go back into hospital?
MRS M. JONES: I don't want her to go back into hospital.
INTERVIEWER: Why not?
MRS M. JONES: I don't think there's much improvement with the
treatment.
INTERVIEWER: How do you see the future for June?
MRS M. JONES: Well I'm worried for her now. You see I can't have
her here all time because I've got to take into account my children.

After having been in outpatient care for three weeks June decided
not to stay at her sister's during the week. She had been advised
by the SHO that this would be in her best interests. Thus from
this time onwards she remained at home permanently.

Two themes gradually emerged concerning June's outpatient care
during the next seven weeks. First, there were the SHO's abortive
attempts to discuss the Smiths' marital situation with both Reg
and June together. On 12 June he wrote in the case notes: 'Mr
Smith tended to be anxious about this approach (i.e. talking about
the marital situation), saying he did not understand it, "too deep
for me", which I suspect was his way of opting out.' Fifteen days
later he wrote to June's GP:

> I saw June once again with her husband who was totally over-
> powering, even answering for her, and telling me what she felt.
> Little response from her other than total agreement. There
> seems little to be gained from pursuing joint interviews and I
> will, in future, see her alone for supportive psychotherapy.

The second theme was to do with a gradual deterioration in June's
condition. On 27 June 1974 the SHO wrote to the GP saying that
June 'was certainly more depressed, being retarded and demonstrating
little spontaneity'. By 25 July June's condition had worsened.
He wrote to the GP saying that, 'Since she has returned to her
husband it seems that she has steadily gone downhill again. She
is moderately to severely depressed, with agitation and expressing
inability to do simple tasks at home.' The only option open to
the SHO, as he saw it, was to offer June inpatient care. Initially
she was opposed to this advice, but by August she had reluctantly
accepted his recommendation.

Mr and Mrs Smith and Mrs Jones were interviewed before June was
re-admitted into the unit by one of the authors.

Mrs June Smith

INTERVIEWER: How have you been feeling since you've been at home?
MRS J. SMITH: I seem to have been feeling ill in myself. I don't
want to go out or anything. Since I've been at home I can't seem
to do the house jobs properly and I can't help my husband around
the house.
INTERVIEWER: How has Reg been towards you?
MRS J. SMITH: He's been wonderful.
INTERVIEWER: Why have you decided to be admitted into the unit,
given your dislike of hospitals?
MRS J. SMITH: I think in the end Mary and Reg have persuaded me
that I'm not getting any better, in fact I'm still going downhill,
and they are both worried about me. They have both said to me
that they think that this is the only thing that will do me any
good. They've said, 'You just can't go on like this.' I don't
really want to go in, but I think they've persuaded me I'm doing
no good going on like I am.
INTERVIEWER: Has the SHO told you how he will be able to help you?
MRS J. SMITH: No he hasn't really. He just said I needed to come
in if I was to get better.

Mr Reg Smith

INTERVIEWER: Has your wife's condition deteriorated since she's
been at home?
MR R. SMITH: Yes, very much so. Pretty grim. No up and go, no
impetus, no will power to do anything, just generally not bothered.
Well, when I say not bothered, with the best intentions in the
world, couldn't bother. And since about three weeks or about a
month ago she's gone downhill, much worse, she doesn't even cry
now, she wails. She'll stand in the doorway and bend up and wail.
INTERVIEWER: So her condition has deteriorated?
MR R. SMITH: Having no parallel and going back to the old adage
compared to what, I would say it's as much as a bloke can put up
with.
INTERVIEWER: In what respect?
MR R. SMITH: Constantly crying, constantly bothering, constantly
calling for you, constantly not believing things you are saying.
INTERVIEWER: How do you see the meetings you, your wife and the
SHO had?
MR R. SMITH: Well quite frankly, at all these meetings I'm only
there to correct statements that are a little bit misunderstood
and that are a little bit, shall I say, offbeat in the answer.
Inasmuch as I don't say anything, I'm not really a participant.
Though I'm there I feel I'm there to protect the interests of both,
i.e. the doctor asks a question, it may not get home in the context he implies it, because shall I say a little bit of bewilderment
on June's part. So I wait for her to answer, then I correct and
that's what I feel is my role in the situation. When there are
three of us together it's not my place to answer for June. Quite
honestly I don't know how she feels, I know what she's like to me
but I wouldn't know how the hell she feels.
INTERVIEWER: When the SHO offered inpatient care to your wife how
did he say he could help her?
MR R. SMITH: Well he gave her the usual story, with undue frankness
between four walls, 'We think we can help you.' OK, this can only
go on so long and if you try to help too many times and you fail,
one of those individuals is going to pick you up on it before long.
And I was a bit worried yesterday to make any comment whatsoever,
unless she realised it was more or less the same words being used.
INTERVIEWER: What are your expectations for her now?
MR R. SMITH: I would be surprised if you people were satisfied
with her inside four to six weeks. I think she is going to be
like this for a very, very long time. You people will be able to
charge her batteries up but they will fail on her again.

Mrs M. Jones

INTERVIEWER: After June went home permanently how often did you
see her?
MRS M. JONES: Twice a week for the first two weeks and then roughly
once a week after that.
INTERVIEWER: How has she been, in your opinion?
MRS M. JONES: She's gone downhill.

INTERVIEWER: In what way?
MRS M. JONES: She's crying and whining all the time and she walks bent in half. She thinks everything is dirty. I asked her, 'Why don't you go out?' She said, 'Because I'm dirty.' I said, 'Who said you're dirty, Reg?' She said, 'No, the house is dirty, everything is dirty.' Everything she looks at she says is dirty. Another time she said to me, 'Look Mary, I've been looking at the gas taps, I can't remember if it's on or off, I don't know nothing anymore.' And she goes on like that for hours and hours.
INTERVIEWER: What other things have been worrying her?
MRS M. JONES: Well this really frightened me. She said, 'If you come down one day and couldn't find me here what would you do?' I said, 'I'd knock and knock and if I couldn't make you hear I suppose I would have to go back home.' She said, 'Would you come again?' I said, 'Of course I would, I would come over the same day if I didn't find you in in the morning and I would call through the letter box like I always do.' 'But,' she said, 'If you didn't find me another day what would you do then?' I said, 'I would come over in the evening when I knew Reg would be home.' 'But,' she said, 'if you couldn't find me and if Reg didn't answer the door, what would you do then?' I said, 'I'd go up his bloody works and I'd go and see his boss, and I'd say, "Go and fetch Reg Smith, I want to know where my sister is".' She said, 'You won't let me go in an institution will you Mary?' She's scared to death she's going to end up in an institution.

THE PSYCHIATRIC UNIT

June entered the unit on 1 August. She was not prescribed any medication, as was the case during her first admission, since the consultant assessed her state as more depressed than agitated.
      The consultant decided to pursue the same treatment plan that he and his team had rejected, in principle, during June's first admission, and that had failed when carried out by the SHO during outpatient care. The consultant and the SHO would interview Reg and June, respectively, with a view to conjoint interviews. The junior members of the team, including the SHO, were pessimistic as regards a successful outcome to this plan. Nevertheless they felt it was preferable to prescribing ECT. The consultant was optimistic. He felt that there were similarities between the Smith case and the situations of patients suffering from bereavement reactions. He noted that these types of patient took a long time to construe the deceased in a realistic fashion. Their initial reaction, always, was to appraise the latter in an exaggerated, positive way.
      As the first fortnight of this admission progressed it became increasingly obvious to all those concerned with June's treatment that their psychotherapeutic attempts would be in vain. June was still not confirming the staff's view that her marriage was a poor one. Reg, said the consultant, had admitted that he was authoritarian towards his wife, but he felt he was too old to change his behaviour. The consultant stated to the rest of his team that he agreed with this, but added that Reg would not be averse to

participating in conjoint interviews with June. Mrs Jones was
interviewed again by the SHO. Although she reconfirmed the team's
view of the Smiths' marriage, this information proved of no value
in trying to stimulate June to talk about the latter.

During a ward round at the beginning of the second week of the
admission the consultant suggested that June would probably have
to be treated with ECT. A general discussion ensued over the
team's use of ECT. The registrar felt that it was illogical to
prescribe ECT given that June's problem was to do with her marriage. He also noted that the prescription of ECT tended to go
hand in hand with staff pessimism regarding the outcome of a case.
The SHO agreed and added that use of ECT would only confirm June's
and Reg's view that June was ill in the brain, when he had been
trying to persuade her that her problem was to do with her life
situation. The consultant disagreed with his junior colleagues.
To begin with, he had taken on the responsibility of helping June.
Second, she had not been amenable to psychotherapy. Third, she
had responded previously quite successfully to ECT. Thus on these
three counts he felt he was justified in treating June in this
way. However, the consultant had failed to remember that the
effects of ECT had in June's case been only temporary.

After a fortnight, as was the case during the first admission,
June received her first ECT.

Mr and Mrs Smith and Mrs Jones were interviewed two weeks after
June had been admitted by one of the authors.

Mrs J. Smith

INTERVIEWER: Do you feel better since you've been in hospital?
MRS J. SMITH: No, I can't say that I do really.
INTERVIEWER: How have you found the interviews with the SHO?
MRS J. SMITH: Well, I know he's been trying to help me but I can't
think of much to say. We seem to have been over everything before.
INTERVIEWER: How have you found occupational therapy?
MRS J. SMITH: I can't see much point to it. I've been doing patch-
work. But I'm finding it like the domestic work I did at home.
When I washed a plate or scoured a frying pan I had to keep on
re-checking them to see if they were clean. When I do the patch-
work I can't tell if I'm sewing the material or the cardboard.
INTERVIEWER: I gather you've been offered ECT.
MRS J. SMITH: Yes I have. I suppose I will have to have it,
because I'm not getting much better. But I'm worried because it
didn't help me that much last time and I've seen many patients in
here who've had it a lot but haven't been cured. Reg thinks it's
for the best.

Mr R. Smith

INTERVIEWER: Do you think your wife's condition has improved since
she's been in hospital?
MR R. SMITH: Not at all. She's still very low and can't do much.

INTERVIEWER: How did you see your meeting with the consultant?
MR R. SMITH: Well, as I've said before if I can do something to
help them I don't mind sparing an hour of my time because this
kind of case is pitiful. He asked me if I would be willing to
join in talks with June and I said, 'Yes'.
INTERVIEWER: How do you think June can be helped?
MR R. SMITH: I think we've got to face up to it, she's got to have
ECT. I gather she's been told this and I've told her it would be
the best thing for her.

Mrs M. Jones

INTERVIEWER: Do you think June's condition has improved since
she's been in hospital?
MRS M. JONES: No, not really. She's still very depressed, and
Reg doesn't help much. He still brings their friends in here.
June doesn't feel this is the place to see friends. He even
brought Vera and her husband in last weekend. It really upset
June. I was there. Reg told them, when June was at the other
end of the corridor, that he had changed his views a bit when he
saw the consultant, so as not to appear too lacking in feeling.
INTERVIEWER: I gather you saw the SHO.
MRS M. JONES: Yes, he told me that there was nothing mentally
wrong with June and that she had to learn to cope with Reg again
like she has before.
INTERVIEWER: What do you think about June getting ECT?
MRS M. JONES: Well I don't like it. I'd rather take her home with
me, but it's up to her and Reg, and I think she'll have to have it.
There's nothing else is there?

June remained a patient in the unit for another fortnight. During
this period she received four ECTs.
    The staff saw June as responding well to this treatment. She
became more spontaneous in her conversation and her behaviour.
She enjoyed occupational therapy. Nevertheless, the registrar
was sceptical as regards how long this improvement would be maintained after June's course of treatment had been terminated. He
also added, cynically, during the same ward round that she had
been given ECT for the sake of the community; if there was a
tragic outcome a coroner would be more benevolent to those members
of staff responsible for June's care if she had been treated with
ECT than if she had been treated by psychotherapy.
    It is pertinent to note that the SHO's term of employment at
the unit ended the day June received her first ECT. June was not
seen by another doctor until after she was discharged.
    Mrs Smith left the unit on 30 August. The consultant made an
appointment to see her in outpatients two weeks later.

Mr and Mrs Smith and Mrs Jones were interviewed a month after June
was discharged by one of the authors.

Mrs June Smith

INTERVIEWER: After you had four ECTs how did you feel?
MRS J. SMITH: I seemed to wake up one morning, whether it was the
first thing in the morning, I don't really remember the days,
but I think I started to joke with somebody across in another bed
and it came to me suddenly that I was doing it and I felt on top
of the world. But I had already started feeling better when the
therapist took us to Good's factory, and looking around there I
felt quite myself that day. I seemed to be my normal self, you
know, joking with other people, it seemed as though a load had
been lifted off me although I didn't know what the load was particularly. I felt that much lighthearted and not worried about anything, even hospital didn't worry me, nothing in the hospital.
INTERVIEWER: How do you see the treatment you had?
MRS J. SMITH: I think it's marvellous that they can lift a load
off you really don't know the cause of. I felt so thankful for
feeling so normal again. I would have done anything for anybody
in those first few days afterwards. It was as though the world
was really a bright place to live in again. Even simple things
made me happy and I wanted other people to feel as well as I did,
the people who were in the hospital with me.
INTERVIEWER: Were you not surprised at not seeing another doctor
after the SHO left?
MRS J. SMITH: Yes, well I thought, 'I wonder why they're not', but
I suppose before he left he had given instructions about what
treatment I was to have and there was a team really all working
together. I imagine they were coping somehow or they were too
busy to interview me.
INTERVIEWER: Would you have liked to have seen someone?
MRS J. SMITH: No, it didn't bother me.
INTERVIEWER: How have you found doing the domestic chores since
you were discharged?
MRS J. SMITH: As soon as I came home I felt fit to get the tea and
put the kettle on. It was just as though I had not been ill really.
As soon as I stepped across the front door things were normal again
and everything seemed bright that had seemed drab to me before I
went into hospital.
INTERVIEWER: Have you been leading an active social life?
MRS J. SMITH: Oh yes. We always go dancing Thursday and Saturday
nights. And we often visit a friend on a Monday night. Also I
have been going to a little bingo session on a Wednesday because
this girlfriend of mine likes to go.
INTERVIEWER: How have you felt when you've been on your own?
MRS J. SMITH: No I don't mind it. I'll admit I felt a bit low
last week, a couple of days, looking out at that very drab weather.
But I went out and did some shopping and had forgotten about it
when I came back.
INTERVIEWER: How did your outpatient meeting with the consultant
go a couple of weeks ago?
MRS J. SMITH: Well I wasn't with him very long, because, I think,
I seemed so on top of the world. I think he was quite flabber-
gasted that I felt so well. My next appointment is in a fortnight.
INTERVIEWER: How do you see the future?

MRS J. SMITH: I feel I'm back to normal, whether or not I shall
look for another part-time job I don't know.
INTERVIEWER: June, in the hypothetical situation of requiring
admission again how would you feel about it?
MRS J. SMITH: I probably wouldn't like the thought of it but I
think the unit is the place to go even if I only went a day a
week to straighten myself out.

Mr Reg Smith

INTERVIEWER: How did you see your wife's condition after she had
ECT?
MR R. SMITH: A spectacular improvement in a very short space of
time. I don't think there was very much improvement in the first
few applications, but certainly the fourth, I think it was the
fourth one, there were some dramatic differences. OK, and that
was the time medical authority decided she was being out.
INTERVIEWER: What was the improvement you saw?
MR R. SMITH: Shall I say normal conversation? Obviously she hadn't
been home then but certainly elevated on what I would say is the
high side to normality. I would say high.
INTERVIEWER: Are you saying she was the person she once was before
all this started?
MR R. SMITH: Yes, that's why I say she was in a little bit of a
high rather than a low because I doubt very much whether you people
with all the availability of treatment and equipment can get people
back up to where they were.
INTERVIEWER: Has June maintained the improvement in her condition
since she's been home?
MR R. SMITH: Oh yes, her activities. What I'm really surprised
at is that she is so physically capable of doing things. Her
physical wellbeing is there, but I still think that mentally she
is not what she was. Now you haven't got rid of the reluctance to
do things and you never will.
INTERVIEWER: How has life been domestically?
MR R. SMITH: The fortnight prior to her going into hospital was as
near to domestic strife as one could be. I'd be doing the washing
up and she'd come and she'd tell me how to wash up. Now I've
stepped to one side and I've stopped doing the things I would normally have done and she copes. No argument. I get the groceries
in and I leave her to do the housework full stop. You people were
confounded that I was making decisions so I don't say anything now.
I just let her get on with the domestic chores. I just make
requests within what I would call a reasonable frame of mind. Instead of saying, 'What shall we have for supper, shall we have so
and so?' I say positively, 'Make me some soup', or 'I'll have some
cocoa.' And I expect it to be done. This is what I gathered the
doctors were implying to me.
INTERVIEWER: How has your social life been since June's been at
home?
MR R. SMITH: She just took it up. She came home on a Friday and
our local dance is on a Saturday night. I didn't say, 'Are you
going?' She knew I would be going for a couple of hours at least.

She had booked then for the hairdresser by phone on the Saturday afternoon, which is the usual. And we went to the dance.

INTERVIEWER: What are your expectations for the future, as regards June?

MR R. SMITH: I don't think, should I say in a brutish frame of mind, one could ever expect improvement, but at least one could say let's hope it stays like this for a few more years.

INTERVIEWER: How do you think June would react if she required hospital admission again?

MR R. SMITH: She's more accepting of hospital treatment now. She's even said a couple of times that as soon as she's under the weather again she's back inside. And I've said, 'Yes you are. I'm not having another fortnight like the last fortnight.'

Mrs Mary Jones

INTERVIEWER: How did you see June's condition after she had ECT?

MRS M. JONES: Oh very much better.

INTERVIEWER: In what way?

MRS M. JONES: I went in and she was on top of the world. She said, 'Mary, I'm going home for the weekend.' I said 'A little dicky bird told me you might be going but I didn't tell you. I had to leave it to the doctor to tell you.' And I saw her again and she said, 'I've been discharged,' and she was on top of the world. I said, 'That's lovely, June.' I went in to see her, and also my other sister Grace was there, oh she didn't want to know us, she was better like. She waved us off, she walked out to the bridge with us, and going home I said, 'That's what I've been waiting to see, June.' She said, 'I feel different.'

INTERVIEWER: In your opinion how's June been since she was discharged?

MRS M. JONES: I didn't see her for a fortnight. Then her and my other sister came over here for dinner last week and she was on top of the world. I hadn't seen her like that since she was a young girl. Everything was lovely. Reg was taking her out for a meal and he was quite kind. She was laughing and joking. Then I saw her a week later and she's different again. I said, 'What's wrong?' 'I've been crying Saturday and Sunday.' I said, 'What for?' Well, apparently Reg is going to skittles one night, he's going to the club another night. She said she don't mind him going out but he don't include her in anything. Anyway I went over there Monday, she was just going out when I got there, so she's that much better.

INTERVIEWER: How do you see the future?

MRS M. JONES: She's still well enough at the moment, but I'm afraid if Reg don't try and coax her it won't take that long for her to be ill.

POSTSCRIPT

After leaving the unit June attended two outpatient sessions with the consultant, and was then discharged from his care.

Towards the end of January 1975 her sister, Mrs M. Jones, wrote a letter to one of the authors. She said that, 'When June was told she was leaving hospital she was like her old self, but now although she isn't so ill as she was at the beginning, I fear she can't go on much longer if Reg doesn't alter.' When Mrs Jones visited her she 'found June very distressed, crying and shaking like a leaf. All she wanted was to go to bed and forget everything, and that was the only place she could get any peace.' Mrs Jones coaxed June into seeing her GP because she said that she felt like committing suicide. The GP prescribed medication and while reading through his notes said to June, 'I gather Mrs Smith that you and your husband are incompatible.' Mrs Jones wrote that 'June nearly jumped out of her chair.'

Mrs Jones wrote to one of the authors again in the middle of March. That is approximately one year after June had come into contact with the psychiatric services. A few weeks earlier June had enjoyed a long weekend with some friends at the seaside. She had gone without her husband. On her return she told Reg that she was upset about something. He decided, so Mrs Jones relates, to send her back into hospital. He left June at Mrs Jones's without any warning and said, 'I am going to work now. I will phone into the sister at the hospital. You get June ready, I will be back this afternoon to take June in.' 'June was in a state, crying and shaking like a leaf', reported Mrs Jones.

Since she had not been referred to the unit by her GP June was not admitted. The next day she went to outpatients and refused an offer of day-patient care. Instead the doctor prescribed medication. June remained in outpatient care for two weeks and was then discharged. During this period she stayed at her sister's home. Mrs Jones wrote that, 'With the capsules they prescribed and by rest and good food with us she was like her old self.'

Mrs Jones saw June a week later, after she had returned home to Reg. 'You should see the difference, bent over crying, coughing with an awful cold. The difference in one week at home with him.' The trouble is, in Mrs Jones's opinion, that June won't tell the doctors about how Reg treats her, although she will tell her sisters.

Thus after two admissions, outpatient care and various treatments, including ECT, marital therapy and medication, June remains the same - depressed and unwilling or unable to express her feelings about her life situation.

SUMMARY

1 The staff failed to clarify the basis of hospitalisation with either the patient or her husband. Thus they unwittingly connived with Mr Smith's plea to cure his wife. This state of affairs was significant when the staff tried and failed to initiate marital therapy with the Smiths. This form of therapy demands that both patient and spouse should participate in the treatment situation on an equal basis. This was not possible in the case of Mrs Smith since the patient had been treated with ECT. Thus Mr Smith was able to confirm his view that his wife was 'ill' and that his involvement in the case was not required.

2 There was a divorcement between decisions made at ward rounds about the diagnosis and treatment of the patient and the day-to-day treatment programme. Although the patient's problem was construed as being interactional in nature, marital therapy was rejected summarily in favour of ECT and drug therapy during the first inpatient phase. But during the outpatient phase marital therapy was introduced on the initiative of the SHO in opposition to the advice of the consultant. During the re-admission to hospital the patient's problem was once more formulated as a marital problem but further ECT was carried out as marital therapy was viewed as nonproductive. A further example of divorcement between theory and practice occurred when the consultant argued that ECT was needed because Chlorpromazine was ineffective, and yet Chlorpromazine was prescribed throughout the first hospitalisation period and outpatient phase. A third example was related to Mrs Smith's sister. Mrs Jones was seen as crucial in understanding the patient's problem but was not interviewed until the penultimate day of the patient's first stay in hospital.

3 There was a lack of professionalism in establishing legitimate ground rules which could form the basis for treatment decisions. For example, a decision had to be made about increasing the patient's dosage of Chlorpromazine. Nobody had talked to her for several days so a nurse was sent out from the ward round to find out 'how she was'. The nurse returned within a minute or two having paid a lightning visit to the occupational therapy department where the patient was reported to be interacting with other patients. On the basis of this report the dosage was increased.

4 There was a lack of contact between the consultant and the day-to-day treatment programme of the patient. This state of affairs was exemplified in the letter he wrote to Mrs Smith's GP after she had been discharged from her first admission. In that letter he asserted that Mr Smith had two sons, whereas he had a son and a daughter; that Mrs Smith was not receiving medication, when she was; and that his SHO was providing the patient with supportive therapy in outpatients, whereas in fact he was actively pursuing a policy of encouraging Mrs Smith to talk about her marriage with a view to marital therapy.

5 After the SHO's term of employment had ended during Mrs Smith's second admission the patient was not interviewed by a member of the medical staff until her first outpatient appointment after she had been discharged as an inpatient. In other words, Mrs Smith received no specific attention from any one member of the therapeutic team for a month.

Chapter 8

The case of Mrs Wright

Mr and Mrs Wright were fifty-seven and forty-seven years of age, respectively, when Mrs Wright was admitted into the unit on 9 May 1974 following a family crisis. They have three children. Tony, who was twenty-three at the time of his mother's admission, was living away from home although he was visiting his parents when the crisis took place. Robert, who was twenty-six and is married, was not present. Mary, who was sixteen, was still living at home.

MARRIAGE

Mrs Susan Wright

During the war I went to nurse at Westchester and I met my husband there. He was a patient of mine actually. I don't think we loved one another as one should love one another in order to marry. I think we were both looking for someone to comfort the other. I have always held sexual intercourse as so sacred and I had vowed never to have sexual intercourse with anyone before marriage. I must have been nineteen and we were engaged and I gave in to Jim before I was married. And you know after that I thought I will have to marry him because I would never be fit to give myself to anyone else.

I feel disappointed in my marriage because I think if I would have married what I feel would have been the right person for me ... I think the basis of true marriage is a spiritual union. So I was disappointed immediately we were married really. In our relationship we were overwhelmed by a grandmother and four spinster aunties of Jim's who all lived, and have always lived, practically on our doorstep all our married life. This is the stupid bit about it, that although he had driven me crazy to get married Jim didn't really want the responsibility of marriage, and would leave me evening after evening for these aunts. I felt pretty rejected by him. I acknowledged this to myself and to our GP once. You see if I had bronchitis I was more or less saying to my husband, 'Well look, I can't look after the children on my own, you'll jolly well have to stay here and care for them.' And I was on Valium and that type of thing for a very long time for depression.

I first of all met David four years ago. I was rather attracted
to him because he seemed to be on a rather more spiritual level
with me than by husband. He came to live in Ashead after his wife
had died. He was in our church the best part of a year before I
had any real contact with him. He used to say to me, 'Oh you are
a dream of dreams Susan.' I must have had an attachment to this
man and I'll tell you for why. I suddenly felt alive. I didn't
think I was sort of falling in love with him but I felt alive. I
felt this marvellous warmth which I seemed to have lost for so many
years. I was very concerned about this, because I kept thinking
why can't I feel this about my husband? This is what I ought to
be feeling about him. I had a certain amount of guilt about this.
As far as I was concerned what I felt for David was more a spiritual
thing. I didn't realise how fond I really was of him until he
became engaged to a girl of twenty-five and he is sixty-seven. That
was last September. I felt how stupid I had been. I thought I was
foolish because I had in my heart felt a deeper thing for him than
what he did for me. I thought how foolish I have been, how wicked
I have been, how disloyal I have been in my heart even though I
haven't done anything to jeopardise my marriage.

I have offered on a number of occasions to part from Jim. I
sometimes feel it would be a relief to him if we could, but I'm
not sure in fact it would be the answer for him or for anyone. I
don't think he ever would because of these aunties. I've often
wondered if we didn't have these aunties whether in fact we would
have done.

Mr Jim Wright

It was while I was in hospital in Westchester, during the war,
that I met my wife. It's silly but it was something that attracted
me. I don't know what it was. I was in the position there, I
seemed to spend my life on social committees, even then I was on
hospital social committees with one or two of the nurses. I had
quite a few nurses. I only had to say to them, 'Do you want to go
out to the pictures?' And they were there. In fact, this seems
crazy, one day I took two. So I can't really think what....
Something different attracted me from the rest of them. Anyway I
don't quite know what it was and that was it. I can't really think
what it was because there was a staff nurse and sister quite fondly
attached to me as well, which was further up the tree than a nurse.
I suppose, if anything, it was probably her nursing qualities, the
way she handled the patients.

I think once a fortnight they had this service in the women's
ward and she was interested enough to attend that, and this was
something else.

There have been occasions when Susan and I have been very, very
happy. Usually when we go on holiday, getting away from the
stresses and strains of everything else, and on the weekends when
we have sort of been able to get out into the garden together.
But I feel in some ways I ought to have put my foot down very much
firmer than I have in the past over certain things. Looking at it
now, I ought not to have asked for permission to do this and to do

that, or to take fruit out of the fruit dish, or stuff out of
the fridge if there was anything in there, or anything like that.
And over the question of drink, for years I have observed her
wishes not to have alcohol in the house. I have now got a stock
in. I keep it there and I don't drink any more than I did, but
it's there.

FAMILY LIFE

Mrs Susan Wright

My husband's aunts were always wanting to tell me what I ought to
do and I have always had this sense of wanting to please, certainly
my husband's people. I think I have accepted, to a very great
extent, that they expected to come first really. You see this is
the problem really, I think to a very great extent my husband has
got himself into endless financial trouble over the years, it's
got into a couple of a thousand at a time, and therefore it has
been behoven to Jim.... Therefore his aunts have a certain power
really.

Mr Jim Wright

There has always been a bit of a bone of contention over the fact
that my aunts have been quite good to us. Originally the first
house we had, they found the money in the first instance to put
down so we could get it, and then we paid them back.
    As I say I think Susan has resented my aunts helping me out.
Of course on the other hand her family have moved in gradually
from wherever they were to Ashead, and I'm surrounded by them. I
don't resent that so long as they ... I mean mother-in-law and
father-in-law were here for umpteen periods.

Mr Robert Wright

I was just coming up to my eleven-plus and mum and dad seemed to
be having a great deal of trouble with each other. He had business
troubles. I think he had quite a lot of financial trouble at that
time because he had quite a lot of help from his aunts. He came
to see them once or twice while my brother and I were staying with
them and things weren't all that happy between them either. It
was obvious that there was some serious friction at that time.

Mrs Susan Wright

When I was younger I had this gift for music and with great per-
suasion my father eventually allowed me to go to Torquay and I
played in the Eisteddfod. I don't know how it came about but it
got into one of the major daily newspapers, and there was this
picture of me with a piano. I must have been ten-and-a-half then.

The headline was, 'PARENTS TOO POOR TO BUY A PIANO'. Well of
course my parents had such hard times that it must have hurt my
father's pride beyond measure.

I think at the time I felt very bewildered. And I know I went
off to boarding school, everyone having seen this in the newspapers, and this wonderful, marvellous chance of coming to this
school and of course I know, and they soon discovered, that I had
not got the ability which the newspaper had made so much of because
I simply hadn't had the tuition. In any case I wasn't a very good
scholar. I was very unhappy and I was homesick. I found it hard
going, because, in a sense, people of our background didn't get
that kind of education.

I've always prayed a great deal that my children would lead
their lives within the will of God. This I think has been the
criterion for my life and for the children. But I felt if they
had potential I wanted to see them use it because I felt I had not.

I've had a lot of fear where my husband's been concerned, and
as we had the children this became very much increased because I
was always so anxious to protect them. When I look back on it I
sometimes wonder if I neglected my husband for the children. I
took more care of the children's upbringing.

Robert is twenty-six now. Well I think I spoilt him a bit
because he was a very difficult baby. And Tony came along and
sometimes I think ... Robert, I tried so desperately not to allow
Robert to feel jealous, but I feel I was over-anxious about everything really. Over-anxious that no one should be hurt and that
Robert should not feel jealous of having another baby in the house.
I wasn't a very wise mother, loving but not wise.

There was always this sort of jealousy over the children, because
my husband I think has got very great ability really, but I don't
think he's ever developed it. He sort of took it for granted that
Robert would just go into the building business with him, but I
felt the child had greater ability. He went to Blacktown Technical
School and he had a very difficult time. At first he was travelling
to and from Blacktown everyday. I wrote to one of the masters and
I said I felt this boy had got this potential and yet I didn't see
how anyone else could help him, although I used to help them with
their homework. This master was wonderful. He took Robert under
his wing and from that moment Robert went ahead like wildfire. He
got two A's and a B in his A-levels. He got his place at university. He got a BSc degree, and he went to another university
as a demonstrator and then he was working for a PhD at the same
time. In the end he submitted for an MSc instead.

I developed a close bond with Tony. I think it was more of a
spiritual bond really. There was a great depth of love I think.
He was a very loving little child. Now I look back I can hardly
bear it because I think I've caused Tony a lot of suffering. He
told me not very long ago he didn't pray very much but one of his
great prayers was that daddy would die. And so he must have suf-
ferrd on my behalf a very great deal and I feel I must have allowed
him to know more of my feelings than I should have done. He's been
getting furiouser and furiouser with me as he's grown up. He gets
mad about people not being allowed to lead their own lives. He
thinks you should be allowed to fulfil yourself and I'm quite sure

he's right. He gets very cross with me. He said to me quite
distinctly when he was in his teens, 'I'm not going to let dad
do to me what he did to Robert.' Oh I can see how terribly anxious
Tony has been, he would say to me immediately, 'My mother's been
such a fearful person.' He's been desperate to overcome my fear
just as if he were my husband, you see.

Tony rejected Jesus Christ. This was when he was sixteen, when
I had a hysterectomy, seven years ago. I didn't realise to what
extent he had done this but he became interested in all sorts of
religions. I was interested, to some extent, in extra-sensory
powers also because I was sensitive to all sorts of things. Perhaps
I shouldn't have started looking into it, but I was interested and
he became interested. He went in for yoga and this meditation
business. As I see it now this meditation thing is an inward-
looking thing, whereas from the Christian point of view one has
an object.

Tony is a very brilliant musician but he has turned his back on
Jesus Christ and he is a homosexual. He has suffered greatly
because of this. But I couldn't possibly condemn him, I mean who
are we to condemn? And my heart bled for him. I wondered what
this poor boy had been suffering all these years. But I do feel
it is not a right relationship and I do think it is of the devil.
That is how I feel about it. I know he could be delivered of it
if he believed in Jesus Christ, because he can deliver us from evil.
My husband does not know about Tony being a homosexual.

I think it's just in the last couple of years that Tony and I
drifted gradually. We were quite close. We could talk for hours
and hours. It has gone rather. I was certainly rather interested
in the occult to a certain extent, but when I felt it was contrary
to the will of God I sort of lost sympathy with Tony because he
continued in that way of being, whereas I felt we ought to be
looking to Jesus Christ. So this caused a lack of understanding.

I'll just tell you about Mary who is sixteen. Now she loves
her daddy very much and she loves me too I'm sure. She says things
to her daddy that I would have loved to have said years ago, but
she gets away with it. In fact she's very good for him. I think
Mary has great ability, but I feel my husband, in a way, could do
more with her than me, because somehow there's a female-male relationship where dads can do more with daughters I think. Of
course if there's anything I can spot that she can do I want her
to do it.

I think my husband felt I was trying to take the children away
from him in some way. I feel in my own heart I didn't do enough
to unite the family. I feel I am to blame there.

Mr Jim Wright

I suppose I was always closest to Robert until he got married and
moved away. We are still very close now. The basis of our relationship is that he is a technical bod. We sort of understand
the same things. And now I still get the power station papers,
even though I've left they send them to me. I sort of save any
articles which are of interest to him. I save that for him when

he comes home. He takes all that lot back with him and we usually
have a chat about it because I know quite a lot about these things.
    I was equally close to the other two. I've been afraid to show
too much affection to Mary. I'm not going to say my wife would be
jealous but there's always the fear that she might be. There has
been a tendency lately, because just lately we have tended not to
bother with set meals. We'd rather save her the work, and she
thinks it's her job as head of the household to get the meals and
so on. Either Mary will cook for the two of us or we will splash
around and get something for ourselves. I've been afraid that if
I show too much attention it will add to this sort of situation
where she feels she is being ousted by Mary. Whether she feels
that or not I don't really know.
    Tony was closer to my wife. I would have said until he went
to university they were very, very close. My wife's relationship
with Tony wasn't unnaturally close, but I sort have felt, at times,
he was getting, well he did get preference over Mary because ... I
can't tell you how much money she spent on him on different things.
    My wife was upset when Tony left for university. She was
worrying about him all the time. Whereas Robert wrote frequently
to us while at university, and he still does now, Tony might miss
a fortnight. My wife would worry if there was anything wrong with
him. I felt he could cope anyway.

Mr Robert Wright

When friction took place between my parents it was expressed
between the two of them rather than on to my brother and myself.
It's difficult to know how I felt about it really. I think when
it got to that summer before I went to Blacktown, I think then it
was quite upsetting because I, then, began to become aware of the
fact that there were fairly serious problems.
    My mother found it very worrying that I had to go so far to
school. I found it very worrying too. I was so unused to travelling you see. We had done very little travelling except for odd
holidays. I got very nervous indeed.
    As regards home life I think the arguments increased or I
noticed them more from the time I went to Blacktown till my O-
levels. I began to be aware that mum used to get worried about
the financial side, and, of course, she used to do most of the
helping with the homework. She claimed she could be more help
than dad. That was in the early days, but I obviously soon left
her behind.
    Up until the time of my O-levels my relationship with my mother
was pretty close. I think it has always been closer than that
with my father up until very, very recently, two or three years.
I think he's opened up a lot, probably because I'm older, and we
talk more on an equal level now and less father to son. Of course
I've got more interests now that he already had an interest in,
but the relationship with my father has been in many ways very,
very restricted. I think, in some ways Tony was closer to mum
than I was. It was because of his music.
    The biggest problem was, and this became more apparent before

I went to university, that my father, although I think he's got
quite considerable abilities himself, up until very recently,
because of his generation, could see very quickly the value of
work that has some physical measure to it. That was the basis
of what he was doing, and studying was something he's found very
difficult to understand as being work. I think he was quite keen
on me doing something in engineering.

I've always been very reserved socially. I suppose independent
really. I've always, particularly when I was younger, felt quite
shy with girls. I managed to go out with one or two at that time.
I'm not really a great socialiser at all. I think one reason for
my being shy was a lack of contact. I think in my early days I
had a fairly restricted social life. My father wasn't too keen
on us going out a great deal.

Miss Mary Wright

Tony is the person I'm closest to in the family. He said to me
that I'm the only one he tells absolutely everything to. I find
this with me to him because I tell him everything.

As regards my parents I think I've probably been closest to
mother over the years. There has been one stage where I've said
'I hate dad', and I've said that to her. I've said that kind of
thing because dad and I are fairly close in our ways, in our
habits, and the ways we get into arguments and things. So that
when we're together we can often have really good rows, and get
it over with and just make up and forget about it. But it's
different when you have an argument with mum because you can't
just drop it straight like that. Neither can dad when they have
arguments.

I used to have a lot of arguments with dad and I still do just
about silly everyday things. Mum never used to because dad gets
really upset if you say anything just to hurt him. Mum has always
let him get his own way. If he came home late for dinner that was
OK. Whereas now, since I've been about five, I've always spoken
my mind as regards him and he has as regards me. Mum would stumble,
unbelievingly, when she hears the things I say to him which she
never dreamt of saying. Also, mum's been tied to the home a lot
because dad is rather possessive in his general ways. It's just
his personality, he's very possessive of mum. Always made a fuss
if mum went out anywhere by herself. But you see right from the
beginning mum let dad overrule her.

Over the years I think Tony was closest to mum because dad was
a bit tough on the boys. You see he never was on me because he
wanted a girl. Tony cared for mum a lot, sort of worried about
her because of her not managing to get out. She always cared for
him a lot.

Mr Tony Wright

One of the things I can remember about my childhood is that my
brother had a very hassly time with my father in the last couple

of years at school. I think there are lots of reasons for this,
conscious ones and subconscious ones. A lot of it was to do with
my father. I think he left school at fourteen. There was a bit
of him that rather liked the fact that we were getting on educa-
tionally, a bit of him that rather resented it, resented my brother
I mean, carrying on to further education, though I suppose it was
just tensions between father and son. There had always been a very
difficult relationship between my father and myself and my brother,
because my father used to be very hairy towards my mother a lot of
the time, especially when we were little. He'd sometimes take it
out on us to get at her, which didn't worry us so much as it
worried her. It was one of those Ronald Laing situations, people
suffering on what they kind of think other people are suffering.
I sat on the sidelines quite a bit and observed this going on. I
thought, 'Well I don't want this to happen between myself and my
parents really.' So I think I made rather conscious efforts not
to polarise with my father but to get along. In fact we had quite
a successful relationship between my father and myself.

My mother and myself there was always a certain amount of
tension. A lot of it is rooted in the fact that I'm gay and she
didn't know this. You see an awful lot of colluding went on between my mother and myself. I would very much be on her side whenever there was a bust-up, not necessarily verbally but inside
myself. I would always talk to her as though there were she and
me and my father was the baddy.

All through my life I was very much affected how my mother was
feeling. If she was depressed it would really worry me. I got
into a real thought track of this. I mean this is really the story
of the relationship right the way through. This got into such a
way of thinking. Sometimes when she would say, 'Don't worry I'm
really happy', then I couldn't quite cope with this because I got
into such a habit of thinking of her as a person who needed my
kind of comfort.

To some extent my mother and I were both close in terms of
music. I think that's true of my father and myself too. He just
doesn't wear his heart on his sleeve so much.

I had the feeling, in a more or less conscious way, that I was
gay from the age of fourteen. My mother, whenever she refers to
it, she talks about it very sympathetically, but 'It's still your
problem, how brave you are to have got through this'. It isn't
so for me really. Because things were unhappy at home I think I
somehow desperately wanted to be free from this home environment,
this family set up. When I discovered I was gay I felt tremen-
dously liberated.

Certainly in my personal situation it didn't cause, at a conscious level, hang-ups. I was quite pleased about it. When I
got to the sixth form I told lots of my friends and they were
quite pleased about it too. A few people came along who were a
bit shocked. But I know at some levels I must have been hung-up
about it because, certainly, the first few times I had sexual
intercourse with people I had tremendous guilt hang-ups about it.

I am sure this feeling of being gay was something I wanted to
keep independent from my mother because it was a way of being
independent for me. Recently I told her I was gay, I think about

a year ago, basically because I started having a relationship
with someone in particular, and I thought this was going to be
something quite permanent. I also knew that he was the sort
of person all mothers would fall in love with. She was pretty
understanding about it. I think she found it difficult at first.
I think she accepted it because she wanted to accept me still. I
still don't think she really likes me being gay.

I feel a bit that because my mother's relationship with my
father has been so unrewarding that she has always looked upon
me as a bit of a substitute. I used to dislike very much any
quasi-sexual tones in our relationship. Yet at the same time I
felt myself being and wanting to be supportive to her. When I
was younger it was much more intimate. More and more as I grew
older I used to find I used to get into very deep conversations
with her, but I always was a little uncomfortable with them.

More and more I began to really like my father's company. I
was quite amazed to find really liking taking dogs for a walk with
him, basically because he and I knew each other so less well. It
was more like two people getting to know each other for the first
time rather than all sorts of assumptions being made about one
another. It was during my last year at school that I began to get
along with my father better.

I suddenly realised I had been so busy, all the time, so-called
protecting my mother from my father that I had never seen that my
father had wanted a relationship with me as much as my mother.
After that I really made conscious efforts during my last bit of
time before going away to university, and whenever I came home,
just to be really a bit more loving towards my father.

RELIGION AND SPIRITUALISM

Mrs Susan Wright

My parents were religious people. I think I have always been the
sort of person that has longed for real love, you know. I know
that when I was fifteen I had a great longing to know what the
Church was really trying to talk about and I had this great yearning
to find Jesus Christ.

About five years ago we had this sort of bother with the church.
Jim had an awful row with the minister's wife. In our church ministers are invited. My husband and one or two others who were in a
position of authority decided that he should leave. It was against
the will of the majority of the people and it caused a lot of upset
and certainly his wife was quite unpleasant towards my husband.
But knowing my husband, I know perfectly well it wasn't all on his
side. My husband said that he was never going to our church again.
I feel, you see, I don't feel you can made decisions like that, I
feel we are in the hands of God and we've got to be guided by him.
This is how I want to live my life, I don't pretend that I do,
this is how I want to live my life, within the will of God. So I
couldn't have left our church without knowing it was the will of
God. That's one thing in our married life I really stuck out over.
I felt that it was too sacred and too important a thing just to

leave the church like that, just because you've had an upset with
the minister's wife.

I had a hysterectomy six years ago. When I had it I was extremely ill. I felt as though I died. Not only did I have a
vaginal hysterectomy but repairs to the bladder and rectum and I
had haemorrhoids all at once. I woke up and I had blood dripping
into me, packages in both departments and a catheter. I was extremely ill for a few days but apparently the surgeon did a marvellous job for me. I certainly think I died because I seemed to
be detached from my body and I seemed to be in the presence of God.
I know afterwards my daughter would say to me, 'Mummy who is God?'
And I knew I had this incredible experience, and I seemed to know
who God was and what God was. While I was in hospital I got to
know a girl who was in the same ward as me and whose mother was a
spiritualist medium. They were very kind to me these people and
they kept slightly in touch with me after we had parted in hospital.

Three years ago, last September, I had this experience where I
was awoken in the night and I smelt insufferable death and I thought
the devil is after Tony. I said to my husband, 'The devil is after
Tony,' and he said, 'For heavens sake go to sleep.' But I was confident that there was something seriously wrong in my son's relationship with God. I prayed about this a great deal during the
night and in the morning.

I didn't say anything to Tony about it but that morning I spent
a great deal of time in prayer before Tony got up in fact. He
went off to university. You see I had this experience the night
before he left. I was able to let him go quite happily actually
but before he went all he said to me was, 'You are very powerful
in prayer mum.' I felt that something had reached him about my
concern for his welfare. But you see the following Friday, it was
when I walked in the back door I was met by this incredible
laughter. It was of a spiritual nature and it was so evil. It
was absolutely terrifying. I was a little bit anxious at the time.
Then I thought Jesus Christ is asking me to call him. I was very
conscious of the fact that this was coming from Tony's bedroom.
I went up to his bedroom and I was conscious of this presence in
the room and I charged it in the name of the Lord Jesus Christ to
leave our home and my son in peace. I would love for you to know
what this meant because a dove of peace descended and the whole
atmosphere of the room was completely changed. I was really conscious of the presence of Jesus Christ, and I know then that this
wonderful peace surpasses all understanding. But I was very shattered by this experience to think that Christ could use me. I
really longed for someone to share this with because I thought,
perhaps, Jesus Christ could use me to help other people. That was
my first real experience of Jesus Christ in my own personal life.

There have been other experiences which I haven't yet mentioned.
I have been searching for help, and I had a feeling within me that
I had a healing power. It seemed to be connected with my left
side. I was concerned about this, and I prayed about it so much
that in the end I was led to these people at Seaway. This Mr and
Mrs Dale are lay preachers and I've known them for some years
through the Methodist Church. I really felt led to go to them
and I went maybe four or five weeks ago.

Well Mrs Dale prayed with me on two occasions and I felt greatly
helped. She gave me guidelines. She was able to tell me, which of
course I knew in my heart too, from experience, that not one of us
is all male and not one of us is all female. Until she put it in
those words I hadn't sort of connected it with my thinking. You
see I've always longed to nurse the sick and we've always been
short of money. I was offered this post at Seaway hospital recently with my sister and we loved it. I only did about four hours
a week, and she did a little more, but my husband made a lot of
fuss about me going because I don't think he cared much for me
having money to call my own. Any way while I was working there
one of the hospital sisters had this enormous passion for me. Well
I didn't feel it for her, but she was desperately anxious for my
welfare. She didn't exactly want a physical relationship with me
but she had this enormous love for me and she was desperately upset
when I left the hospital. In fact it was right I should leave, in
a sense she had this draining effect on me.

Mr Jim Wright

You see I was brought up in a very religious atmosphere. My grandparents were Plymouth Brethren and they were very, very strict.
During the war I was Church of England. At the start of the war
if you weren't Church of England there was nothing else. Personally I would have continued in that way after the war if I hadn't
met my wife. She was a Methodist, so I thought I'll see what this
is like. I suppose at the time I found my way into Methodism I
was in Yorkshire, which is actually the home of the Methodists,
and of course it was a very different church up there than what
it turned out to be down south.
   Until about five years ago I went to the Methodist Church and
so did the children, but there was an upheaval over there and I
pulled out. In the Methodist Church you have society stewards.
Every three or four years they meet from all the churches in the
circuit and decide whether they will ask the minister to stay any
longer. Any way this particular minister had been in Ashead for
five years so the senior society stewards called this meeting and
asked what we thought about him.
   We thought it would be better if we didn't invite him for any
further term of office, and got another man. But when this was
put to a meeting, it was read by the senior steward, there wasn't
a lot said, but at the close of the meeting the chairman said, 'I
don't want you to go, I've got something else to say.' A riot
developed, there's no other word for it. They really went to town
and the things that were said were really unpleasant about us.
Well my wife wasn't in the room, and all she has ever known about
it has been hearsay from other people which could be anything.
The upshot of this was I left altogether. So I went along to the
parish church, I went for eighteen months I suppose and thought
I might as well make a go of this and applied for confirmation
classes. I am now on the local church council and God knows how
many subcommittees and going forward as a lay reader.
   My wife remained in the Methodist Church until just lately.
She came a couple of times with me and Tony used to come with me.

I think it was when she was in hospital with her hysterectomy
that my wife's interest in spiritualism started seriously. There
was a woman in the next bed whose mother was a medium and that's
where it started getting a bit more intense. Although I am convinced these things exist I want nothing to do with them. I tried
to advise her to leave it alone but it was no use.

Then she had a feeling that she was possessed by some spirit or
another. That was partly why she went to Seaway Hospital. I don't
know whether her sister actually got the job for the both of them
to work as nurses. Of course it completely disrupted everything.
I'm not quite sure why she left. I think there was a bit of to-do
with her being too intense with some of the patients. Also she had
to have her father here because he was ill.

After that she took up local preaching. She felt she had to
tell the world something. I never got to hear one of her sermons.
I mean, to prepare a sermon she'd write nearly a whole book of
paper and it used to take weeks and weeks beforehand. Oh, she
was training under all of these people and all of them had problems. I knew nothing about this at all. I've only been told this
quite recently.

You see, the first time I knew anything about her spiritual
experiences was about two years ago. There's a chap who is a widow
in Ashead. David's wife died and he came here to live, and he's
at the Methodist Church. He brought one daughter and a son. My
wife said that his wife used to come to her at night and she was
convinced that she was asking her to look after the daughter. I
don't know whether this was the same as the things I have experienced, but she actually says she's seen somebody who stood at
the end of the bed. She was convinced she was coming back to ask
her to look after her daughter which she tried to do in what way
she could.

When she went on nights while she had this nursing job there
these two things. At night I'd be down in the lounge and I'd
sometimes hear.... Of course the dog spotted these things, they
say dogs have an extra dimension, they can see what we can't see.
He used to get absolutely terrified, you wouldn't be able to get
him to go through the door, he wouldn't stay in the lounge, he
would come upstairs with me. I could walk from the lounge to
the kitchen and I knew that somebody was behind me. Also there
was this absolutely putrid smell and a feeling of terrific evil.
Even with a coal fire and the room very hot you could shiver. It
was as cold as that. You could go through the lounge door and go
up the stairs, and I put those stairs together myself when the
house was altered. They do creak in one place but whenever I walk
up the stairs I know where the place is and I avoid it. I would
be going up the stairs and they would be creaking at the side of
me as if someone was walking up with me. They'd go right upstairs
to the landing. Very often I've spent (this may be daft, they
probably don't prefer darkness to light), but many a night I've
kept the light on all night when I've dropped off to sleep.

Occasionally apart from this other one there was this other
presence which I could describe as perfume. It was absolutely
sweeter than any other scent I have ever smelt and you knew there
was something there. It didn't occur very often but when it did

it was at night. Sometimes it would occur after the other one
had manifested itself in the lounge. Mary got a bit bothered
about this other business. She had it in her room to start with
at one time. I got so cheesed off with this that I made a wooden
crucifix out in the workshop and brought it in. I think Susan
was still on nights, I think she must have been because we were
on our own here. I said, 'Where shall I put it, in the lounge?'
Mary said, 'No dad put it on the landing upstairs,' which we did.
We were far less bothered after that, it didn't seem to like that
at all. We didn't have a lot of trouble after that. We kept it
on the landing.

Miss Mary Wright

I had a great fear of ghosts at one time. I used to do seances
when I was nine but I've packed it in now. But sometimes I feel
there is something in the house. It hasn't happened for ages.
I wouldn't call it a bad spirit. I feel it's unhappy and I'd
really like to be able to do something for it. I think it might
have something to do with the people in the house. You see it
never comes in my bedroom. It's really been in the front bedroom
where Tony and Robert used to sleep.

Mr Tony Wright

I think the most important thing that happened to me was around
puberty. I had a very black sort of period. I was completely
depressed for about three years. This was interspersed with
enormous periods of uplift which, because of my beliefs and so
on, I would call a sort of spiritual experience. It was definitely a real high which momentarily lifted one out of oneself.
I always thought it was a thing I couldn't possibly discuss with
my parents until I discovered my mother had very much the same
sort of experience.
     To some extent my mother and I both became interested in spirit-
ualism because she felt she was fairly psychic, I suppose. Various
things occurred to her which seemed to be of a psychic nature. I
think my mother has regarded me very much as going on in that way,
whereas more and more I've just become more and more centred on
the idea of trying to find the most essential relationship of oneself to Universe or God or whatever you want to call it and to
other people. She is very, I think it is fair to say, she is ex-
ceedingly conditioned by her religious upbringing and I was. I've
regarded the bit of myself that is breaking away from that as the
good bit. She's regarded the bit of herself that tried to break
away from it as her evil bit. She's very much on to a good-and-
evil thing.
     In my first year at university I went to see a hypnotherapist.
You see I used to get very, very nervous when I played the violin.
I used to get so nervous I just couldn't play in public. The
hypnotherapist didn't help me much at all directly but what he did
do was introduce me to a little book called 'Yoga Philosophy'

which has got some good stuff in it. The main thing it did for
me was to give me a tremendous feeling of liberation because it
talked about the sort of experiences I'd felt I had in a non-
doctrinarian way. Through it I got fairly interested in meditation.

EASTER 1974

Mrs Susan Wright

I had this incredible experience at Easter when my son, Tony, was
here. He was very worried about my troubles and was very anxious
for me to overcome them. I think he felt his meditation way of
living would enable me to overcome them. I know what it must have
been, he must have been thinking into this sort of nothingness.
Well he was dragging me into it, this was on Easter Sunday night.
I was awakened suddenly. I think it was about quarter to one. I
hadn't even heard Tony come in. I was being dragged into this
incredible pit. I was virtually dying. My tongue and my mouth
lost all its power and I felt as though I was saying goodbye to
everyone. I was sinking into this incredible pit and I began to
pray with all my heart to the Lord Jesus Christ. To me Jesus
Christ is the saviour of the world, and he is the one that can lift
us out of these horrible pits. Well I had never experienced anything like it ever and it was only by keeping my eye upon Jesus
Christ that I was able to be delivered from this at all. I was
also praying for my family and my son because I felt that he had
really turned his back on the Lord Jesus Christ, and I felt that
it was he who was trying to draw me into what he calls a 'peace',
but you see it wasn't a peace to me.
   The force of it I just cannot describe to you, the blackness,
and it was overpowering this pit, like enormous clouds were encompassing you. In the end I got up and went into his bedroom with
a cross in my hand, which I had taken from the landing. I was
saying to Tony, 'The Lord Jesus Christ is the only way, the only
truth and the only life.' I mean Tony knew I had this healing
power and he was wanting me to use it on other people. But as far
as I'm concerned, and I'm sure I'm right, the healing power I have
within me is not direct from God. I feel it is through this other
power, and I don't think one should heal any other way than through
God.
   I know to the whole family I must have sounded like some mad
thing. I had the cross in my hand and I was praising the Lord, and
asking Tony to give his life to the Lord Jesus Christ, asking the
family to pray, and all the time I was being encompassed by this
enormous force. Absolutely incredulous the power of it, as though
I was being swallowed up by some great force. Well my husband
really got quite cross with me because I was upsetting the family.
He came into the room. I had awakened my daughter. Tony was
wanting me to put my healing power into practice but I was saying
to him not all healing power is divine. He said, 'My dear mother
it is.' I think Tony took the cross from me ... no, no, my husband
didn't think I was fit to hold the cross. He thought I was terribly
evil. I said to him, 'If you want to help me Jim, just ring the

Dales and ask them to pray for me.' But he wouldn't ring them, but he would have the curate in or the rector. The curate came and he was wonderful, but he had no understanding of the spiritual experiences of my life. He just said to me, 'Has anything been upsetting you and worrying you of late?' And I said I have been very concerned about my son, about him being homosexual.

I was still trying to push away all this incredible blackness, and the curate prayed with me. But it seemed to me, I'll tell you how it seemed to me, I was still in this incredible black tunnel but at the end of this tunnel I could see Jesus Christ. He was looking over his shoulder and he was saying to me, 'Follow me, you know in spite of all this agony you're having to endure, follow me.' Then I went to sleep with my mind concentrated on Jesus Christ as the one and great power. I know I went to sleep and I was conscious of this cloud coming back again, but I didn't let it worry me because I was determined to stay peaceful and to concentrate on Jesus. But my husband was awakened by this blackness again, and he heard all these voices coming from the room calling my name. Well I never heard that but I had several experiences during the coming nights of this nature. Any time I felt it encompassing me I would pray and I found through the power of Jesus Christ I could overcome it. But at the same time I was praying very much for my son, because I feel my son has descended into this pit but he has still to climb out and it is going to be very painful. He has descended into this pit in that he has turned his back upon Jesus Christ, he is homosexual, he has suffered greatly because of this.

As I have said I have these people at Seaway who I felt were able to help me. What I felt I needed, I felt I wanted someone to pray with me, to pray me out of this situation I felt I was in, because I felt as though I could easily have been a spiritualist medium because I had this pressure upon me. And these people at Seaway I felt confident could help me. So I went there on these two occasions, and then I had this experience over Easter. On the Tuesday my husband came home at lunchtime and said, 'Where do you think you're going?' You see I had tidied myself up. I said, 'I'm going to see Mrs Dale again,' he said, 'You're not.' I said, 'Oh yes I am, because I know she can help me.' Any way I think he was rather disturbed, and he probably had every reason to be. He knew I had taken a wrong turning because I had been in touch with a spiritualist medium, and I think he had justification in having doubts about my going to see the Dales. Well I went on the half-past-two bus, and when I got there Mrs Dale wouldn't let me in the house. She said, 'You're husband is on the phone forbidding us to help you.' Well this is the sort of thing my husband has done over the years, forbidding this, that and the other. I said, 'Oh but you're going to help me aren't you? I'm beginning to feel liberated from this thing, and I know you can help me.' She said, 'No, I'm sorry, I don't think it is in the will of God. I feel I can only help you if your husband is willing for me to do so.' So I said, 'Can I come in and tell you what's been happening to me over Easter?' So I just told her the story, but she wouldn't pray with me, and so they hustled me out of the house as soon as they could because they had promised my husband they would not do anything for me because he had forbidden it.

I felt a bit resentful towards my husband because I felt on
the brink of being liberated from this awful spiritual anguish
which I had been having to suffer for so long. Then I hung about
in Seaway until half past four, and eventually got a bus home.
My husband was very unpleasant about it that evening, you see.
I was still very distressed because I was still having these
pressures upon me, and in the end he said, 'Will you go and see
the doctor?' Oh, and he was calling in the curate and the rector,
and I think they all thought I was completely mental, and I don't
blame them for that, and perhaps I am. But I knew I needed help
of some kind and in the end he asked if I would see our GP, and
I said, 'Yes I will,' and I told him quite a bit of what had
happened. He said, 'Look my dear, leave it with me, I'll get
you in touch with someone, you obviously need help.' I told him
how my husband had forbidden me to visit these people at Seaway.
The thing is they invited Jim over there, but he refused to go
and talk to them, he just wouldn't even discuss it with them.

I went to see our GP, he was absolutely marvellous. He got in
touch with Dr Case whom my husband had also spoken to and who
suggested I might go and see someone by the name of Black who
lives in Lifton. Well my husband was willing for me to go up to
Lifton, but not Seaway. Well I knew I needed help so I was willing
really. So the GP said, 'I know someone I can put you in touch
with, without you having to go to Lifton.' He said, 'Would you
like to go and see Dr Jones?' I said, 'Yes, yes, but I hope he is
a Christian, because it is certainly spiritual as well as mental.'
He said, 'I feel sure he is the right person for you.' This, then,
is how it came about that I went to see Dr Jones, the consultant
psychiatrist.

Mr Jim Wright

The first thing I knew about what was happening on Easter Sunday
night was when I woke up and found my wife wasn't there, and heard
voices going on in the other room. That evening Tony had come with
me to the parish church. After it he said, 'I think I'll go over
to Seaway to see some of my friends.'

I don't know what time he came back this night. He was in bed
asleep when this started, how long for I don't know. Anyway I
woke up and my wife was at the foot of his bed with a cross calling
for this demon to come out of him. I couldn't get the thing away
from her if I tried and I'm pretty strong. It was held in a fren-
zied grip. Before I knew what was happening he had it got it away
and he was doing the reverse on her.

Then Mary woke up in the commotion. She came in and quietened
my wife down a bit and got her back into bed. I was trying to
get the rector. Unfortunately he had been out late that night.
He had been out late the night before as well. He was dead tired
and he never heard the phone. I tried the curate. I got him on
the phone and he said he would come down in about a quarter of an
hour, which he did. This was something new to him of course but
he did his best. Eventually he quietened her down. He was here
an hour and a half and he said a few prayers. Then he went.

We went back to bed. I feel grim about this when I look back because at one time, when this first started, Tony was clinging to me and crying and he was absolutely dead scared. How much he knows about the spirit world I don't know. I can see now I was tired and exhausted after all this business. It was very callous of me to go back to bed, for all I know he could have stayed awake for the rest of the night. I don't understand these things at all, but at the moment Tony and I are so close although he's in London and I'm here. At the moment I feel I would like to be able to get to him because I'm worried. I'm so perturbed over him, I feel I want to ... sort of get to him and have a chat.

I wasn't unduly worried about Mary. I could see she was at grips with this, whatever it was, and she was taking it as a matter of course. As I said we all dropped off to sleep and an hour later I woke up. This may have been ... I may not have been completely awake, I don't know. I've got a feeling I was and I heard these voices calling. They were calling, 'Susan, Susan', from one corner and then another, from alternate sides. I thought, 'Well I don't know what this is but I had better try and fight this off by myself this time.' Susan hadn't woken up. So I did the best I could with what I knew to try and get shot of it. Stuck the light on and left it on, and I went off to sleep until the next day. On a couple of occasions since, one night I woke her up ... I came to bed and she was in ... she was asleep, she was in real distress. She was writhing around, muttering and moaning, and making terrible sounds.

Anyway I think it was the day after Easter Sunday my wife decided she wanted to see Mrs Dale. She was going on the bus to see her. I asked her not to go. I begged two or three times not to do it. I was convinced that these people had triggered off something of which they could not control the results. They were only lay preachers. The thing is they had always been in the Methodist Church and I had never heard of them in this line of business. When I rang her up on the phone she told me she had been doing it for eight years. I was quite reasonable at first. I said, 'Will you kindly stop seeing my wife over this business and leave it alone?' She got very uppity with me on the phone and started trotting out this business, which I have heard from so many people, that they are the only ones with the gift of the Holy Spirit to deal with these things, and 'I've been doing this work for nine years.' I'd had enough by this time, with the week-end and all. So I wasn't rude, I got very firm and I said ... but before I could I ran out of money. You see I had used a call box on the way home from work. But the upshot of that, apparently was, when my wife got there, Mrs Dale wouldn't see her.

The same day the rector came to see us. He tried to stress the point that Tony was twenty-three and already grown up and should be treated as such. I think what he meant by that was.... Well I suppose a lot of families continue to keep a grip on their families and try to say what they should do. I've experienced this quite a lot through life. They still consider you a child at forty, some people. I think this was probably the case there.

I was so het up about all this business and I didn't really want it widespread at all. I didn't talk to anyone else about it

except the rector, and curate, and this Dr Case. He's at Northern
in Jonstown at the practice there. I've known him over the years.
I said to him, 'There is something I would like to ask your opinion
about. I feel I can talk to you about this situation.' His father
was a Church of England minister.

So we chatted and he said, 'I know a chap who was at college
with me,' and that must have been donkeys years ago because he's
retiring now. George Black. In his opinion he is one of the top
people in the country on this sort of thing. He said, 'If it was
needed I could put your wife in touch with him.' He said, 'I'm
powerless because she must see your own doctor. All you can do
is, if you can get her to see your doctor, if this is needed, say
I am willing to put him in touch if necessary.' Our GP went over
there for dinner, they're on pretty good terms, they chatted this
thing out. Anyway I went over another evening and I had coffee
with him. In the meantime I gather I kept saying to my wife, 'You
must go and see the doctor, you can't do anything unless you see
a doctor.' Oh I know what Dr Case said, 'She must see the doctor
because sooner or later he will have to pick up the pieces and it's
better sooner.' So I kept stressing the point that she must see
the doctor. I think she made an appointment with him and went and
saw him. They had the conference over dinner and coffee as I've
said, and they came up with Dr Jones the consultant psychiatrist.
Our GP wrote a letter to him and made an appointment for my wife.
Then she said she couldn't stick it out until the time of the
appointment so he gave her a prescription of Valium, which I went
over to collect. He was upstairs and sent down a note saying he
wanted to see her again on the Friday morning. That was last week.
The upshot of it was we turned up for the appointment with the
psychiatrist.

Mr Tony Wright

I went home at Easter and I thought ... I decided recently ... I've
sort of got into the positive thinking things as more healthy than
regarding people as in a negative state. So I really went home
thinking, 'Well, if my mother has got her problems, well I'm sure
she has, but I'm really going to believe that she will sort them
out in her own way.' I didn't think it impinged on me terribly any
more.

I was talking to my sister in her bedroom and she said ... I
mentioned something about I was doing some funny yoga exercises
and it was rather fun, and she said, 'Don't tell mum, she's throwing all these books out at the moment because, she says, they're
evil.' These are books on meditation and mysticism, which included
Christian mystics but they went out with the rest. I said, 'Oh
yes', and I thought I'll see what happens. Quite casually the next
day, without meaning to bring up the subject, I said to my mother,
'I feel so stiff, I must get some yoga exercises going again.' She
said, 'Yes, I want to have a word with you about that sometime.'
I said, 'How about now?' Then basically, what often happens, we
got off the subject of me and of yoga as an objective thing, on to
how she was feeling. She just said she had been having these

really funny experiences of pressure on her head and things.
She thought she had got on to this track of meditation and yoga,
and it was not exactly a punishment, but she had got in league
with the devil or something. I said, 'Quite honestly, I don't
think it can be that because you haven't got involved with these
things. You've just about dabbled your toe in them, but that's
all.'

Anyway she was really worried, and she felt that when I came
home things got much worse for her. She really felt all these
pressures building up on her. She said, 'Are you a Christian, or
do you take Christ to yourself?' I said, 'No I don't think I am
a Christian really.' This really freaked her out. The next day
she was washing up in the kitchen, and I thought I must help the
poor soul because she seemed very overworked, because, you know,
she had my grandparents. So I went to help her wash up and I was
just drying the dishes and feeling all right, a little bit tense,
and I suddenly realised my mother was building up this tremendous
tension. Suddenly she collapsed over the sink and started crying,
'Oh God I know I'm going to die, I know I am.' And I thought,
'Oh God this is awful.' I stood there wringing my hands with the
teacloth. It's one of those things I've had to work through about
five times to get it out of my system. Then she sort of turned
round and she said, 'Just say this, you take Christ into your
heart,' and she kept saying this in a really distressed way. I
said, 'Look I accept Christ just as I accept anybody else,' and
I said, 'Would it be better if I went back to London?' She said,
'No we've got to work this thing out,' and she rushed off.

That night while I was asleep, she knocked on the door, and she
came in and said, 'Are you all right?' I said, 'Yes,' and I was,
I had been dozing. She said, 'Oh,' and went out looking very distressed, and went back to bed. The next day I spent most of the
day out because I felt things were really heavy at home, and I
couldn't cope with it. The next night I was asleep and she came
rushing into my room waving a cross at me. She was in a really,
incredibly emotional state, and shaking and crying and shouting,
and trying to exorcise me or the room. I got this incredibly
nervous thing. I started shaking all over. I thought I don't
know what's what. I mean I might be wrong or she might be wrong,
but I wish she could be happy basically and I felt very upset.
She said, 'Please pray with me,' so I did. I don't think I took
the cross out of her hand, not that I remember. I think she hung
on to it.

I felt very upset about this situation. In a way I have felt
that.... My mother's probably said that when she was working in
hospital she used to get tuned into the patient's pain so she'd
be feeling it. It's always been a bit like that with me and mother
emotionally. If she's really got a heavy feeling then I would get
it first-hand. It meant we both created more and more tension.

Anyway that night the curate came round. He was very nice. He
didn't attempt to push anything. The next day the rector came
round. He was fairly sort of open about it. He did say to my
mother, 'You ought to be baptized,' which she hadn't been. He
started spieling on a bit about the priests having a certain position in the Church for doling out certain sacraments and so on.

I knew, although my mother had been pushing the Bible and Chris-
tianity at me, that she couldn't accept that anymore than I could.
She was listening on the sofa, 'Yes you're probably right,' and
looking really drained. I thought what she's really thinking is
sweet fuck-all. 'This really can't help me at all because it's
something inside myself,' which is really all I've been saying to
her as far as I was concerned. Religious experience is inside
yourself and people couldn't provide you with it.

What helped a lot for me in the afternoon was the rector rang
up and said, 'Come round for lunch.' I thought, 'Oh God, what am
I in for now, have I got to start telling him my whole life history?' All he did say was, 'I think your mother is going through
the menopause.' I talked to him about how I felt during puberty,
and he thought this was significant, and to some extent he said
things were so painful for her because of that. He was just very
objective with me.

I felt really awful about the whole thing, mainly because I
could see my mother felt totally alienated. She felt my father
had got the rector in because she was going mad. She really saw
herself as the person who was alienated. Everybody else was not
exactly ganged up against her, but everybody else knew what they
were doing but she didn't know where she was. That's why it was
so awful for her, because she was the one person who felt out of
joint. It really did make me feel very, very sad because I felt
that she did have this awful feeling of alienation, and that in
some way I contributed to it really. You see when the rector came
round I was able to be very calm and objective at the time and she
was totally fucked up about it.

My mother and I had a really nice talk the next day, and it was
still very much polarised. She said, 'You know you are on the
wrong track and you've got to sort this thing out.' But it was
all very calm and nice. I suppose the thing that really counted
in the end was that we both loved each other, and because of that
she was able to accept me in spite of not being a Christian. We
left really quite friendlily.

When I left I didn't know that my father was going to get psychiatric help for my mother. I knew that he was very frightened
by things. But one of the great things that happened actually was
that the night my mother was so upset and waving the cross at me,
I was really feeling weak after this. My father was on the landing
looking really shattered and we had a nice cuddle. I said, 'Just
hold me, I feel very weak.' That was really nice because it was
the first time I had any real physical contact with him for years.
I really felt that was one good thing that grew out of the whole
situation. He and I really got so close on that occasion.

OUTPATIENTS

A summary of the general practitioner's letter written on 1 May
1975 to the consultant psychiatrist in charge of Mrs Wright's
initial outpatient appointment.

The GP thanked the consultant for seeing Mrs Wright. He had
received a letter from Mr Wright three days earlier. Mr Wright

had felt that his wife would not come to see the GP but, in fact, she had turned up in his surgery on 22 April. The GP felt that Mrs Wright's problem was a very difficult one and yet she had told him that he had helped her more than the clergy. Nevertheless the GP admitted that it was way beyond his scope.

The GP related the events that led to Mrs Wright consulting him. Her son Tony had become interested in spiritualism and she felt that a spirit had invaded her home some weeks ago. Using her power as a Methodist lay preacher she had commanded the spirit to leave the house. Following this there had been a feeling of tranquility and it had seemed incredible to Mrs Wright that the 'Lord could use her to do this'.

She told the GP that she had been overcome by it all and had wanted to talk the matter over but had gone to the wrong person. Apparently she had come under the power of that person who had had a hypnotic effect on her and she had become possessed of an evil spirit.

The GP went on to say that Mrs Wright felt that she could have become a spiritualist medium but knew that this would have been wrong since she is a true member of the Church. A week before her consultation Mrs Wright's son had gone back into one of his mystical phases and she had felt a terrible pressure in the head and ears. Mrs Wright had gone to see a minister because she had been concerned about the voices she had been hearing and he had prevented her from hearing them, 'although they were hammering at my ears' (in Mrs Wright's own words).

On Easter Sunday night she had awoken from a dream in which she felt she had been in a great abyss - she had gone into Tony's bedroom, and from Mr Wright's letter the GP understood that she had tried to cast out a devil - in Mr Wright's own words she had been 'practically raving' and had been holding a crucifix so tightly that they had been unable to get it away from her; Mr Wright went on to say that the next thing he had known was that Tony had taken hold of the crucifix and had tried to cast out a demon from his mother and Mr Wright had felt that later he had to fight off this 'presence' himself.

Following this Mrs Wright had got help from a Mrs Dale in Seaway but Mr Wright had now forbidden her to see this woman.

The GP said that Mrs Wright had a past history of anxiety depression, in 1964 with domestic upset at that time. He commented that Mr Wright had always wanted to seem to tear the house apart but had never seemed to replace it.

Mrs Wright had also suffered from a spastic colon and in 1967 she had had a hysterectomy which had been followed by anxiety and depression and had been treated with Nortriptyline as before, and in 1968 she had been given Parstelin. One of the GP's colleagues had seen her in 1970 with abdominal pain and she had written in the notes that Mrs Wright 'probably had marital troubles'.

Also, the GP assessed that Mrs Wright had been under some strain looking after her parents and had been rather depressed and now had a psychotic illness as well. The GP had given her some Valium 10 mgm noct. 5 mgm. b.d.

A summary of the consultant psychiatrist's reply to the general

practitioner written on 2 May 1974 after his initial outpatient
consultation with the Wrights:

The consultant thanked the GP for referring Mrs Wright to him.
He commented on what an interesting problem Mrs Wright's was. He
said that Mr and Mrs Wright had talked at length to him and his
colleagues about the various difficulties there had been, and it
seemed quite clear that there had been a fairly clear onset five
or six years ago soon after Mrs Wright's hysterectomy. Whether
there were such things as demons and devils, the consultant felt
quite unqualified to say, but in psychiatric terms he thought
Mrs Wright was depressed and that delusions about feelings of
presences arose out of her depression. He thought it was important
to admit Mrs Wright into hospital and had put her on the waiting
list. He hoped to admit her in the near future. He invited the
GP to join his team in discussions about the case at a later date.

Mr and Mrs Wright were interviewed by one of the authors in the
time between Mrs Wright's outpatient appointment and her admission
into the unit.

Mrs Susan Wright

INTERVIEWER: How did you feel about being asked to come into the
unit as an inpatient?
MRS S. WRIGHT: I must confess when I came back into the room and
I was told by the consultant that he wanted me to be admitted into
hospital I was a bit taken aback. I thought maybe he thought this
girl is very mentally ill, and maybe I am. I resented a little
being asked to come into hospital because over the years whenever
we've had little upsets in the family my husband has said things
like, 'Well you're mentally sick in your family', that sort of
thing. I thought that when the consultant said that to me, this
is exactly what Jim wants of the doctor, to confirm that I am a
mentally sick person.
INTERVIEWER: Do you see yourself as mentally sick?
MRS S. WRIGHT: I see myself in that I have not been able to concentrate on my work because I have felt pulled by other forces.
And I'm sorry to say that every time this poor man, David, becomes
my victim. I feel, to some extent, that he has opened up some
channel that I have been vulnerable to.
INTERVIEWER: In what way do you expect the hospital to help you?
MRS S. WRIGHT: People who pray in the Holy Spirit, they can virtually lift an evil spirit out of you, through prayer, and command
it never to enter you again. In fact, this is what Christ gave me
the power to do in this house but because I've got into this tan-
gent thing I've lost this direct power of Christ. Therefore I'm
the one who needs help now. Mrs Dale has delivered many people
through the power of Jesus Christ, drug addicts, all sorts of
people she and her husband have been a wonderful help to. I don't
think I can get that kind of help in hospital. I don't know.
INTERVIEWER: How did you understand what the consultant said in
terms of the way he felt he might be able to help you?
MRS S. WRIGHT? He was talking about psychology wasn't he? I wasn't

quite clear what he meant. He obviously realised that there was
something between my husband and myself which needed adjusting.
I felt he was wanting to have further communication with me, and
with my husband and daughter. What I feel about my daughter ... I
think that if you have psychic powers I don't think you should
ever attempt to develop them, and this is something I would like
to be able to put over to her now before she gets ... I think my
husband is psychic too, and because we both are the children are
bound to be. I don't really want her to follow it out because
I think you can get led into very great depths. So I think she
can be helped too.

Mr Jim Wright

INTERVIEWER: Did you attend the outpatient appointment with your
wife?
MR J. WRIGHT: Yes.
INTERVIEWER: In what way do you expect the hospital to help your
wife?
MR J. WRIGHT: I haven't got a clue because I'm not familiar with
this sort of thing. The only thing I know about, and that is only
loosely though ... once or twice, as an ambulance driver I took a
couple of patients but they were quite passive and normal. As far
as I am concerned we want help desperately. As I see it this is
one of the points I stressed to Mrs Dale on the phone. 'Through
your agency,' I said, 'You've practically caused a tragedy.
There's no knowing what possibly could have happened.' I quite
think somebody could have had a heart attack as a result of this.
As I say I want something done and the GP recommended the consultant, Dr Jones. As far as this goes this is alright by me. He
knows what to do, that's good enough. What he does I don't know.

THE PSYCHIATRIC UNIT

Mrs Wright was admitted into the unit on 9 May 1974. She was
placed under the care of Dr Jones's team.
    A ward round and team meeting that took place during the first
five days of Mrs Wright's admission were important in the management of this case. The consultant decided on a treatment policy
that would pursue problems to do with the Wright's marriage. He
conceptualised Mrs Wright's problem as one where she was involved
in a chronic marital situation and suffering guilt feelings owing
to her relationship with David.
    The team agreed that it was important not to approach this case
on a spiritual level. It was felt that Mrs Wright would use her
spiritual experiences to avoid talking about her marriage and thus
protect herself against the team.
    The consultant instructed his SHO to interview Mrs Wright and
a student social worker to interview Mr Wright with a view to
marital therapy in the future.
    The SHO was doubtful whether the unit could help Mrs Wright.
It seemed to her that Mrs Wright wanted a spiritual healer and not

a psychiatrist. The SHO was aware of the fact that the patient's husband had forbidden her to see Mrs Dale and had persuaded her to see the GP. The GP had advised Mrs Wright to consult Dr Jones since he was a devoted Christian. But now Dr Jones had left Mrs Wright's treatment to the SHO, and she felt that she was not a Christian in the image that Mrs Wright desired. When the SHO voiced these doubts to Dr Jones she told one of the authors that he replied, 'Are you a Buddhist?'

The issues that the SHO was raising were important. Underlying them was her assumption that Mrs Wright had accepted inpatient care expecting that she would be helped by someone whose religious beliefs more or less coincided with hers. The GP had arranged her outpatient appointment on this basis. But it was the case that, although the consultant leading each team held ultimate responsibility for his inpatients, typically their care was always passed on to the junior members of staff. In the case of Mrs Wright this meant that her expectation of who was to treat her would not be met.

During the first few days of her admission Mrs Wright kept a daily record for one of the authors of how she was experiencing hospital life. The following extracts are taken from what she wrote.

9 May

Very tiring day, great deal of work to do in order to prepare the departures of myself and father to prospective hospitals. Felt bewildered and rather resentful on arrival. First impression of ward poor but many kindness shown by admissions secretary, nurses, doctors and other patients.

My head aches and I am so very tired, wonder if I should have asked for sleeping tablets.

10 May

Restless night inspite of Mogadon, so much disturbance. Wonder why the night nurses put the main lights on in order to attend to individual patients. Very good breakfast. Number of young people disturbed concerning 'some' problem. It is true that it is best to stay silent on many matters and have the Lord to undertake them. In my effort to find some quietness away from all the tension I am wondering again what am I doing here! Had better try the keep fit classes. I feel very deeply for young people here; some of the young men remind me of my sons.

Jim rang me tonight. He has seen our GP who has explained to him that my trouble is due to the fact that I had a hysterectomy six years ago; I wonder! I know I was very ill just then and had the strange experience of being separated from my body for some days or maybe the complete fusion did not take place for weeks. It was an experience of dying and it was so beautiful, I really knew what God was and we smiled at each other as we looked back over my life and were able to view it in perspective; but I soon lost my wisdom! It was at the other extreme to my experiences over Easter!

11 May

One or two young people for whom I prayed are looking a little
better today; how wonderful is the power of the Holy Spirit.
    Jim and Mary and her boyfriend came at 3 p.m., and I was very
happy to see them; Jim brought me some flowers from the garden
and 'Readers Digest'. Mary brought me some tulips and a loving
card; so I was greatly blessed, I was glad Jim brought me a gift.
He also brought me some money for which I am glad. I think Mary
found it a bit oppressive here as she was apologetic about her
eagerness to go, but maybe it was me. There is something still
which affects my left side and especially my throat and this
something there wants to come away and I suddenly find myself
wanting to vomit. It has happened often of late but quite suddenly about 5.30. Maybe someone was praying especially for me
just then because I still believe the Holy Spirit has the power
to release from this. It will be good when I am free and perhaps
I can then help others.

12 May

Felt an urge to ring my sister during the early afternoon and
found they were about to contact me concerning my father. He is
deteriorating in hospital and the family have been summoned.
Sister gave me permission and Jim took me to see him. Dad has
greatly changed but he still knew me and I am very thankful that
he is peaceful and well cared for.

13 May

I am more than ever convinced that spirits harrass or even possess
us and the Holy Spirit can release us. Had an interesting chat
with Simon, we both agreed that above all everyone wants to be
understood and some of the experiences we have are too ludicrous
to admit to ourselves let alone expect others to understand! However we also agreed there is an Almighty Power.
    Have rung about my dad on two or three occasions; he is still
alive, mainly asleep but so peaceful.
    Praise the Lord.
    Mary and daddy have big upsets over Mary's boyfriend but I
cannot do anything from here and no doubt he is extra concerned
for her welfare.
    Better go to bed. There is much to be thankful.

The initial interviews held by the student social worker and the
SHO with Mr and Mrs Wright, respectively, both revealed a poor
marital situation.
    The student social worker wrote in the case notes on 5 May
that
    Mr Wright presented a picture of 'parallel' lives led by him-
    self and wife. Little feeling for his wife came across. Seemed
    to have 'rubbed along' because of mutual religious observance
    of 'until death do us part'. Sees his wife as dominant.

The SHO wrote that

> Meeting her lay preacher, David, meant someone for the first
> time who said she should stick up for herself. Therefore she
> stood up as regards splitting in going to church.... She
> rationalised this by saying God told her to.

Between 13 and 20 May there was a team meeting and a ward round.
The consultant was present for the former but not for the latter
because he was otherwise engaged for a week. The consultant,
having heard the SHO's and the student social worker's reports on
their interviews, revised the treatment plan for the Wrights. The
principal PSW suggested that the whole family ought to be involved
in treatment, but Dr Jones rejected this on the grounds that Tony
was living in London and Robert was happily settled. But he decided that it would be necessary to involve Mary in the treatment
programme since she had experienced spirits. The consultant did
not delegate the responsibility of interviewing Mary to any of his
colleagues, and Mary was never interviewed while Mrs Wright was in
contact with the psychiatric services. As a result of this omis-
sion the team failed to monitor how Mary was coping with her
parents' distressing relationship. At a later date Mrs Wright
told one of the authors that Mary had felt under considerable
pressure while her mother was in hospital.

The SHO and other junior members of staff were anxious for Mrs
Wright to be discharged. They expressed the view to the consultant
during the team meeting that while she was an inpatient it would be
difficult to set up marital therapy. On the one hand Mr Wright was
required to join in the treatment plan on an equal basis with his
wife. On the other hand the fact that Mrs Wright was an inpatient
allowed her husband to perceive her as 'ill' and himself as 'well'.
The consultant rejected the idea of discharging Mrs Wright immediately. In his opinion she ought to remain an inpatient until
therapy for Mr and Mrs Wright and Mary had been set up. This would
initially require a number of individual interviews and the complexity of the case would have to be unravelled. Dr Jones asserted
that he would review the case a week later after he had returned
from his engagement.

From 13 May until 20 May Mrs Wright kept a record of how she was
experiencing events for one of the authors. This record was not
a daily one. The following extracts are taken from what she wrote.

I am sorry not to have kept my promise to keep this diary daily.
So much has happened and there is a great deal of pressure, little
time for quietness. Many very kind letters and visitors so my
time has been well filled....

We have been awaiting my father's death and rejoiced that he
found his peace with God and everyone I feel sure, since he changed
from being in so much distress to complete peace....

It has been good to talk to people here, especially those one
felt an immediate affinity. Maybe that, and the release from
domestic responsibilities, makes this into some kind of haven....

The statement that we were 'born in sin' is becoming clearer,
for there are spirits within us which may lie dormant until triggered off by some channel and the Lord waits for us to be willing
to renounce those forces within us and since He knows the heart

will then lead us to the people whom he has chosen as His channel
for us....
   I am grateful for all the kindness and patience I have received
here but how can the spirit be left out (of my discussions with
the SHO), for we are three dimensions. I do see things in better
perspective since speaking to the SHO, for while I came from a
large family in which each individual was expected to consider
each other, my husband was the centre point of attention from one
grandmother and four spinster aunts. We must have pursued our
usual way of life until I was challenged by God when Jim left our
church four to five years ago, and for the first time my faith in
divine guidance was put to the test. Although I am now happy to
worship with Jim at the parish church I am still mindful that God
gave me a direction at that time, and wait for Him to reveal the
future....
   I believe within me there is an active spirit of healing and
another of homosexuality, perhaps, which has aroused desires in
another woman, the sister from Seaway hospital, no matter by how
small a degree. Through His channels and in his time the Lord
will deliver me....
   This is a great place for testing faith.

Mr Wright was interviewed by one of the authors eleven days after
his wife had been in the unit.

Mr Jim Wright

INTERVIEWER: Have you been visiting your wife since she was admitted?
MR J. WRIGHT: Yes I have visited her quite regularly.
INTERVIEWER: How do you think she's been coping with hospital life?
MR J. WRIGHT: I'm quite worried because, in my opinion, she's been
mixing with suicidal maniacs. But this might be good for her. As
a friend of mine pointed out she might be shocked out of the state
she's in by being in the company of such patients. But actually
I don't think they're having this effect on her. I don't think
she's been behaving any differently here than she has done for
years. She feels sorry for those in distress and sees herself as
someone who they can unburden themselves to. I mean she lent a
sum of money to a patient who didn't have a pair of shoes and
wanted to buy some. What perturbs me even more is that she wants
to return to the unit after she's been discharged in order to
visit patients.
INTERVIEWER: Has her state of health improved in your opinion?
MR J. WRIGHT: Well she's still a bit touchy. When we were driving
back from her father's funeral I mentioned some plans about a
holiday for her after she's been discharged. She just said she
didn't want to talk about it while she was in hospital.

Individual interviews held with Mr and Mrs Wright provided further
evidence to the interviewers of marital discord. On 22 May the
student social worker wrote in the case notes that Mr Wright 'admitted to religious conflict stemming from marital problems.

Talking in terms of longstanding marital conflict - and described his wife and himself as "operating on a negative plane, point-scoring" etc.' On 23 May the SHO wrote that Mrs Wright 'confesses that her joy to be in here is because she is free. No husband to object to her seeing friends, phoning up, spending money for what she wants. Dreads what will happen when she goes home.'

A team meeting held the next day was attended only by the junior members of staff since the consultant was absent. The consensus was that, while Mr Wright agreed that religious disagreement between himself and his wife stemmed from marital conflict, Mrs Wright would not admit this.

The student social worker added that she felt Mrs Wright dominated and manipulated her husband.

The SHO, with the agreement of the PSW present, decided that Mrs Wright should spend Whitsun weekend at home, returning to the unit on the following Tuesday. She also decided that Mrs Wright would be discharged once the consultant had been presented with the information to do with the case.

Mrs Wright was interviewed by one of the authors fifteen days after she had been admitted into the unit.

Mrs Susan Wright

INTERVIEWER: Having been in the unit for over a fortnight, what do you now see as the purpose of your stay?
MRS S. WRIGHT: For a rest. Now I am here I know just how tired I was. I realise I did need a physical rest and I needed a rest from the pressures of home, and, of course, now that my father is gone I realise that was an added pressure apart from the horrible experience I had over Easter.
INTERVIEWER: What has being in the unit meant to you?
MRS S. WRIGHT: It's been wonderful to be free, in that I've loved being able to join in all sorts of things without wondering whether Jim would approve, or whether it would upset the family harmony.
Also I've enjoyed everything that's been done for me - the meals.
Although at first when I came in I felt the same intensity about other patients. I sometimes do feel great suffering on behalf of other people. But now I seem to be a little bit more constructive or objective in my view.
INTERVIEWER: Has your husband changed in any way since you've been in the unit?
MRS S. WRIGHT: Yes. I feel he's been very humble in many ways.
Well he actually said to me, 'You haven't had much of a time with me, have you?' And I have said the main thing is the future really, to try and have more understanding towards each other.
But how much I have to adapt and how much he has to adapt I don't know, because the SHO said, 'Is your husband going to expect you to make all the adjustments?' I have yet to find out really.
INTERVIEWER: You have said to me recently that since you have been an inpatient your husband has become more independent.
MRS S. WRIGHT: Yes independent of me, but Mary has said that she is not going to let him latch on to her. You see she was sitting

on my bed and she was talking very freely and she said how she
had quite a few rows with daddy. She said how she's got this new
boyfriend and she wanted to bring him in to see me yesterday. She
said, 'But for him I don't think I could have enjoyed it while
you've been in here.' I said, 'What do you mean?' She said,
'Because I couldn't have stood it with daddy.' I said, 'You love
each other really,' which they do. They have a certain amount of
fun which I feel is more of an understanding than I have with Jim.
She said, 'Well I'm not hanging around keeping his meals hot like
you've done.' You see this is what Jim has wanted of her. This
is what he has done to me and he expects her to cope in the same
way. We've had quite considerable rows. Jim would choose to come
in at five for tea, or half past four, or seven. So whereas I
would put things so as to be at home for when Jim eventually came
in, Mary said, 'I'm not going to do what you have done.' She's
right of course. On the other hand I expect her daddy has got a
certain amount of concern for her because he doesn't want her to
get herself into any unhappy situations.
INTERVIEWER: How do you see the treatment you've been having?
MRS S. WRIGHT: Well it's been very helpful to talk definitely.
And it's been helpful to be here because you find a certain affinity
with the patients. You realise you can say things to them and they
don't think you are completely mad because they have had the experiences too. This is why I think it is valuable to be in a place
like this. But I don't feel we've reached the root of my problem.
I've referred to this on this side of my face before. From time
to time this becomes very much apparent. It's as if there is a
part of my face which lights up so that I can almost feel that
the left-hand side of me is different. That has not been dealt
with. What I want plucked out of me is this which I feel entered
my life three or four years ago, this open channel.
INTERVIEWER: How do you see the hospital helping you in the future?
MRS S. WRIGHT: I don't think I can get the help here that I feel
I need.

Disagreement over how Mrs Wright had been progressing arose between
the consultant and his junior colleagues during a ward round that
took place after the Whitsun weekend.

    A staff nurse reported that Mrs Wright had spent a satisfactory
time at home and had not returned to the unit talking about demons
and spirits. The junior members of staff felt that this assessment was superficial. To begin with, the SHO pointed out that
Mrs Wright still viewed relationships in religious and spiritual
terms. Second, a senior PSW asserted that weekend leave was not
a satisfactory situation for judging a patient's progress. It was
more like a holiday for the patient than living at home because
he knew that he would be returning to the unit. The SHO agreed
and added that Mrs Wright ought to be discharged immediately so
that she could face up to living with her husband. While she was
an inpatient she was protected from this situation. The SHO recommended that marital therapy should be set up on an outpatient
basis.

    The consultant was opposed to the views of his junior colleagues.
He was of the opinion that Mrs Wright's situation had altered

radically since he had first interviewed her as an outpatient.
Inpatient care had been a constructive experience for Mrs Wright
for she no longer experienced spirits or other matter of a similar
nature. Second, he felt that weekend leave was an appropriate
testing ground for a patient's state of health and that Mrs Wright's
time at home had been a satisfactory one. Third, both Mr and Mrs
Wright had been prepared for marital therapy by the SHO and the
student social worker. The object of the latter would be to help
them arrive at a position where they could speak honestly and
openly to each other about one another. The consultant decided
that Mrs Wright should not be discharged immediately. He recommended that marital therapy should be set up during the week. The
SHO and the student social worker would be the interviewers.
Finally, the issue of Mrs Wright's discharge would be reviewed at
the end of the week.

The consultant's assessment was clearly quite removed from the
facts. It was an example of how distanced the consultant was from
the day-to-day events of the unit. Although the Wrights had been
made to examine their marriage, Mrs Wright was still having experiences of a spiritual nature. Furthermore, the SHO's view that
Mrs Wright to some extent avoided issues to do with her marriage
while she was an inpatient was true. She saw the unit as a place
where she could rest from the pressures of home life, and be free
to act as she pleased without having to seek her husband's ap-
proval.

A day after the ward round, on 29 May, an interview with both
the Wrights and the SHO and the student social worker took place.
The SHO wrote in the case notes that

Both very wary of each other and not willing to admit any of
the things they'd been talking about separately. Mrs Wright
very meek and proper, using religion in the discussion. Mr
Wright after initial reticence, more willing to admit to their
failings.... It appears Mr Wright is probably more willing to
discuss personal failings than Mrs Wright, but he was quite put
out by the thought of his wife being discharged and further care
being directed to both of them.

Two days later the SHO reported to the rest of the team, at a team
meeting, how the marital interview had fared. There was a concen-
sus among the members of staff that this first interview had been
quite successful. The consultant decided to discharge Mrs Wright
and instructed that further interviews should take place on an
outpatient basis.

Mrs Wright was interviewed by one of the authors towards the end
of her stay in the unit.

Mrs Susan Wright

INTERVIEWER: How did you find being at home over Whitsun weekend?
MRS S. WRIGHT: I felt there was some oppression in the home. To
some degree I wondered if it was connected with my father because
he had been so very distressed.
INTERVIEWER: How did you enjoy being with the family?

MRS S. WRIGHT: Well my husband made it very tight for me.   On
Friday evening he said, 'If you want to go and see your mother you
better go tonight,' so I went on the Friday night.   Then I never
went outside the garden all day Saturday.   Oh yes we just went
briefly to the village but he stayed with me close by the whole
time.   I wasn't all that sorry to come back to hospital on the
Tuesday.
INTERVIEWER: How have you found the last week you've spent in the
hospital?
MRS S. WRIGHT: I've loved being here in many, many ways.   I've
loved the freedom, you see.   A lot of people wouldn't agree with
that, but I've found a great sense of freedom in the hospital.   I've
been free from having to please mainly my husband.   And of course
I've got this little fear thing of meeting this man, David.   I
think he's been anxious about me, the fact that I've been in hospital.   He's obviously been very much wanting to talk to me.   On
the weekend I came home, on the Sunday, he came to church without
his wife.   It was quite clear he wanted to have a chat with me
afterwards but he just didn't get the opportunity.   I am quite sure
that he has been concerned about me, but then I may be absolutely
wrong.   It might be entirely my imagination.

OUTPATIENTS

After Mrs Wright was discharged from the unit she and her husband
continued to participate in marital therapy on an outpatient basis.
    From the point of view of the SHO and the student social worker,
little was being achieved by this form of treatment.   Although they
found Mr Wright willing to examine his marriage, Mrs Wright was
less inclined to do so.   She tended to retreat behind her religious
beliefs and spiritual experiences.   On 24 May the SHO told me,
'It's a real effort to make her, more than him, say anything personal.   It's all very pious and if anything it is referred back
to the spiritual level.'   The student social worker was of the
same opinion as her colleague:
    Mrs Wright has retreated into 'I am possessed, I know I have
    influence on other people'.   Mr Wright has physically retreated
    into his chair, and in fact he has emerged, particularly over
    the last two interviews, as trying to get his wife to discuss
    on a more personal level, and as he's tried to do this she's
    retreated and he's become angry and hasn't been able to express
    his anger.

Mr and Mrs Wright were interviewed by one of the authors approximately one month after Mrs Wright had been discharged.

Mrs Susan Wright

INTERVIEWER: How do you see your problem now?
MRS S. WRIGHT: The problem is related to these pressures.   I'm not
sure what it is.   I can't really put my finger on it.   Something
has to come away from me and either someone is praying for me, or

what is happening I'm not quite sure, whether someone is renouncing
me, or what it is I can't say but it makes me vomit. I feel when
I have vomited, and whatever this is, as far as I am concerned some
kind of spirit, then I shall be free of that.
INTERVIEWER: In what way did the hospital help you?
MRS S. WRIGHT: I think, perhaps, the greatest thing that helped me
was to be able to talk to people without being treated as if I was
mentally ill or completely mad. You see my husband has this sort
of attitude towards me, and I think certain other people had
become almost a little bit frightened of me if I tried to share
my experiences with them with my earnest desire for help. The
other thing that was a great help to me, I could listen to other
people and when they said things to me I wasn't shocked at all.
Because I had such incredible experiences I could understand them.
INTERVIEWER: How do you see the marital therapy you and your husband have been participating in?
MRS S. WRIGHT: I didn't bother too much about it. I knew it could
be quite painful. The second time I went I was quite strung-up
about it. The first time I was quite calm and collected because
I had been at the hospital then. When I went back after being at
home here I was a little bit agitated about going because it was
quite clear to me that the SHO was so point-blank in a sense. I
was a little bit agitated the second time we went because I did
feel it could be one thing or another. One's marriage could be
absolutely destroyed or brought together. It could be one thing
or the other as a result of being forced, in a sense, to talk to
each other. I do believe the whole object of this is that my husband and I should communicate better. But as far as I am concerned
I made my vows before God and that is final. My marriage must last.
INTERVIEWER: Has your relationship with your husband improved since
you've returned home?
MRS S. WRIGHT: No, not much.
INTERVIEWER: How has Mary been affected by your hospitalisation?
MRS S. WRIGHT: I'm really distressed about my daughter. I think
the poor little thing has had so much bewilderment. It's been very
difficult for her. People still do not understand psychiatric hospitals and she's obviously had a bit of a problem, I feel sure, at
school. She's had to do so much at home. She hates for me and
her daddy to have this sort of ... I know she doesn't want us to
part because she loves us both. You see she has been terribly
worried because she has decided in her own mind that daddy and I
are going to part. She said, 'I love you both but you two are
tearing me pieces,' which, of course is the last thing I would want
to do. She said, 'It is I who is going to end up in that hospital.' Well, of course, that's the last thing I want for Mary or
any of the children. I said, 'I have no intention of leaving your
daddy.'
INTERVIEWER: Are you still concerned about Tony?
MRS S. WRIGHT: I feel my relationship with Tony isn't what I would
like it to be. Although we still love each other we can't quite see
eye to eye in some senses. Now those people who are baptised in
the Holy Spirit and are being used as channels are able, in fact,
to deliver people from this situation. I am saying someone could
deliver Tony of his homosexuality. I wouldn't dream of suggesting

who Tony should go to, but first of all Tony has got to want to
overcome it. I think he is at the point now where he does, because
he said to me that he felt he would have to try and live a celibate
life.
INTERVIEWER: How do you see the future?
MRS S. WRIGHT: I'm just having to live day by day. Someone once
said to me you can't. In the Gospels it talks about Jairus'
daughter being healed by the Lord Jesus Christ and it says this,
you see, that, 'There came to Jesus', because he was delayed by
this woman who had the haemorrhage, and this person came and said,
'Don't lose heart', and Jesus went on. Now as far as I can see
this is my situation. I feel I am up against the mountain but the
power of the Lord Jesus Christ goes on in the hearts of men because
he said this, 'If I am lifted up I shall draw all men to me', so
nobody in the long run can resist the magnetism of the Lord Jesus
Christ. It may take some people a whole lifetime, but other people
will come to it sooner, and sometimes we're completely broken before
we come to it. And I have been greatly broken of late. I expect
that He will open the door for me but for the moment He's asking
me to suffer for Him, and if I'm right in thinking this then I've
got to be willing to do so.

Mr Jim Wright

INTERVIEWER: While your wife was in hospital did you change the
way you saw her problem?
MR J. WRIGHT: Yes. At the time she went in I would have said it
was a purely spiritual thing or whatever you call it. But I began
to look at it in a different light after going in and out for a
while and seeing other cases, I suppose. And the other night I
watched a programme on this and I realised the number of hospitals,
up and down the country, involved in just this. It needn't necessarily be all spiritual, it could be medical. You know it could
respond to that type of treatment, let's put it that way.
INTERVIEWER: How did you see your wife's stay in hospital?
MR J. WRIGHT: In my own way I thought this is not doing her a lot
of good especially when she was downstairs surrounded by the type
of people that were there. In any case from my point of view I
would have thought ... she was getting involved with all these
people's problems and it wasn't probably improving hers. She seems
to do this wherever she takes on other people's worries.
INTERVIEWER: Did your wife's stay in hospital help her?
MR J. WRIGHT: Oh yes, I would say she's tons better.
INTERVIEWER: How do you see the marital therapy you and your wife
have been participating in?
MR J. WRIGHT: Well it was all right until I met the SHO. First of
all I was told the social worker wanted to see me. I saw her on
two occasions. She said on the next occasion, 'I would like all
four of us to meet.' Some people you get on with, some you don't.
I get on very well with the social worker but with the SHO I don't,
I'm afraid. There's something about her that gets my bristles up.
That's the effect on me.
INTERVIEWER: What issues have been brought up in the interviews?

MR J. WRIGHT: As I could gather, the SHO seemed to think that a lot of this was attributable to home background and this needed sorting out, from what she said. The SHO trod right on my toes the first night because she gave me the impression that one solution was to give up the Church of England. I said, quite frankly, if it came to that I would give up altogether. So we didn't get very far on that question. Issues have also been raised to do with the marriage. Mainly about problems that had occurred. We have never got on in our social life together and this was one of the issues that was raised. This is one of the things me and my wife are not all that compatible over. Especially now I would be very inclined to join a country club or something like that and have somewhere to go on an occasional evening, with the wife I mean, to give her a break from things.

INTERVIEWER: How has your wife coped with home life since she's been discharged?

MR J. WRIGHT: Her main thing, I don't know whether this is a symptom or just a reaction to someone else running the house, but when she came back from the hospital Mary had done all the washing, put clean towels out. The next day she went round and did the whole thing again even though we said it's all been done.

INTERVIEWER: How did Mary cope with home life while your wife was in hospital?

MR J. WRIGHT: As far as I was concerned very well, because she's been doing her CSEs and O-levels and perhaps she's been at school two hours a day or something like that. She's been able to get meals and so forth and as far as I am concerned things have run along on wheels. But the effect on Mary I don't know. We did get a remark from her this morning that she would be needing psychiatric help, because of the tension. She said 'I'm quite happy to live with one or other of you but I can't stick it out with the two of you.'

INTERVIEWER: How do you see the future?

MR J. WRIGHT: I don't really know, I hesitate to think. I feel already I have to cut down on some of my activities. I don't really know until tomorrow night anyway. Last Wednesday night ... I've had some sort of turns over the years, on and off for quite a while. Could never seem to get it out of the doctor what they were. I had a pretty hard day on Wednesday and I came in and this was upstairs in one of the rooms. I thought I'll make a cup of tea. I went into the cupboard to pick up the tea bag and stood up again and that was all I knew. I had landed full length on my back straight through the door. How long I was out I don't know. Anyway I called Mary and she said, 'Don't get up,' and I said I wasn't going to anyway. We weren't at all sure what it was and still don't know. Anyway I'm going to see the doctor tomorrow night, I might be able to get some sense out of him.

A summary of a letter written by the SHO to Mrs Wright's GP on 12 July 1974:

The SHO thought that she should let the GP know the situation as it stood as she and Miss Moore, the social worker, were both leaving and were arranging for new people to get to know Mr and Mrs Wright. She said she and Miss Moore had participated in several

joint interviews with the Wrights and had really found it quite
hard work 'to get over to look at this rather cover up with the
spiritual situation'. She felt that Mr Wright was much more amenable to discussing the Wrights' long-term problems than Mrs Wright.
It had been fairly obvious to both therapists that over the years
the Wrights had had almost a complete lack of communication between
and understanding of each other, and Mrs Wright had obviously been
the dominant partner of the relationship. The SHO went on to say
that a fortnight previously Mrs Wright had gone to see yet another
minister who had told her that she had committed adultery and
various other sins that were the cause of her falling away from
God and of allowing evil influences to take over.

The SHO was unsure of what influence she and her co-therapists
had made on the outcome of the case. She said that Mrs Wright was
now trying to reverse the roles and had made her husband dominant
in their relationship. In the SHO's opinion this had very effectively removed all responsibility from Mrs Wright to Mr Wright,
but she felt he was rather floundering and felt that further
interviews with the Wrights would probably be along the lines of
supporting Mr Wright and less probably encouraging some form of
equilibrium in their relationship.

POSTSCRIPT

After the SHO and the student social worker had left the unit Mrs
Wright was not seen by any of the medical staff until the beginning
of August. In fact, it was a letter she wrote towards the end of
July that precipitated her coming into contact with the psychiatric
services again. She wrote to the consultant saying:
    Forgive me for writing to you directly but I know that the SHO
    has left the hospital and I have not seen anyone since. Al-
    though I have received help and guidance from someone acquainted
    with spiritual matters I am still suffering a great deal.
The letter provided further evidence that Mrs Wright was still very
troubled by her son's homosexuality and her relationship with him:
    My son has felt he has to accept his condition but I am praying
    the Lord will reveal to him that He is the one great authority
    in heaven and upon earth and is able to pluck out of him that
    familiar spirit which has caused him so much distress, just as
    I am trusting the Lord Jesus Christ to deliver me in his own
    good time.
When she commenced therapy in August with a new doctor, much that
had been discussed with her old therapist was discussed again.
For the first three months she continued to place a lot of stress
on the spiritual experiences of her life and also the poverty of
her relationship with her husband. By November the doctor wrote
in the case notes that Mrs Wright was becoming calmer and had
been helped by medication. Although both the doctor and Mrs Wright
attempted to persuade Mr Wright to join them in therapy, he was
reluctant to do so.

On 20 December Mrs Wright was discharged from care. The doctor
wrote to Mrs Wright's GP saying:
    I am pleased to say that Mrs Wright is now very much improved.

We have talked at some length about the experiences she had in
the spring and have related them to her feeling about her marriage and other men who have come into her life. She is now
off all medication and is working a few hours each day nursing.
I had an opportunity to see Mr Wright last week who told me
that he felt that his wife was back to her normal self. There
are various conflicts still within the marriage, in particular
Mrs Wright feels that her husband does not allow her to be free
in her activities outside the home.

Since she was discharged from care Mrs Wright has had no further
contact with the psychiatric services. In letters she wrote both
to the doctor and one of the authors she has said that she no
longer feels pain and pressure upon her brain. She feels her
relationship with her husband has improved and she is less concerned about Tony's homosexuality. She still feels she has some
way to go in becoming fully healed: 'Of one thing I am confident,
that Jesus Christ is the answer to all our problems and His power
is limitless. He must have a good reason for delaying my healing.'

SUMMARY

1 The unit was organised in such a way that the consultants rarely
treated inpatients. Mrs Wright was led to believe by her GP that
she would be treated by a doctor whose religious beliefs were
similar to hers. Although the latter would have been true of the
consultant, the only occasion he was in contact with her was during
the initial outpatient appointment. Ultimately she received psychotherapy from a doctor who was not sympathetic to her religious
beliefs. This issue of therapist-patient incompatibility also
arose between the SHO and Mr Wright, again owing to the former's
lack of sympathy towards religious beliefs.

2 Although the consultant made the treatment decisions at ward
rounds and team meetings, he had no day-to-day contact with the
patient. This distance from the patient resulted in him ignoring
the SHO's assessment that inpatient care protected Mrs Wright
from facing up to her marriage. This assessment was clearly
correct.

3 Although the consultant decided that Mary should be involved
in the treatment programme, this decision was never carried out.
This led to a failure to monitor or support her at a time when she
was undergoing considerable emotional distress owing to the frac-
tious nature of her parents' relationship.

4 The staff quite rightly assessed the case as a marital problem. But the autobiographies of the patient and her family,
taken by one of the authors, suggest that the dynamics of the case
were far more complicated. Although one of the members of the
team speculatively suggested that other members of the Wright
family should be involved in the treatment programme, this was
never taken up. Indeed, on no occasion did the team attempt to
understand the important and complicated relationship between Mrs
Wright and Tony. The autobiographies lead the authors to believe
that at one time Tony provided considerable support to his mother
and that the weakening of this relationship resulted in considerable

stress for Mrs Wright. In the opinion of the authors, the relative
poverty of the team's assessment stemmed from the lack of diversity
in the models used by the team to assess psychological disturbance.

5 Mrs Wright's religious beliefs were treated as epiphenominal
by members of the staff. The team justified this on the grounds
that she used these to avoid examining issues to do with her marriage. Thus the team members believed that by not discussing these
beliefs with the patient they would discourage Mrs Wright from
mystifying her relationships. The evidence contained in this
chapter suggests that the team's decision in this respect was
unrealistic, since Mrs Wright continued to see her life situation
in religious terms. She did so because this was fundamental to
the way she construed it.

6 The consultant told one of the authors privately that he admitted Mrs Wright into the unit because he wished to break up the
crisis situation in the Wright family that had arisen over Easter.
The authors question this decision, since Mrs Wright entered the
unit over one month after Easter, and by that time the immediacy
of the crisis was obviously over. This decision to admit her is
further questionable when one realises that the team embarked on
a treatment plan aimed at persuading both husband and wife to
examine their marriage. Although Mr Wright was ultimately willing
to do this, initially he construed his wife as 'ill' since she was
an inpatient, thus tending not to see himself as requiring treatment on an equal basis with her. This is essential in marital
therapy.

7 The consultant was aware that the SHO's and the student social
worker's term of employment ended at the beginning of July. Yet it
was predictable that the duration of Mrs Wright's care would take
longer than the two months these junior members of staff were in
contact with her. The authors question the decision to pass on
the care of Mrs Wright to them in these circumstances. When she
resumed treatment at the beginning of August the new doctor found
it necessary to go over much of what she had discussed with her
former therapists in order to acquaint himself with the patient
and the case.

Chapter 9

The case of Mrs Davis

When Mrs Davis was hospitalised she was twenty-eight years old.
She had married at sixteen and by now had five children.

Unlike the cases of Mrs Smith and Mrs Wright, Mrs Davis had
received psychiatric help before coming into contact with Porchester
Hospital. But she had never experienced inpatient care.

Like Mrs Smith, Mrs Davis is typical of the kind of patient who
receives treatment over a long period of time.

THE PROBLEM

Mrs Kathy Davis

MRS K. DAVIS: When I look back it's always my father. I think it
must be my father now.

I've just got no feeling. I feel if I don't get away I'll just
give up and stay in bed all day. I can't breathe when I go out.
I just want to stay in bed. The fear, I just can't understand it.
Why should my father have such an influence? After I had Rosy,
ten years ago, I was becoming like my father and I would accuse
Roy of adultery and such things, and I would get in terrible tem-
pers and smash things.
INTERVIEWER: What effect does your father have on you at the moment?
MRS K. DAVIS: He just criticises. You know you just can't have a
conversation with him.
INTERVIEWER: How do you feel about that?
MRS K. DAVIS: Well, you know, I laugh it off whereas somewhere down
in my mind I'm not laughing it off. This is what is upsetting me
so much. You know everything I love he has said this, that and the
other, and I have found myself saying the same things.
INTERVIEWER: When?
MRS K. DAVIS: Say two weeks later, not straight away. Then I
started dreading him coming down, but now I seem to want him to
come but I don't want him.

In the past year, over the months I have lost contact with my
husband and my children. I feel I've lost everything I love and
I do want to love my children the way a mother should. I want to,

also, love my husband the way a wife should. A wife should love
her husband in a different way from her children, by that I mean
with sex. I know I'm not sexless as something happened a few
months ago, but now it's gone again. There is so much more behind
it than just sex. There is a fear. This fear has come back in me
again. I had it before. I don't know why it's come back again,
maybe it's to do with my father. I'm no good to my family any more
because my mind has gone wrong again. I don't want my father and
I don't want to be like him.

My father has been coming down every week, on a Friday at first,
and then on a Tuesday. He would say things to me but I would
think, 'Here he goes, never a good word.' Then after a few weeks
went by I began to row and get violent towards my husband and say
he was no good and a lot more. Then afterwards I was sorry, and
I would think to myself about what I had said and it was things my
father had said to be beforehand.

I don't want to give Roy what my father gave my mother, and I
don't want to give my children what my father gave us.
MRS K. DAVIS: You know if I thought to myself tomorrow I had to go
on the bus all the way from Porchester, I couldn't do that.
INTERVIEWER: Why?
MRS K. DAVIS: I couldn't, I don't know why, because I'm afraid.
INTERVIEWER: You're afraid.
MRS K. DAVIS: Mm. But that's how it affects me, just afraid to go
a great big distance. But when we go on holiday I can go from
where we are staying down to the beach. You know I can travel that
far, or I can go and do my shopping.

I've become more upset. I wasn't like this before. I feel shut
up in a corner. I'm mentally exhausted, not physically. I get
this feeling when I wake up in the morning of breathlessness.

Mr Roy Davis (29 years old)

MR R. DAVIS: She's got this fear of her father. I don't really
know what it is. I should think it is something down inside her
because she says she don't like him on the surface but, underneath,
she's sort of drawn to him like magnet. Seems strange, outwardly
she hates him yet underneath she seems to want some kind of affection from him.
INTERVIEWER: Kathy told me that for a long time sex, for her, was
just to do with babies.
MR R. DAVIS: Yes, and you know she said the father has got it over
to her that sex was something which was dirty, if you like. More
or less she accepted sex as something to have children. She comes
in patterns, sometimes she likes sex and at other times she doesn't.

Her father, he tires her out mentally. He comes over to here,
he rubs his finger along the chair. He says you haven't done so
and so, you haven't done the garden. This sort of gets under
Kathy's skin and she feels run down and depressed when he's gone.
MR R. DAVIS: He's such an aggressive sort of person. He puts the
fear of hell up her. But this is no good at all. She's phoned
up the GP, phoned up the health visitor. They're worried up at
the surgery. The way she's feeling now she could take a dose of

tablets.   Of course her fear is also to do with travelling on the
buses, travelling any distance.   This is another problem which
she has.
INTERVIEWER: Why does she have this problem?
MR R. DAVIS: I don't know.   She gets it if she goes about a mile,
two miles on the bus, then she starts wanting to get off.   She
gets frightened.   She's had this problem for quite a while.   I
can remember going on a bus while we were courting, on a bus for
Porchester.   I found she couldn't do it.   She would either have
to get someone to bring her around or she would have to get a taxi.

Mr and Mrs Frank Fletcher (62 and 61 years old, respectively, and
Mrs K. Davis's parents)

INTERVIEWER: How do you see Kathy's problem?
MR F. FLETCHER: My wife and I feel that she is depressed and this
is because she became a Jehovah's Witness.   Before she became a
Witness she was always a gay girl.   We feel it is a harsh religion,
look you can't even give the kids Christmas presents.   She's definitely changed for the worse since she became a Witness.
INTERVIEWER: But Kathy became a Witness five years ago and her
problems seem to go back further than that.   I gather from her
that she was receiving treatment for the same ones over nine years
ago.
MR F. FLETCHER: Well she was becoming a Witness then.
MRS I. FLETCHER: You may be right but she's become even more depressed since she became a Witness.
INTERVIEWER: Do you think that these problems of hers might be
something to do with events in her childhood?
MRS I. FLETCHER: Well, all the children were treated equally when
they were younger, in fact Kathy was treated better than the
others.
MR F. FLETCHER: She's far too sensitive.   Whenever we talk about
religion and anyone disagrees with her she can't accept it.
MRS I. FLETCHER: You see dad says a lot of things he doesn't mean,
For example when he goes and visits Kathy he complains about the
garden but he doesn't mean anything bad.   We all know this and
accept it.
MR F. FLETCHER: I gave Roy and Kathy some leeks and cabbages to
grow but they cooked and ate them instead.   She's far too sensitive.
MRS I. FLETCHER: I wonder if she might not be feeling guilty about
the circumstances in which she got married.   You know she was
pregnant when she got married.

FAMILY LIFE

Kathy comes from a large family.   She is the middle child of five
children.   Liz, at thirty-six years old, is the oldest member of
the family.   She is married and has two children.   Simon is thirty-
three years old and is also married with children.   Kathy's younger
brothers, Tim and David, are twenty-three and twenty-two years old

respectively. Tim is married with children, while David is single
and was still living at home with his parents at the time of the
study.

In this section, apart from Kathy and Roy, the authors present
how Simon and Tim saw family life before they married and left
home. Thus the reader will be able to sample the opinions of a
sibling older than Kathy and of one younger than her.

Mrs Kathy Davis

INTERVIEWER: How did your father bring you up?
MRS K. DAVIS: Mum was called a prostitute and a whore. Well he
didn't really call me that when I was little but that was what I
understood I was.
INTERVIEWER: You're father called you that.
MRS K. DAVIS: One night I came home from work and I was going out
again and he called me a whore and he told me that I had been with
every man. I was so upset that I came downstairs and I said, 'I
am not what you are calling me.' I said I would go to the doctors
to prove it because I must have been old enough to know that you
could prove it through a doctor. He'd accuse my mother of committing adultery with my uncle.
INTERVIEWER: Had she done this?
MRS K. DAVIS: No. He would go out to the pub and get drunk. He
would then go to bed and he would go on and on to my mum until
two o'clock in the morning.
INTERVIEWER: About what?
MRS K. DAVIS: Adultery.
INTERVIEWER: And she had done none of this.
MRS K. DAVIS: No. My uncle lives a couple of doors away, and my
father would say that I belonged to my uncle and so did my elder
brother because we have fair hair. The other ones have dark hair.
INTERVIEWER: Why did he believe your mother was like that?
MRS K. DAVIS: It's his temper. I mean he would get up in the
middle of the night and get hold of the paraffin stove and say
'I'm going to burn you all.' Then one day he hit me. I've got
the scar over here on my head now. I was starting to wear stiletto
heels and they had worn down a bit. He sort of kicked me to the
floor and my shoe came off and he picked it up and whacked me
across the head with it and it bled. That was the only time, more
or less, he picked me up because he was frightened, because all
the blood was gushing everywhere.
INTERVIEWER: Did you feel anything for your father?
MRS K. DAVIS: No. I hated him, he frightened me.
INTERVIEWER: Was that the same for all the children?
MRS K. DAVIS: You know the others didn't seem to worry about it.
He picked on me and my youngest brother more than the others.
INTERVIEWER: Why do you think he did that?
MRS K. DAVIS: Because we were always mummy's pets. When I was
young mummy used to take me to the town, and David was the youngest
and I suppose she doted on him a lot.
INTERVIEWER: How did you feel about your mother when you were
living at home?

MRS K. DAVIS: My mother was always there when I needed her. But
she never talked to me about different things that you should
talk to your children about. Nevertheless we always stuck by mum.

Mr Roy Davis

When I was younger I never used to have to go through what Kathy
used to go through. I never used to have to take what she used
to take.
   Up at her house there was always a free for all. Her father
used to come back drunk. He'd come in and take it out on his
wife, and his children who were living there. One time he came
in and started on Kathy. Her mother and I had to pull them apart
and they both picked on me then. I said never again. If he wants
to get on with it let him get on with it.
   He sort of beats the place about. He runs up and down the
stairs! A normal person's not like him, you know.

Mr Simon Fletcher

MR S. FLETCHER: Father is a pretty loveable person really. He
used to like a lot of drink sometimes. Sometimes father used to
go on the drink at weekends. Mother used to say to me that he
was affected by the moon. I don't know whether you've heard of
this expression, I don't know whether there's any truth in it.
It seemed like it would happen when the moon would change, which
would be about once a quarter. Father used to get a bit wild
then, once he had been on the drink, and sometimes he used to make
life impossible.
INTERVIEWER: For whom?
MR S. FLETCHER: For everyone in the family. I don't know why
really. But he's a lot better now than he used to be. When he
was younger he was quite violent I suppose, although he never
physically hurt us badly. He may have given us a smack as any
father would but he was aggressive when he'd been on the drink.
He used a lot of bad language. Father was the only one who used
bad language in the house. It was all right for him to use bad
language but no one else must do this sort of thing, which is
silly really.
INTERVIEWER: So how was he to you as you grew up?
MR S. FLETCHER: Well, we found him difficult. He was very demanding. He was always trying to assert his ideals in life but I
can't say they were right. He thought they were right for him.
Father was a miner. He demanded that we be in at certain times
and things like that, and then he'd say you mustn't mix with so
and so because they are a bad influence, which probably had no
foundation at all really. Just because he didn't like the people.
   When I was at home I used to sit in the background. Mother
used to ... she said I was too ... I wouldn't speak up enough, I
always tried to avoid a confrontation with father but there were
times when I did have a confrontation, like the time I threw the
tin at him.

So it has been a rather rocky road, our family life. Mother has often said she thought she ought to have left father at times, but they're very happy together now. People get mature when they get older I suppose. I think they have definitely in their case.
INTERVIEWER: How do you feel about your father?
MR S. FLETCHER: I could see some of the things he used to do were wrong but I never used to hold it against him.
INTERVIEWER: Were you closer to your mother than your father?
MR S. FLETCHER: I don't think so. I think I hold the same affection for both of them. I don't say one's got more faults than the other. I just sort of think that's the way he is.

Father was always accusing mother of carrying on with uncle Bernard. He would do this when he'd been on the drink. She used to get very upset over this but I don't know why he used to say that. As far as I know he didn't have any proof.

Father was never more bad-tempered towards Kathy than the rest of us. I think in his eyes we were all the same. I think mother had a very good relationship with Kathy.

Mr Tim Fletcher

INTERVIEWER: Will you tell me how you saw your parents' relationship?
MR T. FLETCHER: Their relationship was as any other normal one as I saw it, except for the times when my father did drink and get into these moods. And obviously as a child I saw things differently as I do now.
INTERVIEWER: Will you tell me how you saw things as a child?
MR T. FLETCHER: I saw my father as being very strict on morals and things like smoking. But apart from when he was in a bad mood we received as much love and affection from them as any other child would or probably more so than some children. I probably had more or had to put up with more bad temperedness from my father, and hidings, which some children don't get, but I don't think they affected me.
INTERVIEWER: How did you see the way your father treated your mother?
MR T. FLETCHER: I never approved of it.
INTERVIEWER: What were the things you disapproved of?
MR T. FLETCHER: Well he would swear and call her names, have rows and that, but this was only at certain times. Other than that he would treat her as any other husband would treat a wife. It upset me when he was violent but as he did give us his love; this, of course, did over-rule his violent moods. You know I judged him more for the good times rather than the bad.

As a child I resented him at times but I accepted this as being normal and I accepted he couldn't help himself when he was drunk or when he had been drinking. My mother used to say it was the moon but obviously I knew, as I grew older, that something was wrong. You know, he couldn't help himself. But when I was younger I was the same as any other child who had a hiding. If I did something wrong I got the punishment, or when he was drunk I probably couldn't comprehend why he was like it anyway. As I grew older I

realised he was right or ignored him and carried on with what I
was doing.
INTERVIEWER: Was what Kathy had to put up with any different from
what the rest of you put up with?
MR T. FLETCHER: Well as she is a girl obviously she may feel it
more emotionally and her getting hidings were probably worse than
what I received but they probably even affected her more so because
she was a girl. I don't think she helped matters you know, because
she was more ready to argue the point out whereas I would rather go
out than argue. One of the main things I can remember she used to
get bullied for smoking. She would be more open about her smoking
and her behaviour than I would be and I think this aggravated him
much more than what I did.

     I think this is one of the main reasons why she was kept on at
because she was more like father than what I was. Because he was
always right and she was always right and there would be friction
between them.

     My father worked down the ground and he was hit on the head
underground and he had meningitis and then he had a haemorrhage.
Which followed what I don't know. I know he was hit on the head
first, this must have been about twenty years ago. Whether this
had any effect on his behaviour I don't know, but obviously I
should think it did, but I didn't attribute it to that when I was
younger because obviously I couldn't understand it. As I've grown
older I've realised it was just not normal behaviour.

MARRIAGE

Mrs Kathy Davis

INTERVIEWER: When did you meet Roy?
MRS K. DAVIS: When I was fourteen.
INTERVIEWER: When did you get married?
MRS K. DAVIS: When I was sixteen.
INTERVIEWER: What were the circumstances surrounding your marriage?
MRS K. DAVIS: My father kept bullying me all the time. He hit me
after I left school. I had a great weal across my back when I was
going out with Roy and I wouldn't let him put his arm around me
and he was curious. So we thought, well, that we would have a baby
and get married. That was the only reason why we had intercourse.
INTERVIEWER: In other words you became pregnant in order to get
married.
MRS K. DAVIS: I loved Roy. I didn't want to sleep with him just
for sex. I wanted to have intercourse for a baby.
INTERVIEWER: Will you tell me what happened when you announced
that you were getting married?
MRS K. DAVIS: I never announced I was getting married. My mother
found out.
INTERVIEWER: How did she find out?
MRS K. DAVIS: Well I'd been to the GP because I was pregnant, and
I suppose he filled in some forms and the district nurse heard
about it. She found out that I lived in the area and so she called
on my mother. She must have thought it was my mother who was

pregnant. So my mother found out who was pregnant in the end
and when I came home from work that day, they said, 'Eat your
tea,' and so I ate it, but I could feel they were looking. Then
she said, 'I want to see you upstairs,' and so we went up into
the bedroom and sat on the bed and she lectured me. She said,
'What are you going to do about it?' And I said, 'Get married
to Roy.' She said, 'You've made your bed of nails to be in,' and
'What will the neighbours say?' And stupid things like that.
Anyway I didn't answer her back all that much. She said, 'You
better see to it that his mother knows.' So I said, 'Roy will
deal with that.' I went downstairs and my father just looked at
me and he said, 'Do your hair and go out.'
INTERVIEWER: In what year did you get married?
MRS K. DAVIS: In February 1962.
INTERVIEWER: Will you tell me about your living arrangements after
you got married?
MRS K. DAVIS: We went to live with mother-in-law. After Mark was
born, and just before Christmas 1962, we moved back up to my
mother's, because I had a row with Roy's mum. We stayed there over
Christmas. That was a very bad year for the weather - the snow was
very high and Roy was laid off for about six weeks. Anyway my
nerves went to pieces up there.
INTERVIEWER: Why was that?
MRS K. DAVIS: Because father would come in and he would moan and
groan, and say, 'Hasn't she washed the nappies?' Or ... we weren't
living in their part of the house, we had a separate room.... But
then one day he came home after being on the drink and he was
shouting and kicking at mum, and I got afraid and I went out there
and said, 'Stop it!' He was shouting at me and then Roy came out
in a furious temper and I said, 'You go back in there, you go back
in there,' because he started pushing the table at my father. He
had the devil in his eyes and I pushed him away. I didn't want
anything nasty. So we moved back to mother-in-law's after Christmas, in 1963.
INTERVIEWER: So you stayed with your parents for only a very short
while.
MRS K. DAVIS: Yes, and then we started looking for a house of our
own after we moved in mother-in-law's. Well father-in-law saw
one, this old cottage behind theirs, and they borrowed us the
money to buy it. We moved in there before the summer of 1963.
INTERVIEWER: During this period was it possible for you to make a
break between being a daughter and a child, and having to be a
wife and presumably a little more grown-up? Did you become a
different person in this respect at that time?
MRS K. DAVIS: Things stayed the same. I was living in dream land
I suppose.
INTERVIEWER: What did that mean?
MRS K. DAVIS: I was away from the big bad wolf and had someone to
protect me.
INTERVIEWER: Who was the big bad wolf?
MRS K. DAVIS: Father.
INTERVIEWER: And was the protector Roy?
MRS K. DAVIS: Yes. I loved babies and so therefore I had babies
and they were very pretty. I'd keep them all pretty clean.

Especially when we went up to see my parents and father would
always inspect their ears, so I would clean them, and I would
clean my teeth because he would inspect those to see if I had
been smoking too much. So on and so on, that's all. Somewhere
deep down I knew it was wrong. It should be different from what
it was.

MRS K. DAVIS: I just knew it was supposed to be different.... I
wasn't going to become like my father, I just didn't want to become
like him and I was becoming like him at that time. But I fought
against that, after I had discussed these problems I had with
Dr Marks. This was after I had Rosy in 1965.

INTERVIEWER: Why did you decide to go to Dr Marks?

MRS K. DAVIS: I was losing control of my temper and sex wasn't any
good. Then we decided to move from Mineway to Blacktown. Dr Marks
said it was the best thing. He did say my father had this influence
and Roy said it was worth moving because if we moved away I wouldn't
come into contact with my father so much.

INTERVIEWER: In what year did you move to Blacktown?

MRS K. DAVIS: In 1967.

INTERVIEWER: How was life once you moved there?

MRS K. DAVIS: I was on top of the world for a length of time. I
got closer to Roy.

INTERVIEWER: Why did you decide after that to leave Blacktown and
move back to Mineway?

MRS K. DAVIS: Because I didn't understand why I was like it. I
couldn't understand it, I'd been through all of this before with
Dr Marks. I knew that my father was like he was and so therefore
he had no influence over me any more. But the fear was there. I
began to fear going out. I couldn't go out anywhere. This was
after I had Barry in 1968.

INTERVIEWER: Do you know why the fear started again?

MRS K. DAVIS: No. I got so bad that Roy thought, well, I had close
friends at Mineway and we moved back there. You know, it was more
compact. The shops were near, the children would only have to
cross over the road to school and so on and so forth. I got shocked
out of that dreaded fear, but not completely.

INTERVIEWER: When was this?

MRS K. DAVIS: When I was pregnant with Fiona, in 1971. We had moved
from Blacktown in February and this American woman started work
about Easter where Roy worked. Roy would come home and talk about
her all the time. She used to bring him in sandwiches and he even
changed his brand of cigarettes to hers. He used to feel sorry for
her because she said her husband treated her bad. Whether he did
or not I don't know. I told Roy he was a stupid fool and a bloody
liar.

INTERVIEWER: You got angry and upset about it.

MRS K. DAVIS: Aggressive. But he used to bring her a couple of
times along for a cup of tea. Then she asked us both out to her
place with her husband to have a meal. So naturally enough I
thought I better ask them back but I didn't feel like it. I
wouldn't change my clothes and I wouldn't even do my hair when
they came. Roy sent the children up to bed and he made them cry
because they had to go up to bed. I wasn't going to have that
either so I said Barry could come down and sit on my lap if he
wanted to.

INTERVIEWER: Did all this happen while you were pregnant?
MRS K. DAVIS: Yes. I was just extremely jealous I suppose. She
was about forty but she tarted herself up. Anyway Roy knew how
I felt and before I had the baby he said, 'Well the only thing to
do is to get out of temptation's way, if that's how you feel I'll
leave my job,' because by then he was missing days at work because
I'd nag him so much. So I had the GP in one day because I was so
sad. He said they knew who it was. Anyway I wanted Roy a fortnight before I was due to have Fiona ... and I thought I was as
good as her anyway. He made love to me and then I had to stay in
bed that week because of my legs and the nurse came in every day.
So on Friday the waters broke and I went into hospital but nothing
happened. Then I had Fiona on the Sunday. When I came home after
having Fiona I was very shaky and upset. But Roy did come to see
me every night while I was in hospital even though it was pouring
with rain.
INTERVIEWER: Did this relationship he had with the other lady fade
out?
MRS K. DAVIS: Yes.
INTERVIEWER: Was its effect to get you out of the fear for a while?
MRS K. DAVIS: Yes, but it was still there, though it wasn't as bad
as it had been. The whole business made me wake up short. It made
me realise I would lose Roy.

Mr Roy Davis

INTERVIEWER: When did you meet Kathy?
MR R. DAVIS: When I was fourteen I think. She's got a better
memory about these things than I have.
INTERVIEWER: Was Kathy your first girlfriend?
MR R. DAVIS: Well I'd been out with a few girls before. I didn't
have time for a lot more.
INTERVIEWER: She told me that you both decided that she should get
pregnant in order to get married.
MR R. DAVIS: She told me this afterwards. It was more her idea
than mine.
INTERVIEWER: Oh I see. Did you want to marry her?
MR R. DAVIS: I did want to marry her, but I would have rather
waited till I was much older before I married her because we getting
married meant we had to live with her parents and live with our
parents, which isn't good for any marriage. I didn't get on with
her parents very well because of her father. I don't think a lot
of him for someone who has sort of upset people as much as he has.
Well we couldn't live with them very long so we came down and lived
with my parents.
INTERVIEWER: How was that?
MR R. DAVIS: It didn't work out well because I found that if we
had any arguments my mother and father would come and side with me.
    When we went to live in Blacktown, things got better until Kathy
started having this problem of not being able to go out. You see,
her father couldn't come in to see her very easily because he
didn't have the transport. But then his youngest son passed his
driving test and her father came in more frequently. Our sex life
wasn't too good once Kathy started seeing him again.

RELIGION

Mrs Kathy Davis

INTERVIEWER: Has religion been important to you?
MRS K. DAVIS: I have always believed in God. I was a Catholic,
but I changed my religion.
INTERVIEWER: What did you change it to?
MRS K. DAVIS: Jehovah's Witness.
INTERVIEWER: Why?
MRS K. DAVIS: Well you know the people who call round at your door.
I was a Catholic, a practising Catholic, and I was in a mood one
day and I thought I had better go with them. I just studied into
it and I found it was the truth and that what the Catholic religion
taught wasn't. I knew it was teaching a lot of old traditions
which were not true that I could back up from my beliefs and the
encyclopaedia.
INTERVIEWER: Did Roy also change?
MRS K. DAVIS: He didn't have any religion really before. He was
a sort of Protestant.
INTERVIEWER: How did your parents feel about you becoming a Witness?
MRS K. DAVIS: My father didn't say much to me then, which was about
five years ago. But I wrote a letter to my mother telling her
because I thought it was only right that I should tell her and not
for her to hear it from somebody else. She came in and she was
very upset and said, 'Will you go to hell?' And all that sort of
business. I said, 'You've got to do what you think is right.' My
father didn't say anything to me directly. He just said what my
mother said and he wouldn't hold Barry because I hadn't had him
baptised or christened. He said he's not clean. What a thing to
say. Then a few months ago he had a go at me over religion. Not
that I wanted to have a go but it was brought up by them and father
had been down the pub. I thought he was going to hit me and I was
just about to go and get my brother to drive me back home....

PSYCHIATRIC CARE PRIOR TO PORCHESTER

There were two periods before 1973 during which Kathy received
psychiatric help. In 1965, when she was nineteen years old, Kathy
was referred by her present GP to a doctor who had retired from
London to the Mineway area. Previously he had been a GP and had
been trained in psychotherapy at a major clinic in London. Mrs
Davis was in contact with Dr Marks until the middle of December
1966. In 1967 she moved to Blacktown, and three years later she
was referred by her GP there to a psychiatrist at the General Hospital. She was in contact with him for approximately three months.

Mineway

At the beginning of 1965 Kathy was referred for treatment because
she complained of feelings of frigidity, and of, consequently,
being unable to enjoy sexual intercourse with her husband. By the

end of June 1965, having undergone six psychotherapy consultations
with Dr Marks, Kathy was discharged, considerably improved. They
discussed a number of issues: first, her inability to find a
suitable contraceptive; second, the lack of feeling and guilt she
experienced during sexual intercourse; and finally, her relationship with her father. After their first session, Dr Marks formulated that: 'This simple and attractive girl seems to have the
right basic instincts; she comes from a home where the parents
have not made a good match, but I shall be surprised if she does
not soon do better.'

During their next three meetings more material emerged about
Kathy's father. Dr Marks construed his prohibitions against sex
as inhibiting Kathy's enjoyment of the sexual act. He felt she
needed to grow from a daughter into a wife. In May and June Kathy
reported considerable improvement in the physical side of her
marriage. He interpreted that 'She is now able to feel that Roy
is the most important man in her life, and that father's dislike
of sex, and his prohibition of it to her, no longer operates.'
He decided that she did not require further consultations.

A year later, in June 1966, Kathy was referred again to Dr
Marks by her GP. She had been unable to maintain her independence
from her father and was becoming aggressive towards Roy and the
children. Dr Marks assessed that:

Her father still exercises a strong love-hate pull. Sex relations much better, he withdraws. She is confused about her
aggression and afraid she is repeating the pattern of her
father and grandfather (in part she may be). The fact that
she is afraid of making Roy's life a misery, and apologises
to the children is hopeful. She has not yet changed from the
rebellious daughter to the contented wife, but it is hopeful.
One cannot say how much she has inherited the violent temper
of the male side of her family.

Towards the end of 1966, and after six consultations, Kathy reported to Dr Marks that she had overcome her fear of being like
her father, and that she was putting Roy and the children first,
and was less irritable towards them. The Davises decided to move
to Blacktown so that they would not be living so close to their
respective parents. Dr Marks discharged Kathy and concluded in
the case notes that 'She has matured considerably.'

Blacktown

In November 1970, after a number of appointments with her GP,
Mrs Davis was referred by him to a psychiatrist at the General
Hospital in Blacktown. She complained that she felt depressed,
and that she was unable to go out anywhere without her husband.
Kathy was pregnant at the time with Fiona and the psychiatrist
recommended that her pregnancy should be terminated on psychiatric
grounds. She refused this. The psychiatrist also encouraged her
to consider having a sterilisation operation. Kathy took up this
recommendation, and was sterilised in 1973 following the birth of
her fifth child. She had returned to Mineway by that time. The
psychiatrist treated Kathy's complaints with medication. She was

prescribed Nardil, 15 mg p.d., in combination with Librium, 5 mg
t.d.s., although from the fourth month of her pregnancy the medication was halted on medical grounds.

It is interesting to compare the approach of this psychiatrist
to Kathy's problems with that of Dr Marks. The former made little
attempt to relate Kathy's symptoms to her interpersonal relations.
He construed her problems in terms of the 'medical model' and thus
emptied them of their personal content. The reverse was true of
the way Dr Marks conceptualised them. Consistent with the psychiatrist's formulation was his prescription of medication, and
consistent with Dr Marks's assessment was his use of psychotherapy.

The following are extracts from a letter written by the psychiatrist at the General Hospital in Blacktown, on 20 November
1970, to Kathy's GP:
> She presents with a phobic anxiety state of some two years
> duration and following the birth of her youngest child. Prior
> to this she had a history of rather atypical puerperal de-
> pression following the births of the first and second child
> during the second of which she was referred to a psychiatrist....
>
> The patient herself showed some evidence of early neurotic
> traits in fears of the dark and temper tantrums, as well as
> school phobias, and mild behaviour disturbances....
>
> The present symptoms consist of fears of going out of the
> house, particularly into crowded places or public transport.
> In such situations she feels shaky and panicky and fears she
> may be incontinent of urine. At times she experiences symptoms
> of derealisation, nausea, butterflies in the stomach, and
> shaking of the legs. There has been some impairment in con-
> centration, libido and sleep, particularly initial insomnia.
> Overall she has felt increasingly tense and restless and has
> bouts of compulsive eating....
>
> Personality examination shows evidence of hysterical and
> neurotic traits. I believe her pregnancy should be terminated
> on psychiatric grounds....
>
> Treatment - 2 week prescription of Nardil 15 mgms p.d. in
> combination with 5 mgms t.d.s. Dietary restrictions. If
> pregnant should stop pills from 2nd-4th month.

The psychiatrist wrote again to Kathy's GP on 19 January 1971:
> As you know this girl is 16 weeks pregnant and has therefore
> reduced her medication. There has been a recurrence of all
> her phobic symptoms, so that she is almost completely house-
> bound unless she goes out with her husband. However, at this
> point, I do not think we can do anything more, except to allow
> her to take Valium p.r.n. One hopes as the pregnancy pro-
> gresses things may improve but in any case I would like to see
> her once more when the baby is born.
>
> She is now definitely considering a sterilisation operation
> and I think could be well encouraged in this.

Kathy did not see the psychiatrist after Fiona was born because
she had returned to Mineway, and she was not in fact sterilised
until after the birth of her fifth child, Sally. Her fear of
going out lessened after Roy's relationship with the American lady
had ended, but nevertheless was still present in 1973 when Kathy
had cause to seek psychiatric help once again.

OUTPATIENTS

A summary of the general practitioner's letter written on 12
December 1973 to the consultant psychiatrist in charge of Mrs
Davis's initial outpatient appointment:

The GP thanked the consultant for seeing Mrs Davis, whom he
described as having long psychiatric problems related primarily
to her relationship with her father. She was the middle child in
a family of five and had an extremely demanding father, and in
spite of the fact she now had five children herself she still was
unable to make a satisfactory relationship with her husband.

Apparently the relationship with her father was now such that
she left the house rather than be at home when she knew he was
likely to visit. She had made a few gestures of independence,
having revoked her Catholic religion and become a Jehovah's
Witness. The GP commented that when she had told her father this
he had said that the children would go to hell. She found intercourse a waste of time and after her last pregnancy she had had
her tubes tied. The GP felt that she resented this as she had
liked being pregnant and had enjoyed all the emotions relating to
childbirth.

The GP went on to describe Mrs Davis's past contact with the
psychiatric services. Between 1965 and 1966 she had had a dozen
sessions of psychotherapy in his practice and then had moved to
Blacktown where for a while things had been better, but she had
become connected with psychiatrists at the General Hospital who
had tended to treat her with drugs and she was now 'hooked' on
Librium. The GP thought that Kathy was a not unintelligent girl
with a considerable degree of insight into her problems and thought
that she might be helped with further therapy. He wondered therefore if the consultant would consider taking her on.

A summary of the consultant psychiatrist's reply written on 12
December 1973 to the general practitioner after his initial outpatient consultation with the Davises:

The Consultant thanked the GP for referring Mrs Davis to him.
She had presented her problem as one of being sexless and had
indicated to the consultant that she needed to be admitted into
hospital in order 'to have things put right quickly'.

On taking a slightly fuller history the consultant had come to
the conclusion that Mrs Davis had experienced major difficulties
with her parents and with her husband for the past twelve to fourteen years. He went on to say that Mrs Davis was raising the
stakes and had tried to determine the form of treatment and also
what her husband would do in the situation.

The consultant did not think there was a lot to be gained by
admitting Mrs Davis unless his team could have access to Mr Davis
two or three times a week. Then the team might be able to get
something going between the Davises. He felt that this was likely
to prove the key to her recovery.

Mrs Davis had threatened the consultant that if he did not do
as she said she would kill herself in six months' time. Finally
he asked the GP if they could speak about this case on the phone
in the near future because the Davises were making very great
difficulties regarding coming to outpatients.

Mr and Mrs Davis were interviewed by one of the authors after Mrs Davis's outpatient appointment.

Mrs Kathy Davis

INTERVIEWER: What made you go to outpatients to see Dr Jones?
MRS K. DAVIS: When I went to see the doctor I told him the problem was sex. You see I had been sterilised after the birth of Sally and there was nothing else, I might as well not have bothered, and so I just put it to him bluntly how Roy said I was sexless as well as useless.
INTERVIEWER: What did Dr Jones say to you when you told him that?
MRS K. DAVIS: He said quite bluntly back, 'You are not sexless,' and I don't suppose I am and after I went back home something wonderful happened. Roy and I really hit it off well for the first time. For two nights running, which is record-breaking. I found out there was something else to intercourse, that it wasn't just like doing the weekly washing, that it was something wonderful. But then my father started coming down again and it was gone.
INTERVIEWER: What effect did he have on your sex life?
MRS K. DAVIS: He made it ten times worse than it's ever been, just no feeling.

Mr Roy Davis

INTERVIEWER: Why did Kathy go to outpatients to see Dr Jones?
MR R. DAVIS: Things have come to a point. She's been getting worse gradually but we've talked a lot more about our sex life. We've had appointments with the GP and he's come down.
INTERVIEWER: Is this recently?
MR R. DAVIS: Yes, in the last six months. Well as I've said, her father has got it into her that sex is something evil but after we'd seen Dr Jones she liked sex for a while and then her father started coming down and put a stop to that.

OUTPATIENTS

A summary of the general practitioner's letter written on 21 January 1974 to the consultant psychiatrist in charge of Mrs Davis's second outpatient appointment:
    As the consultant had suggested, the GP had not intervened in the Davis case until Mrs Davis came to see him earlier in the week. At this meeting she had indicated that she would be happy to accept psychotherapy for herself on an outpatient basis with her husband.
    The GP went on to say that, since seeing her Mrs Davis had gone to see the health visitor, he suspected following a visit from her father, in a dreadful state demanding that something should be done urgently and saying that she could only keep going until the weekend. The health visitor had been somewhat concerned about Mrs Davis and had discussed the situation with the GP that morning. The GP felt, like the consultant, that this might just have been Kathy increasing the heat.

The GP asked if the consultant would see her again and arrange for outpatient therapy.

A summary of the consultant psychiatrist's reply written on 30 January 1974 after his second outpatient consultation with the Davises:

The consultant wrote that he had seen Mrs Davis again and thought that she should be admitted into hospital as soon as this could be arranged. He hoped that this would be the following week.

Mr and Mrs Davis were interviewed by one of the authors in the time between her second outpatient interview and her admission into the unit.

Mrs Kathy Davis

INTERVIEWER: Why did you go to see the consultant for a second time?
MRS K. DAVIS: My brother came down on the Saturday and brought my father's pair of trousers for me to put some zips in; my brother wanted me to put two zips into two pairs of trousers. I was so livid, I've got enough work to do.
INTERVIEWER: So you were very angry about this.
MRS K. DAVIS: Yes. He said he would come down at 1.30 after lunch. He's got no ties you see. I'd done the washing and I thought he wouldn't be here till two or three. Well, he wasn't here by three so I thought I'd wash the floors and clean up before Roy came home and then I'd go shopping. I thought to myself, 'I bet he comes down tonight.' I was tired, I'd been working all day, and Roy was tired. I still felt I wanted Roy. About 7 o'clock, bang on the door, my brother comes in and he says, 'Here's two pairs of trousers. Put the zips in. While I'm here I'll fix your washing machine for you.' Roy kept saying to me, 'When's he going, when's he going? I bet he'll stay till 12 o'clock.' You see, this is my youngest brother, the one that lives at home. He's got nowhere else to go, only to me and my brothers. I then said to Roy, 'I'll go to bed, and he'll probably go.' But no, I was reading and I heard the door bang and then the television went off and they started talking. I suppose Roy thought he couldn't really be rude and say Cheerio because my brother had done the washing machine. You see, Roy didn't know about the zips.
INTERVIEWER: Why?
MRS K. DAVIS: He would've been upset. And so half an hour went by and I was getting more cross than ever. I then got up and came down and swore in front of David. I said to Roy that I'd been waiting for some tea. Of course, Roy won't usually show his feelings in front of a person, he waits till they've gone. I then marched upstairs and David said, 'Oh, I'll go home now, I've got you into trouble.' I came back down and I was in a furious temper and made some tea and sort of sloshed it around. Then I went back upstairs and Roy went to bed. I wanted Roy but I was so cross because he wouldn't tell David to go home. He got out of bed and he hit me but I didn't care. Usually if I've provoked him and he's

hit me I would've hit him back, but you know, the experience of
that love-making after seeing the consultant, I just couldn't hit
him. I wouldn't get up the next day. But Roy got up and he put
the dinner on and saw to the children. I smelt the cooking and
thought I'd better get up and make the gravy and so I did. I felt
a bitch and I said to Roy, 'Where are those trousers?' He said,
'What trousers?' I said, 'Those trousers that were in the chair.'
He said, 'That bag, I've chucked it in the cupboard. What was in
there?' I told him and he got in a temper and said, 'Why didn't
you tell me about the trousers? I didn't realise the trousers
were down here. You can pack them up and send them back, you
aren't mending them.' But I couldn't. I said that I'd got to
mend them and I mended them. My brother came down for them last
Saturday.
INTERVIEWER: How did you react to your brother when he came down?
MRS K. DAVIS: I wouldn't talk much and he said, 'Got the miseries?'
I was very depressed. Of course, during the week my father had
come to visit me and pester me. I was just very depressed. I had
called the GP in on the Friday and I called him again in the week
after my brother had come again and told him I wanted something
done.
INTERVIEWER: So the GP made the appointment for you to see Dr Jones.
MRS K. DAVIS: Yes.
INTERVIEWER: Did Dr Jones say how he could help you?
MRS K. DAVIS: No.
INTERVIEWER: How do you think the hospital will be able to help
you?
MRS K. DAVIS: I hope they will be able to sort me out. If it is
this fear of my father I hope that they can help me to face up to
that so that I can write a letter and tell him not to see me again.
INTERVIEWER: What kind of treatment out of the following three do
you see as the most valuable for you: taking medicine, talking to
people who can understand you, or electrical treatment?
MRS K. DAVIS: I don't want medicine or electrical treatment. If
they talk to me it will help me.
INTERVIEWER: How long do you expect to be in hospital?
MRS K. DAVIS: Not long, it's inconvenient for Roy.

Mr Roy Davis

INTERVIEWER: Did you attend the outpatient consultation with your
wife?
MR R. DAVIS: Yes.
INTERVIEWER: In what way did the consultant say he would be able
to help your wife?
MR R. DAVIS: He didn't say really, except that she had to come into
hospital.
INTERVIEWER: How do you feel about her going into hospital for a
while?
MR R. DAVIS: Well I'd rather her stay here. Of course I would.
But we've got the children living amongst it all the time. It's
six lives that are being affected. We don't want her to go but
that's the only thing we can do I think.

INTERVIEWER: She told me that she was keen to go into hospital
before next Tuesday. Why is this?
MR R. DAVIS: Well her father didn't come down this Tuesday but
it is pretty guaranteed he'll come down next Tuesday. You see,
he usually visits her then because he's in the area to collect
his miner's pension. She's terrified he's coming down on Tuesday
and that's why she wants to go into hospital before then.
INTERVIEWER: That's why she's so keen.
MR R. DAVIS: Yes, I think so. As I said, things ought to be done
owing to the fact that she keeps getting the GP in and I'm worried
she's going to take some overdose. She says she's going to shut
herself in the toilet. It upsets me. It upsets the kids. I'm
at work wondering if everything is all right. I phone up everyday during my breaktime to see if everything is all right. Half
the time it wears you down as well.
INTERVIEWER: What kind of treatment out of the following three do
you think would be the most valuable for your wife: taking medicine,
talking to people who understand her, or electrical treatment?
MR R. DAVIS: This could go on for ever if she goes on tablets and
pills. I think she got a lot out of the doctor who she saw before
we went to Blacktown. He seemed to have understood her problem.
She seems to have got a lot of confidence out of him. So I think
talking to someone would be the best thing. They should sort out
what's bugging her about her father. I think it's the main problem
and possibly this will help her with her fear of going on buses and
all these other things. I think the big problem is her father and
I think some of the other problems stem from this. I want to write
him a letter to tell him to come down only when I'm here or else
stay away.
INTERVIEWER: Why don't you do that?
MR R. DAVIS: Well, she went to the doctor and he agreed but he said
how Kathy was at the moment it wouldn't be the right thing to do.
She said she felt a bit bad about it. She said how would I feel if
one of my children sent me a letter saying I should stay away.
Also she said if I were to write a letter he might come down here
and throw a fit or chuck stones through the window or something.
This is what she fears, you know.

THE PSYCHIATRIC UNIT

Mrs Davis was admitted into the unit on Tuesday, 5 February. Thus
she was able to avoid her father who she thought would visit her
at home on that day. She was joined in the unit by her youngest
child, Sally, who was ten months old. Mrs Davis felt that it was
unwise to be separated from her daughter.
    Members of Dr Jones's team had great difficulty in assessing
Mrs Davis's problem. What emerged from the ward round and the
team meeting that took place during the first week of Kathy's admission was that the consultant disbelieved Kathy's formulation
of her relationship with her father. He claimed that on any
learning theory perspective she should have learnt to cope with
him by now. He could not understand why the crisis had taken place
when it did. His puzzlement over this case was reinforced when a

staff nurse told him, during the second ward round of the week,
that Kathy only occasionally appeared distressed. Dr Jones felt
that her behaviour in this respect was unlike that of other inpatients, whose distress, typically, was enduring. Significant,
in the consultant's opinion, was the fact that Kathy hardly ever
spoke about her husband or mother. He construed Mr Davis as being
a 'doughnut' i.e. as being passive and being dominated by his wife.

Dr Jones decided that his SHO, who was newly employed in the
unit, should interview Mrs Davis. He directed her to encourage
Kathy to talk about her husband. He also asked his principal PSW
to interview Mr Davis twice with a view to marital therapy.

The SHO found it almost impossible to direct interviews in the
way the consultant had instructed. Mrs Davis was preoccupied by
her father and his aggressiveness towards her. The other part of
the treatment plan was not pursued vigorously. The two interviews
between Roy and the principal PSW, which were supposed to have
taken place during the first week of Kathy's admission, were can-
celled. Roy was unable to arrive at a suitable time for the social
worker on one occasion, and on the second occasion she was absent.
As Kathy's admission wore on it became a feature of this case that
interviews arranged between Roy and the social worker failed to
materialise on a number of occasions, principally because the
latter was periodically absent from the unit.

As a result of the team's inability clearly to assess Mrs
Davis's problem, the consultant decided that this case should be
the topic of a case conference. This was held at the end of the
first week of the patient's admission. Staff members from all the
teams in the unit participated in this meeting. A number of people
were of the opinion that Kathy's sterilisation might be responsible
for her present problems. It was felt that she might regret not
being able to have any more children. Also, Kathy's conversion to
the Jehovah's Witnesses was construed as significant by some members of staff. They wondered what this change of religion meant
to her. These issues were explored by the SHO with Mrs Davis after
the case conference.

During the first week of her admission Mrs Davis kept a daily
record for one of the authors of how she was experiencing hospital
life. The following extracts are taken from what she wrote.

5 February 1974

I was upset when the children went to school but I just kept
shutting it out of my mind.

I still don't believe I'm in here. Tell me Geoff I won't end
up mad as I want to love so much. I try to think of Roy and want
him but again I shut it out. Why?

When Roy left me he was upset and as the family were leaving I
walked away as I was getting upset but I just told myself I have
to stay here because if I go back home I'd go mad with fear. I
hate it.

We had dinner at 12 o'clock but I didn't want it. I don't want
any food, just love. Then I phoned up Roy to see if he had got
home alright.

6 February 1974

I had a pill to make me sleep last night but I kept waking up.
Then at 4 o'clock I got out of bed and had a cup of tea and took
it back to bed. But then I got out again and sat down outside
the ward and read for an hour. Then the head nurse kept telling
me to go back to bed. So I did but kept crying. I kept trying
to think of Roy and the children....
    When Roy and the children came in I didn't pretend. I took the
children upstairs and talked to them. I told them how much I love
them. After I had been with them I saw Roy on his own. Oh I do
hope the doctor can help me tomorrow....
    When I saw you I was very upset but when I got talking to some
of the other patients it was not so bad. I like talking to them
because lots of them don't know why they're like it. When I'm on
my own I want to cry so much because I know I can't go on with the
show. I want sex with my husband as it was seven weeks ago. Nothing less will do. I've come back to my bed. My baby is asleep.
I want to hold her. I love her but my father will make me hate
all of them.

8 February 1974

Got up at quarter to four as I could not sleep. I dreamed about
you and Roy and after that I couldn't sleep. First you as a friend
asking you if you would get me some Woodbines. I was upset about
something. I don't know what but you were kind. Then it went on
to Roy, my husband. I won't say anymore. I thought about you and
Roy. Roy as my husband and you as a friend. You see, always
before if Roy had looked at another woman I'd have jumped at him
because then I had never known what love, I mean real love with my
husband, was. I would say, 'You like her', and row with him, but
now I know you can have a friend or say hello to a man, if you are
a woman, or to a woman, if you are a man, without meaning what I'd
say it meant. Then all I thought of was Roy but I'm afraid if my
father was to see me I'd be cold again. I'd just go mad.
    Why can't they give me an answer to my fear?

9 February 1974

Roy came in. He made me feel good. I got so afraid that that
lovely feeling that has come back since I've been in here will go
when ... I just keep thinking of Roy, in that way I love him.
    Now I'm going to bed but my father, I'm afraid.

10 February 1974

I gave the pram a good clean for Sally but it's been a long day,
too much time to think. After dinner I put Sally in the cot and
thought about Roy while I was lying on my bed but then I thought
about my father and got very upset. The nurse came and talked to

me and I felt a little better but still afraid. But when Roy came
in I knew the feeling was still there. I think if I saw my father
just once ... I don't know. When he came down he would go on and
on. Then when he was going he would put 50p down and say, 'Buy
some chips for the children.' I would tell him I didn't want his
money but he would leave it all the same. But I don't want his
money.

12 February 1974

I saw the SHO and told her I was upset about what we had been
talking about the day before, about why I married Roy, but also
there was too much talk about my father. When I got up today I
felt dead inside, so when I talked to her today it was about Roy,
all about Roy and the children. I told her about trying to sell
the house this time last year because I wanted to get away from
dad but by the time we came back from our holiday we gave up the
idea. I hate my father for what he has done but after the talk
with the SHO I felt better as I'd been talking to her about all
the things Roy has done, and other things like my sister and her
boys, my faith and so on.
     I was glad to see my brother and his wife tonight but would
like to see more of Roy on his own. When I had to tell Simon a
little about what was going on it was about my father, nothing
about Roy and myself, not about sex.
     When they had gone home I was upset. It was because I had been
talking to Simon about my father and I don't want to talk about
him. Do you think I should? Do you think it will help in the end?
But it doesn't now. I just go dead inside and I can't understand
it. I want someone to tell me. All I want is my husband and children. Where can we hide?
     When will I get better?
     I do so want Roy but if I go home my father may come and cut me
off from Roy again, just like he did before. I don't understand
how.

The SHO reported to the ward round that took place after the case
conference that the issues of sterilisation and religious conversion held no significance in relation to Mrs Davis's problems.
She wrote in the case notes on 12 February that Kathy had 'No
regrets re sterilisation apparently. Definitely doesn't want any
more (children).' She also wrote that Kathy was converted to the
Jehovah's Witnesses 'via door to door visitor. Several questions
in Roman Catholic faith never answered for her - answered by
Jehovah's Witnesses.'
     The assessments of Kathy's state of health presented by the SHO
to the team in ward rounds during the three weeks that followed
the case conference were increasingly optimistic. The SHO told
her colleagues that Kathy was thinking of writing to her father in
order to ask him not to visit her in the foreseeable future. She
was also thinking of confronting him about his conduct towards her
when he came to visit her in the unit. The SHO also explained to
the team that the Davises had decided to put their house up for

sale and move away from the Mineway area.   Another reflection of
Kathy's improvement was the fact that she was looking forward to
going home and rejoining her family.
  The consultant was pleased by this state of affairs.   Nevertheless he remained sceptical as regards Mrs Davis's belief that her
father was the cause of her problems.
  During this period the principal PSW managed to interview Mr
Davis only once because of her recurrent absenteeism from the unit.
This situation was seen as critical by the consultant when the
team decided during a ward round that Mrs Davis should be allowed
weekend leave over 2 and 3 March, that is three and a half weeks
after she had been admitted into the unit.   The consultant considered it important that Roy be interviewed a second time and that
there should be a conjoint interview before Kathy went home.
These plans were not carried out by the team, although there were
members of staff available.
  In any event, the SHO reported to a ward round that took place
after Kathy's weekend leave that she had enjoyed a satisfactory
time at home.   The consultant was satisfied that matters were resolving themselves with this case.   He looked forward to the next
ward round when he would learn about the outcome of Mrs Davis's
meeting with her father.   This was due to take place the next day.

During the second, third and fourth weeks of her admission Mrs
Davis kept a daily record, for one of the authors, of how she was
experiencing hospital life.   The following extracts are taken from
what she wrote.

13 February 1974

I'm fed up.   I want to go home with Roy but can't just yet.
  I love Roy but tonight my two friends were with him.   I only
wanted to talk to Roy, but when we were alone after my friends had
left all we were talking about was how to get my mother in and so
on.   I got rather upset and I know that must have upset Roy.   Then
he had to go.   He had a sweet in his mouth when he kissed me.   I
wanted so much more but where can we go?   I'd rather go back and
just be happy like before, only sex every two weeks, than how I
feel inside now.

16 February 1974

My mother and sister came in.   I was upset that they were coming
as I would have to tell them.   When they came in I put on a good
face and took them upstairs.   I asked them if they knew why I was
in here.   They said, 'No.'   I said to mother, 'But you do, I told
you a long time ago that father upset me when he came down.   But
you told me not to take any notice as he always says things to
every one that are not true.'   Then she said, 'Kathy, my child,
that's not true.   If you're always going to get upset about things
like that then I don't know what.   I've always put up with him
over thirty years but I've learnt to live with it.   It's never

made my nerves bad.' Then I shouted at her and got upset and was crying. I told her I was no longer a little girl, that I was a woman. I told her I didn't understand it and I didn't expect her to but to please listen. Then I told her. At first she listened but she kept trying to butt in, saying I should feel sorry for him and 'You know what your father is like.' But I just told her to shut up and listen. When I went into all of it, about having intercourse to have a baby and all of that, she said she didn't understand it. But my sister was different. She was much better. She said she could understand. We calmed down after that.

20 February 1974

All my life, it's been one big show, even in bed. I'd hate to have to go back to that. The show can't go on. I love Roy and want to be a good wife, not to row with him over nothing or what my father has said to me, and to be a mother to my children.

24 February 1974

I hate the mornings when I wake up because of the fear. I can't breathe and feel sick. My hands are sweaty. I must get up and get the feeling away. I hope it will go soon.

26 February 1974

I get afraid most of all when I wake up. My hands shake and it feels hard to breathe, but if I make myself get up it helps a little. Then if I'm sitting down too long I sigh a lot because I feel as if I may run and jump out the window or something like that. I get very nervous. I feel I must get away, but I tell myself to stop thinking and talk to Sally. I don't like the fear, it's like when someone jumps out at you in the dark and you don't know they are there. It's just like that, it takes your breath away.

27 February 1974

The fear has not been so bad today. I'm looking forward to the weekend, but we will have to see Monday how I feel.

28 February 1974

I phoned Roy this evening. I told him David, my brother, had been in and that he had asked me whether mother and father could come in next week. I said yes and asked him to phone me at 6.30 on Monday in order to let him know definitely. I don't really want to see them but I must.

Well I'm going home tomorrow for a nice weekend. I hope every-thing will be all right.

3 March 1974

It was so good to be at home. I never went out as I didn't want
to see any one as they only ask you how you feel and I wouldn't
know how to answer them.

     But I've got to tell my father. If I don't he would only come
down again week after week and I wouldn't say any thing to him as
he doesn't know why I'm in here. Mother has told him something
but not the truth. I don't have to tell him every thing only what
I think he should know. I shall write it down tomorrow and try to
remember what I have to say. I don't really want to but I must,
there is no other answer.

4 March 1974

We had a lovely weekend but now I know I have to face up to things.
So I didn't feel too good today. I kept saying to myself, 'What
shall I say to my father when he comes in tomorrow?' But then I'd
shut it out of my mind. After dinner we went to Occupational
Therapy. I sat next to someone, she is nice, but all the time I
sat there I could smell my father. I wanted to run, it was just
like a pub. I was glad when it was tea time but I only felt bad
or sick so I went downstairs and got on my bed and cried but soon
put on a good face and went up and had tea as I knew crying
wouldn't do any good.

     I want to be free. I believe that if someone is doing some-
thing you don't like you should tell them that and I'm going to
tomorrow. All that matters to me is my husband and our children.
I know how much they miss me and need me. I'm no good to any one
in here. I don't want my family in my life and I don't want to
worry about what my father says. I'm glad it's tomorrow and not
Thursday as that would be so long to wait. I'll think of something
to say. I won't tell Roy as he will worry about me and I don't
want him to. He is lonely on his own at home. That's what he said
to me. Well he won't be lonely much longer, not just for my
father.

Four ward rounds took place in the fortnight after Kathy confronted
her father. The outcome of this meeting marked a turning point in
the assessment and treatment of Kathy's problem. Three days after
it occurred the SHO reported to her colleagues that the confrontation had not gone well for Mrs Davis. Her father had failed to
react in the violent and aggressive manner she had expected and
thus she was unable to reject him.

     This state of affairs further reduced the credibility of Kathy's
formulation of her problem in the eyes of Dr Jones and his team.
During subsequent ward rounds the team advanced a number of other
hypotheses as regards Mrs Davis's problem. When the SHO reported
that Kathy had asked her for Valium injections the consultant
wondered whether this request was motivated by a desire for a
truth drug in order to unveil a deeper reason for her problem.
Related to the consultant's speculation, the principal PSW put
forward the idea that, possibly, Mrs Davis's problems stemmed,

literally, from an incestuous relationship with her father. This
assessment met with agreement from the consultant and he advised
his SHO to pursue this thesis, in a cautious manner, with Mrs Davis.
By now the SHO was at a loss as regards how to approach the
patient's problem, since Kathy seemed further away from resolving
her relationship with her father than when she entered the unit.
In fact, the subject of incest was never raised with the patient.
   By the fifth week of Kathy's admission the principal PSW had
interviewed Mr Davis for a second time. She reported to a ward
round, towards the end of that week, that Roy had confirmed the
team's suspicion that Kathy was exaggerating the extent of her
father's violent conduct towards her. Now Kathy's version of her
problems held no credibility with the consultant and his team.
Dr Jones decided that a conjoint interview should be arranged for
the beginning of the next week. The two therapists, the SHO and
the principal PSW, were directed to discuss the state of the
Davises marriage with Roy and Kathy.
   Imperceptibly, Dr Jones's team had moved towards construing Mrs
Davis's problem as a marital one.

During the fifth and sixth week of her admission Mrs Davis kept
a daily record, for one of the authors, of how she was experiencing
hospital life. The following extracts are taken from what she
wrote. Also included in this section is a letter written by Mr
Davis, with the permission of his wife, to Kathy's parents, and
an interview held with Mr Davis by one of the authors.

5 March 1974

I thought I'd be on top by this time, but I'm not. I'm dead all
over again. I can't understand it but I've got to get better to
get back to what we had at the weekend because it's gone now.
   When the three of them came in I asked mum if she would have
Sally and said I'd like to talk to dad alone. So I did. We
talked. I told him some things. All right I wanted him to get
cross with me but he never. He never wanted me as a child, why
does he want me now? If he had got cross I could have said, 'All
right if that's how you feel we had better not see each other
again.' But he said, 'You don't want to stop your mother coming
down, it doesn't matter about me.' Then he went on about coming
down himself in the week to bring the children some chocolates
but I told him Roy and myself wanted to be on our own for a time,
but he didn't understand. I'm fed up. I want them to leave me
alone. When they went I phoned Roy, but as I was going to the
telephone I saw the woman who had earlier told Sally to shut up.
I looked at her and thought, 'You say another word and I'll smack
you right in the mouth,' and I would have. That's the old me. I
spoke to Roy and got very upset. He asked me if I was crying. I
told him I was. He got upset and said, 'That's it, I'm going to
write them a letter, I've been sitting back too long, not being
able to do anything.' I said, 'No don't, you can leave it to me,'
but I was crying and I knew my feelings were dead. Later I phoned
Roy again and said I felt a bit better. I told Roy to write the

letter but that we would talk about it when he came in. I didn't
want to leave him at home thinking about me crying, so I'm glad I
phoned him again.

Well it's all gone wrong so now I have to say it's Roy and the
children. I'm sorry but my father just does something to me,
because he never said much tonight, only a few little things. I
thought if he was nice I wouldn't get like that. I don't understand, my eyes are sore. Why does he make me dead inside and
also violent? I don't want to be like that.

7 March 1974

What a day. I hope I get up feeling better tomorrow than what I
do now. All I can think about is that I must get home even if I
feel the way I do inside. Roy seems so upset and I feel it's all
my fault. I wish it would end one way or another but I have to
go on. When I lie down I will think of Roy and the children then
I may feel better in the morning.

I've felt so afraid today. Sometimes when I was sitting down
I'd feel as if I'd do something mad if I didn't get up. The fear
gets on my nerves. I want it to go away so I can have a life like
everyone else. I had better soon. Everyone says I'm always happy
and talking. If only they knew how I felt inside, but I won't
have a long face.

9 March 1974

The day hasn't gone as slow as I thought it would. After dinner
I went out. I wanted to go to Woolworths but I couldn't make it
so I came back. I was cross with myself. I may as well be dead
than be like that, afraid to go very far and not knowing why.
After I got back I talked to the nurse. I like her but I still
don't understand. Do you think I am still afraid of my father?
If so how can I stop myself, as I'm always telling myself that he
can't hit me in any way now. So where does that leave me?

When I'm out and have this fear I just feel I have to get back.
I hate it. So I have to tell myself I have to get back to how I
was last week, just thinking of Roy and the children, just to love
them. I feel I'm not giving myself to them as I should at the
moment, and I hate myself for that. I don't know how my father
kills all my love in me and makes me feel so afraid but he does.
It must go soon so I can go home.

12 March 1974: a letter from Mr Roy Davis written to his wife's
parents

Dear Mum and Dad

I am writing to you because Kath says she would like to be left
alone when she comes out of hospital and left to put her whole
mind and thoughts to me and the children and we want to do what's
best for her and whatever she needs to be able to get her back to
herself.

It would be pointless not to do as she wants because it would only mean her going back to the hospital for I don't know how long and I can't let that happen for her sake and for me and the children.

So I am asking you all just let her come home and settle down and get back on her feet for about four months or so and Kath will write to you in between these four months and afterwards you can come down as a family when Kath feels herself again.

But I ask you all not to come down until Kath writes to you and asks you to come down after four months or so.

Because I think she's suffered enough and I won't have her hurt anymore.

Lots of love from
Roy and the children. X X X X

14 March 1974

I think I feel a little better, well happier but still afraid. Let's hope it won't be long now before the fear goes. Then I will have to see in four months what I'm like when I meet my father again. I don't know what I'm supposed to think about him. I wish I knew. I don't feel so violent today.

15 March 1974

When Roy and the children came in I felt happier but Roy said, 'You've been crying.' I don't like to say this but when Roy kissed me I felt nothing. I feel upset about it because I can't go back to him like that as I would want no part of it because I would be no good to him. It would hurt him and myself. It's no good that way. I will have to think about him more. I know sex is not everything but it bloody well helps a lot. I want to want him also, but since one week I've been talking about my father and know it's about time I thought of Roy. He means more to me.

17 March 1974

The last two days have been hell. I've been so nervous. When Roy and the children came the fear inside me made me so bad tempered with them. I wanted to talk to Roy but couldn't as the children were there. They could see I was upset.

I've been in my room most of the day. I don't want to talk to anyone.

Mr Roy Davis

INTERVIEWER: How do you see your wife's progress since she's been in the unit?
MR R. DAVIS: As I said to the principal PSW the other evening, Kathy was coming along pretty well until her father came in last Tuesday and I've noticed a sort of decline in herself since then.

INTERVIEWER: How do you feel the hospital has helped her up until now?

MR R. DAVIS: I think she's come closer to us in a sense, me and the children. She's had a different feeling towards us than she did before she went in. She wants to show more affection for me for a start. And I think sexually-wise she's happier.

INTERVIEWER: Kathy told me that you decided to send a letter to her father asking him not to visit you all for a while.

MR R. DAVIS: I wanted to do this before she went into hospital. Anyway she sort of agreed for me to do this. The hospital must have accomplished something for her to allow me to write the letter. She wanted to see it, so I thought it was better for her to see it because she might think I've put something there which mightn't ... As far as I know she's posted it.

INTERVIEWER: Why did you decide to write the letter?

MR R. DAVIS: She wanted her father to come in there to tell him how she felt and sort of have it out with him, but he came in and sort of took her by surprise. He was all sort of nice. It didn't seem to sink into him because he said he would see her again. So I thought I shall have to write a letter now and explain it to him, not to come down for a while and after than only come down as a family. If he comes when I'm here he's different, he won't keep on all the time.

INTERVIEWER: Will you tell me what you've talked about with the principal PSW?

MR R. DAVIS: About this physical thing with her father, and how he used to treat her when she was a child. It's probably gone on until now you know. As I said to the social worker she seems to have this sort of fear for him, and a fear that I can't protect her from him. Of course I said to her a man of sixty-three, he just hasn't got what it takes. All right, he may be able to say he's going to do this or he's going to do that, but at that age you just haven't got it to be able to come down and push your weight around. He might have been able to ten years ago. I think his bark is worse than his bite.

The marital interview between the Davises and the SHO and the principal PSW was the topic of discussion during the first ward round of Kathy's seventh week in the unit.

The principal PSW reported to the rest of the team that the interview had been a failure. The Davises had been reluctant to discuss the state of their marriage with the therapists. They steadfastly maintained that Kathy's relationship with her father was at the root of her problem. The social worker added that Roy had used the meeting in an inappropriate manner. Instead of exploring issues to do with the marriage he had spent most of the time attempting to elicit from the therapists the 'medical' reasons for his wife's problems and the date of her discharge from the unit. The social worker also described a situation where Kathy and Roy had been flirting with each other, in an adolescent way, during the interview. In assessing this case the social worker was of the opinion that the Davises marriage was of such a fragile nature that it needed Kathy's relationship with her father in order to survive. Without this relationship the marriage would crumble.

Marital interviews were abandoned, principally on the insistence
of Mr and Mrs Davis and also because the social worker construed
Kathy and, especially, Roy as being too rigid to change.

The consultant was astounded and angry at the way the interview
had fared. As had been the case during previous ward rounds, he
implied that Mrs Davis was malingering because she did not constantly exhibit bizarre symptoms like those of other inpatients.
In his opinion the staff were no nearer understanding the nature
of Mrs Davis's problem than when she had entered the unit over
one and a half months before. On the basis of his principal PSW's
assessment of the interview he viewed Mr Davis as being an incom-
passionate husband as well as being insensitive and lacking in
understanding. The consultant instructed his SHO to discharge
Mrs Davis from inpatient care immediately and to follow her up in
outpatients. It was as if the consultant was punishing Kathy and
her husband for not co-operating with his team.

The consultant's impetuousity placed his SHO in a compromising
situation with Mrs Davis. In an interview held a day or two before
the ward round she had agreed with the patient that Kathy should
spend a weekend at home and then be discharged from the unit during
the following week. Thus she either had to break her agreement
with Mrs Davis or reject the consultant's instruction. In fact,
she decided upon the latter course of action and carried out her
own treatment plan.

Kathy enjoyed her weekend at home. She returned to the unit on
the Sunday evening and was discharged three days later. The SHO
wrote in the case notes on 28 March 1974 that,

> In view of the diarrhoea outbreak (Mrs Davis) is to go home
> today especially in view of baby. Happy to go. Seems to be
> intent on starting 'new' life, throw away old clothes and fur-
> niture when moves to new house. No further progress with house
> buying and selling. To be seen in outpatients weekly.

During the last ten days of her admission Mrs Davis kept a daily
record, for one of the authors, of how she was experiencing hospital life. The following extracts are taken from what she wrote.

18 March 1974

I am still afraid in the mornings but hope to overcome that as time
goes by. I want to talk to Roy and not in front of the SHO and the
social worker. Roy never liked it. I agree with him. If he wants
to talk about sex he said it's with me or the consultant but not
two women. You can understand that can't you? I kept saying it
was my fault, then the social worker said the meeting of the four
of us was to see into our family, that meant Roy and myself. Do
they think we don't love each other? Anyway I know I love Roy and
I don't care what they think. If I lose him that would be the end,
that's why I don't want to hurt him again and want to make him
happy. Why have I been cold?

19 March 1974

I've been feeling so down. I just felt I would have to die if
any thing turns bad again. But I felt down all day, my first meal
was at supper.
    I phoned Roy tonight. We had a good talk and we're going to go
out Saturday night and have a meal. So I said I will go on the
bus. I hope I'll make it, I think I will.

20 March 1974

I'm so glad I can feel for Roy now. I shall have to think of him
and the children all the time. Sometimes it's hard as sometimes
my father comes back again and then I'm afraid but I soon tell
myself to stop it and just how I love Roy and how wonderful it is
being with him, then I'm happy again and feel good.
    I do hope we sell the house and move away as I long to be on our
own and I know Roy will do every thing he can to sell it as he
wants to move as much as me.

22 March 1974

If I go home and have a good weekend, which I know I will, they
will think every thing is better but it won't be. And I get afraid
because it's my father I've got to get over not sex. I know I've
always thought it's no good just to have babies but it's not like
that any more. I never want to be cold to Roy again or a bitch.
What will happen if I am. Oh bugger, I'm going to get a cup of
tea, if I stay here I'm going to cry.
    I was very afraid to go to the park today but I made it there
and back so I was pleased with myself. When we were walking, on
about four occasions, I became afraid. I thought I wanted to go
to the loo. I get so afraid but then I made myself think of good
times with Roy and it would go away. I'm so glad I'm going home
tonight. It will be so good. I hope we don't row any of the time.

25 March 1974

I feel so fed up. I don't want to talk to anyone as in the end I
don't know what to say to them. When Roy and the children came in
I wasn't very good as far as talking went. I told Roy I wanted to
come home now. He said, 'Why don't you ask?' But I shall see. I
want to be with him. Barry said, 'Only nine days now mum and you're
coming home.' I said, 'Only four days Barry.' He looked at me.
You know I miss them so much. It's not the same in here without
them running round me, saying mum this and mum that, jumping up and
down the stairs and being with Roy and talking and so on. We have
to live for today and be happy. Oh I don't want anything to go
wrong again. I hope we can move soon.

27 March 1974

Woke up today at four so I feel tired tonight. I was not very
happy today. It was fine when I was talking to Roy or you. I
shall be glad when I'm home.

Mr and Mrs Davis were interviewed by one of the authors towards
the end of Mrs Davis's admission. The following extracts are concerned with their views of the marital therapy in which they participated.

Mrs Kathy Davis

INTERVIEWER: I would like to talk about the interview you and Roy
had with the SHO and the social worker. Did you know you were
going to have such an interview when you came into hospital?
MRS K. DAVIS: No, nothing was said to me about it.
INTERVIEWER: Did the consultant ever say anything about it to you?
MRS K. DAVIS: No.
INTERVIEWER: What did you think it was for before you had it?
MRS K. DAVIS: I just thought you had to talk about how you got on
together, whether you probably could talk to each other, I suppose
probably about some of the subjects we can't talk about. Perhaps
I ought to have brought them up then, but I didn't think of it then.
INTERVIEWER: How did you see what happened then?
MRS K. DAVIS: They were trying to say that we couldn't communicate
and that they wanted to help us, such that we should talk about
things like sex, but you know we can talk about that on our own.
So it was pointless.
INTERVIEWER: How did that interview affect you?
MRS K. DAVIS: Roy wasn't going to go to another one and I thought
it may help and he said, 'If you want to agree with them instead
of me it's up to you. You can side with them.' So I thought,
'Crikey, it's making another issue,' and I said all right, we won't
go, because he got cross. He doesn't like talking. I told them my
problem wasn't Roy's fault.

Mr Roy Davis

INTERVIEWER: How did you see what happened in the interview you
and Kathy had with the SHO and the social worker?
MR R. DAVIS: I saw it as a waste of time, that's putting it bluntly.
I didn't think we got anything out of it really because we sat there
most of the time staring at one another almost and I didn't really
know what they were trying to get at. If they would have asked me
a question, like you're doing, and I would have given an answer, it
would have been easier. They didn't do it that way ... whether they
wanted us to talk sexually-wise I don't know because I felt a bit
embarassed. There were two women (the therapists) and I feel a bit
embarassed about talking about sex in front of women you know. I
didn't feel we achieved anything. It just got all four of us
irritated.

Summary of a letter written by the SHO on 3 April 1974 to Mrs Davis's GP:

The SHO wrote that Mrs Davis had been admitted on 5 February following increasing difficulty in coping with the situation at home. She said that Mrs Davis had complained of being nervous and frightened 'to the state of being shaky'. Mrs Davis had not been sleeping well and had been failing in her housework and the emotional care of her children.

The SHO assessed Kathy's problems as centring around an unresolved relationship with her father. She had left home at the tender age of sixteen in order to get married and immediately start upon a family, and since then had had a fairly up and down marriage with little communication between her and her husband. The SHO went on to say that the Davises had made Kathy's father responsible for failures in their marriage and in Kathy's motherhood and that the team had almost felt that it had been the father who had been keeping the family together in a 'roundabout sort of way'. When Mrs Davis had been discharged her sexual problems had seemed to have been resolved to a certain extent but the SHO was of the opinion that she was still clinging to the source of her problem being her father.

Mrs Davis would be seen in outpatients at regular intervals.

OUTPATIENTS

Mrs Davis resumed contact with the SHO in outpatients two weeks after she had been discharged from the unit as an inpatient.

During that admission she had steadfastly clung to the notion that her relationship with her father was responsible for her unsatisfactory sexual relationship with her husband, her bad-temperedness towards him and the children and her fear of open spaces and travelling. She had refused to capitulate to the staff's view that fundamentally her marriage was fragile and unsound, and more specifically that there was a gross lack of communication between her and her husband.

It is ironic to note that when she came to her first outpatient appointment she withdrew her conception of the problem. Instead she confirmed the staff's marital thesis. The SHO wrote in the case notes on 10 April 1974 the following:

Came in and poured out her problems - not father at all - husband - he's had two affairs, though not sexual, but lied to her about them. She feels terribly insecure - he's threatening to leave and she's threatening to divorce him. If he has another woman friend (last one three years ago), will she forgive and forget - never sorted these things out between each other before and still he's very reluctant to talk i.e. won't co-operate with her. Obviously he's had to look at himself again - hurt re her not enjoying sex - now making a great show of eyeing up other women and saying Kathy might be a lesbian. She laughs and says she hates women because of the threat to her re Roy, but could there be some truth in this?

Wanting to get into hospital again - discussed - no answer to the problem which must be solved at home.

It is worth speculating how this reversal of views came about. Undoubtedly the staff were correct in assuming that the Davises' marriage had its problems. They were aware of Roy's so-called affair with the American woman while Kathy was pregnant with Fiona. But it is not unreasonable to suppose that the staff amplified the problematic nature of the marriage such that the patient's view of her problem was accordingly influenced. They did so by paying more attention to the state of the marriage than to Mrs Davis's feelings and views about her father. Thus in the opinion of the authors the change in Kathy's conception of her problem was as much a product of a self-fulfilling prophecy generated by the staff as it was a reflection of reality.

Mr and Mrs Davis were interviewed, by one of the authors, approximately one month after she had been discharged from the unit as an inpatient.

Mrs Kathy Davis

INTERVIEWER: While you were in hospital did you change the way you saw your problem in any way?
MRS K. DAVIS: No. I went in because my father was interfering with our marriage; if it hadn't been for my father it wouldn't have occurred.
INTERVIEWER: Did going into hospital help you in the way you expected it to? I would like to remind you of something here, I think you expected to be provided with answers.
MRS K. DAVIS: I don't really think it was a good idea myself, but still. It doesn't answer anything, not really. By talking to others who have the same situation, the same trouble, that helps. Even the doctors don't really understand you fully unless they've had it themselves. There was a lot there that were worse than I was. But it helped in a way because it helped me get away from my father. In there I was protected. If I would have stayed here he would have still come down. I shouldn't have been able to say, 'I don't want you to come down for a little while, just leave me alone.' And it would have gone on and on.
INTERVIEWER: Would you evaluate the treatment you had?
MRS K. DAVIS: I saw the SHO four times a week when I went there. It gradually went down. I did most of the talking while she sat back and sometimes she would get a bit impatient because she didn't know how to answer my questions. I couldn't blame her, I couldn't answer them if she had asked me, and she didn't know.
INTERVIEWER: In what way didn't she know?
MRS K. DAVIS: Because she didn't understand how my father could affect me. Don't suppose anybody would. I don't. But when I went in Wednesday (i.e., to outpatients), the subjects I was talking about she was quite nice about and answered quite sensibly.
INTERVIEWER: Kathy, how has it been settling down again since you left the unit?
MRS K. DAVIS: Quite hard really. Coping with Roy is the hardest.
INTERVIEWER: In what way?
MRS K. DAVIS: Because I get possessively jealous.

INTERVIEWER: Why?
MRS K. DAVIS: I always was like that but I learnt to control myself.
Then I found out that certain incidents were true and it all started
again.
INTERVIEWER: When did you talk about that with Roy?
MRS K. DAVIS: On the Tuesday before I went to see the SHO in out-
patients.
INTERVIEWER: What led up to you speaking about that?
MRS K. DAVIS: When we had the leaflets about the houses in
Blacktown.
INTERVIEWER: Will you go on and explain what happened?
MRS K. DAVIS: I read them and got upset and thought I didn't want
to go back there.
INTERVIEWER: Why?
MRS K. DAVIS: I didn't know really, just the name, her name kept
going through my mind.
INTERVIEWER: Whose name?
MRS K. DAVIS: This woman, Doris.
INTERVIEWER: Will you explain what happened in Blacktown?
MRS K. DAVIS: I'd just had Barry and Roy had had an accident and
he was at home for a little while. Then he went back to work. I
didn't know what I was looking for but I found a letter in Roy's
pocket saying she wanted him to prove his love, that there are lots
of men in the same situation as him and she wanted to meet him at
9.30. I was in such a rage I took the children to the phone box
and phoned up Roy at work and asked if he was there and they said
yes, so I thought good. So I waited until he came home and questioned him about it and he said a boy gave it to him on the bus,
that he'd picked it up off the floor, bloody fool. And so I
thought, can't say much about that and then a little while later I
found the same writing in an envelope in the back of the cupboard
and I knew it had been in Roy's pocket because it had his indelible
pencil on there and so I cross-examined him about that. I was very
upset about it. He didn't care, he wouldn't admit to anything. He
didn't care what I did. I threw myself on the floor and screamed
and so I then went up to see Dr Marks and he said, 'You'll have to
try and put it to the back of your mind.' I didn't like what he
said much but I thought I suppose I shall have to put it to the
back of my mind. But I couldn't because I didn't know whether it
was right or wrong. Anyway I never mentioned much more about it,
but gradually I couldn't go out anywhere and this woman, silly
bitch, she just looked at me in Tortan.
INTERVIEWER: Where?
MRS K. DAVIS: In Tortan, he says it wasn't her. Roy still says it
wasn't her.
INTERVIEWER: Was it after this that you got this fear about going
out?
MRS K. DAVIS: I'd go so far and I'd think I must get back home.
INTERVIEWER: Why?
MRS K. DAVIS: I'd want to go to the loo, I was frightened.
INTERVIEWER: So this was brought up again....
MRS K. DAVIS: Before I went to see the SHO.
INTERVIEWER: Had you and Roy not been getting on?
MRS K. DAVIS: He kept looking at other women. I think he was only

doing it to annoy me. I just lost my temper. He said he felt
sorry for this woman Doris.
INTERVIEWER: What has all this to do with why you came into hospital?
MRS K. DAVIS: It has nothing to do with it. It is in me this
terrible thing about adultery; there is something there that is
distasteful to me. I suppose I've just got to learn to control
my temper and accept it.
INTERVIEWER: Are you going to be moving house in the future?
MRS K. DAVIS: Roy says that if he doesn't move by the summer he's
going to get another job. So therefore I think if he gets another
job it's because there's no women up at Roystons.
INTERVIEWER: You don't want to move now.
MRS K. DAVIS: Yes I want to move. It's no good for us staying
here.
INTERVIEWER: Have you heard from your parents since you've been
back?
MRS K. DAVIS: No. I wrote my mother a letter, I posted it today.
All I've been wanting to do is talk to Roy and get his attention.
He doesn't want to give it much and I just want to be able to go
out and not be afraid and be able to control my temper and not be
afraid of bloody adultery. I've always been jealous. When I was
going out with Roy I used to write letters to him and on the bottom
tell him to make sure he behaved himself. That's partly why I saw
Dr Marks. I was accusing Roy of adultery for no reason at all and
I was becoming like my father. He used to accuse my mother of
adultery and say she's got a fancy man.

Mr Roy Davis

INTERVIEWER: Do you see Kathy's problems differently from the way
you saw them when she first was admitted to hospital?
MR R. DAVIS: She seems to see two problems now. It's just not her
father, it's partly me as well, and it's something that has just
come up recently which Kathy thinks is the problem why she can't
go out or won't go on the bus. And this was a problem when I was
in Blacktown and I was on the buses and a woman wrote me some
letters and this sort of thing although I never went out with her
or anything like that. Kathy found them in my pocket and it upset
her and she used to think that when she was going on the bus people
used to look at her and this sort of thing.
INTERVIEWER: Were you working on the buses?
MR R. DAVIS: Yes. And this problem has come up recently since she's
been at home and she's asked me to talk about it. I did, as much
as I could remember, and she said by me explaining it to her, by
going into all the details, it would help her. This is a thing
which, I'm afraid, she throws at me now, so I don't know whether I
should have said it or not really. You see Kathy said I told her
that the letters I had on me was what I found on the bus. She
didn't really believe it but she never sort of said much about it
until now, when she's been thinking about it a bit recently
apparently.
INTERVIEWER: Since she's come out of the hospital.

MR R. DAVIS: She said she was thinking about it a bit while she was in hospital, but it's sort of piled up on top of her since she's been home.

INTERVIEWER: Given this state of affairs and the trouble Kathy has had with her father, what effect has all this had on you in relation to your marriage?

MR R. DAVIS: Since Kathy's been home she's flared up a few times and told me to pack my case. But you know, I think I wouldn't go because of the children and they're sort of what really holds you together. Probably if it would only be me and Kathy we'd have probably split up and lived separately for a time but we probably would have come back together again, but when she sort of packs my case and this sort of thing you feel you'd like to; well, she wants me to clear off for a couple of weeks, it would shake her up a bit. I haven't felt like leaving through other women. I wanted to leave because it's really on top of me. For instance, if we go up the street together, there's a woman walking by, I daren't sort of look at the woman, I'm frightened she's sort of going to speak to me. Because I've been born here there's a lot of women I know in Mineway. I haven't sort of been out with them but I went to school with them. They say hello and if I say hello back to them our Kathy will swear blind I've been out with them. And it's this sort of thing which puts you on edge.

INTERVIEWER: Do you think being in hospital helped Kathy?

MR R. DAVIS: It helped her sexually, she enjoys sex now whereas she didn't before. She wants more affection taken over her than she did before. She wants a lot more understanding, more concern. She feels more sorry for herself is her way of putting it. She's sort of very possessive, as I say I haven't got to look the wrong way and I've had it. It's an awkward position to be in really, it gets you very fed up and ends up with a lot of rows.

INTERVIEWER: Would you elaborate on how life's been for both of you since Kathy's been discharged?

MR R. DAVIS: There's been a lot of difficulties with a lot of rows. Life is quite difficult at the moment because we've got the house up for sale and since I've had time off from work I've gone a bit low on cash. I suppose if it was just Kathy alone without having to worry about the house it would be bad enough.

INTERVIEWER: How have you found going back to work?

MR R. DAVIS: Killing. It makes you feel a bit tired the first couple of days until you're settled back again. I don't like working there very much.

INTERVIEWER: What are you hoping to do in the future?

MR R. DAVIS: It's up to what Kathy wants to do, really. If she wants to move away then we'll move away. If she wants to move to another house then we'll move. We wanted to move to Wontsea and she said that since that happened with the woman in Blacktown it might happen in Wontsea and she doesn't want to move away from people she knows down here.

INTERVIEWER: Will you change your job if you stay here?

MR R. DAVIS: Yeah, I don't feel I'm achieving anything working there. I'm just on the end of a machine banging books on a table. It drives you crackers, it really does. It's just wasting time, it's wasting your life really. I like mixing with people. That's

why with the bus work, I used to like mixing with people on the
buses. I should like to do things where I achieved things. I
like artistic painting quite a bit or the social side of work where
you would feel you were doing something useful, whereas up there
you're in dead man's shoes.

During April, May and June Kathy continued to be interviewed by
the SHO on a fortnightly basis. The material that emerged during
this period was mainly to do with Mrs Davis's views about the
relative poverty of her relationship with Roy. Indeed, towards
the end of May a second marital interview took place, between the
Davises and the SHO and the principal PSW, after a particularly
violent row beteeen Roy and Kathy.
    But suddenly, at the end of June, Kathy was discharged from out-
patient care apparently 'cured'. This remarkable improvement had
little or nothing to do with the therapy she had been receiving.
For some time there had been a growing conflict between Kathy and
the elders of her local branch of Jehovah's Witnesses. They had
told her repeatedly that she had to give up smoking or she would
be disfellowshipped. She did not comply with their demands and
was sumarily disowned by the sect. Coincidental with this freedom
from the Witnesses was an immediate improvement in her relationship
with Roy, a new-found ability to go out and travel without experiencing any fear, an improvement in her relationship with her
parents and a less urgent desire to move away from the area.
    These changes resulted in Mrs Davis reappraising the nature of
her problems, in terms of her relationship with the Jehovah's
Witnesses. She described the religion as one that generated fear
in its members. In an article about her conflict with the Witnesses
that appeared in a local newspaper it was reported that, 'Her personality was happy-go-lucky before she became a Witness ... but
when she became a member she had to keep herself apart from the
world and became a "cabbage".' She now claimed, speculatively,
that her affiliation to the Witnesses before Roy became a member
(four years after she had joined) was responsible for his 'adul-
terous' behaviour. It was the duty of every Witness to persuade
non-converts to join the sect. In carrying out this practice in
relation to Roy she must have alienated him from her. Likewise she
claimed she must have alienated her parents from her.
    It is sad to write here that this dissipation of her problems
was more apparent than real. Shortly they were to re-emerge with
increased severity.

POSTSCRIPT

Mrs Davis's liberation from the Jehovah's Witnesses did not free
her of her problems for long. Within a month of being discharged
from outpatient care most of them had returned. While under inpatient care she had located her father as the source of her problems; after she had been discharged she had blamed first Roy and
then the Jehovah's Witnesses. But from July 1974 to March 1975
she did not attribute responsibility for her problems to anyone or
anything. She was frustrated and depressed because she was unable
to find a solution to them.

In February 1975 she wrote to one of the authors saying,

I feel so depressed. I don't feel like doing anything, only to go to bed and hide. Why won't the fear go? I'm still so afraid. I think I know why but everyone says, 'Don't be silly, you must put it out of your mind. Forget.' But I've tried to do it, but I just can't. (How can you forget something that hasn't happened?)

All I do is smoke and drink but that's all right I can live off my fat.

All I want to do is cry because no one knows how I feel inside. I don't want to be like a cabbage.

It was a year ago when I went into hospital but I feel just the same inside as I did then.

From April 1975 Mrs Davis's frustrations gradually centred around her inability to achieve orgasm with her husband. As her frustration worsened her relationship with Roy deteriorated and he became identified as the 'problem' - 'I've blamed myself for too long' (Mrs K. Davis).

In May she wrote to one of the authors, claiming that she felt 'So depressed and frustrated about Roy. I don't know what to do about it. I can't really believe he hates me for the past, or put it another way, that I stopped him from playing around.' She was adamant that he treated her cruelly and abused her.

Some days when I get up I could break everything in the house, but that wouldn't do much good. Roy would only say, 'You're bloody mad, the doctors know it, everyone does. No one likes you, you're sexless, fat.' For God's sake why doesn't he say nice things? If I'm really like my dad I'd be on at the children. But I'm not my dad, I'm not good, I'm not bad, I'm me, KATHY. If Roy doesn't love me why stay and hurt me all the time?

Her contact with the unit since she was discharged from outpatients has been minimal. She and her husband were occasionally interviewed by the consultant and the principal PSW, but little was achieved by these meetings. On one occasion she sought admission into the unit on an informal basis. She arrived at Porchester demanding inpatient care but was turned away by the staff.

Recently she has strained the resources of the general practice in her area by occasionally taking small overdoses of tablets and medicine. Her GP, who has an exhaustive knowledge of Mrs Davis's problems, has been participating in marital therapy with the Davises. He believes there are indications of some improvement. Roy and Kathy are beginning realistically to appraise the state of their marriage whereas previously they had been slandering each other.

SUMMARY

1 The length of Mrs Davis's admission in the unit, seven weeks in all, was not in keeping with the policy of general hospital psychiatric units of short-term admissions.

2 As in the case of Mrs Smith, the staff failed to clarify the basis of hospitalisation with either Mrs Davis or her husband. Thus the patient and her spouse were unaware that they would be

expected to participate in marital or conjoint interviews.   Another consequence of this failure to 'contract' the patient was that Mrs Davis was allowed to assume, for most of her admission, that the staff agreed with her conception of her problem.   Clearly this was not the case.

3 As in the cases of Mrs Smith and Mrs Wright, there was a divorcement between decisions made at ward rounds about the treatment of the patient and the day-to-day treatment programme.   For example, on many occasions the principal PSW failed to interview Mr Davis after the team had decided that this was necessary. Another example was related to the implementation of marital interviews.   The consultant decided that it was imperative that a conjoint interview should take place before Mrs Davis went on her first weekend leave early on in her admission.   Mrs Davis went home but the interview failed to materialise.

4 The staff were partially correct in assessing the patient's problem as a marital one, but the evidence suggests that the nature of her problem was more complex.   There is little doubt that the relationship between Mrs Davis and her father was such that it had a disturbing influence on her and her marriage.   In the opinion of the authors the limitation of the staff's formulation stemmed from a lack of diversity in the 'models' they used to understand psychological disturbance.   In general there was a bias towards formulating patient's problems in terms of the marital dyad.   One explanation for this bias lies in the social background of the staff, which was exclusively middle-class.   The staff were unable to understand that Mrs Davis's extended family continued to play an important part in her life.   The patient's parents lived in the same locality as Mrs Davis and her brothers, and regularly visited all of them.   In fact, Mr Fletcher visited his daughter more frequently than the rest of the family because she lived near the place he went to collect his pension every week.   Given this, a basis existed for the continuation of the relationship the patient had experienced with her father when she had been living at home.

5 The staff failed to carry out domiciliary visits.   Had they done so the social distance between the patient and the staff might have been bridged.   It would have been possible for them to experience some of the 'flavour' of Mrs Davis's home background.

6 The consultant often pointed out, during ward rounds, that Mrs Davis did not display distressing symptoms of an enduring nature like those of other inpatients.   But this is not surprising, since the patient construed the unit as an asylum.   As an inpatient she felt protected from the demands her father made on her.

7 As in the cases of Mrs Smith and Mrs Wright, there was a lack of contact between the consultant and the day-to-day treatment of the patient.   Thus, he intervened in the case in such a way, after the conjoint interview had taken place, that he placed his SHO in a compromising situation.   He instructed her to discharge the patient immediately, when she had agreed with Mrs Davis that she should spend a weekend at home before leaving the unit permanently. The SHO therefore either had to break her agreement with the patient or ignore the consultant's instruction.   She chose the latter course of action.

8 As in the case of Mrs Wright, the issue of patient-therapist

compatibility was evident in the case of Mrs Davis. The failure of
the marital interview stemmed from the unwillingness of Mr and Mrs
Davis to discuss the nature of their marriage. They were unwilling
to do so partly because they disagreed with the therapists' formulation that the state of the marriage was responsible for the
patient's problem. But another factor related to the failure of
the interview was to do with Mr Davis and the two therapists.
Understandably, he found it extremely difficult and embarrassing
to discuss the physical side of his marriage with two women who
were virtual strangers to him.

   9 After Mrs Davis was discharged from inpatient care she re-
appraised her problem as a marital one, whereas previously she had
vigorously denied the staff's suggestion in this respect. It is
worth speculating about how much this reappraisal was generated
by the staff and how much it was a reflection of reality.

Part four

Conclusion

Conclusion

The case histories we have presented in the last three chapters
indicate that the psychiatric unit at Porchester Hospital experienced a variety of problems in discharging its diagnostic and
therapeutic functions. The salient weaknesses of the unit as a
diagnostic and therapeutic setting can be briefly listed as
follows.

1 Ironically, the unit was situated within a large and foreboding nineteenth-century general hospital which was geographically
isolated from the community it serves. The unit's relationship
with the community was so weak that many of the specific problems
that psychiatric units are meant to avoid were depressingly still
evident. The unit's staff members were effectively 'institution-
alised' – they rarely made domiciliary visits to their patients
and they were not involved in the communities from which their
patients came, so they could never develop an understanding of the
patients' way of life or devise methods for using community resources to help the patients.

2 The complexity of the patients' problems was revealed by
interviewing in depth, particularly in the patients' own homes.
The findings of these interviews contrasted with the relatively
shallow and anecdotal formulations made by staff members who were
often operating from hearsay or from very partial and misleading
contacts with the patient.

3 Since the unit was staffed by personnel with very different
social and professional backgrounds, staff attitudes to patients
were often mutually contradictory. Thus the overall therapeutic
philosophy of the unit was belied by the very obvious fact that
staff members could not agree about basic diagnostic and therapeutic issues.

4 Due to the hierarchical structure of the treatment teams within
the unit, decision-making was often heavily biased by interventions
from the senior medical staff who had virtually no contact with the
patient during the period of hospitalisation. This often led junior
staff members to act on their own initiative and go against decisions that they saw as arbitrary and unhelpful for their patients.

5 Even when agreed diagnostic and therapeutic formulations were
established at decision-making meetings, they normally conflicted

with the day-to-day treatment of the patient so that there was a
divorcement between theory and practice.

6 The staff failed to establish the true basis of hospitalisation
with the patients and their relatives. This often meant that the
expectations of the patient and significant others with respect to
the purpose of hospitalisation were incongruent with those of the
staff. This state of affairs often limited the prospects of effective treatment.

We have already discussed some specific aspects of these points
in the earlier chapters, but in this chapter we are concerned primarily with the relationship between the structure of the unit and
its decision-making processes. However, we begin our discussion
by examining the sixth point first, since in many ways the unit's
inadequacies in dealing with the process of hospitalisation established a mode of dealing with the patient which tended to set a
pattern for later developments.

THE TREATMENT BARRIER AND THE NOTION OF CONTRACT

The process of hospitalisation itself cannot be fully understood
and evaluated without in turn analysing first the culturally derived
definitions of mental disorder that influence patients' behaviour
and second the nature and content of the sick role which the patient
enters as a prelude to being hospitalised. We seek to establish
that it is the culturally derived expectations associated with the
sick role that form a barrier that makes all forms of psychotherapy
extremely problematic. But at the same time we would argue that
these expectations are conducive to other forms of treatment -
especially physical treatments and drug therapies, which require
a passive-dependent type of patient who will follow the doctor's
instructions.

Our views are based partly on the work of Scott (1973), who has
argued that a treatment barrier will exist inevitably whenever a
person has been labelled as being mentally ill by a doctor or
another form of authority. The barrier arises because the culturally accepted view of mental illness does not allow that the
relationships between the patient and his relatives are crucial
since they influence both the nature of the disorder and possible
therapeutic outcomes. Scott therefore insists that the treatment
barrier has to be penetrated before effective treatment can begin.

Scott assumes that the cultural view of mental illness can be
best understood by examining first Parsons' classic work on the
sick role (1951 a and b, 1952) and second Mechanic's more recent
exploration of the illness behaviour (1962), i.e. the actual behaviour of individuals when they enter (or run the risk of entering)
the sick role. Parsons assumes that the sick role involves both
rights and duties as the following formal definition indicates:

1 The sick person is exempted from certain of his social obli-
gations and commitments which are taken over by others.

2 It is a condition that he is unable to recover by a conscious
act of will; i.e., he cannot help it. Thus his disability is
regarded as something for which he cannot be held responsible.

3 He is obligated to want to get well. That is, he is

responsible for seeking and accepting treatment. He must regard
the sick role as an undesirable one.

4 He is regarded as being in need of competent help, and since
he is obligated to want to get well, his status as a 'sick person'
is conditional on his becoming a patient.

Parsons argues that entry into the sick role is dependent upon
adequate evidence of the presence of a disease process that would
justify this role. This immediately causes a difficulty in relation to mental disorder since the presence or absence of disorder depends as much upon subjective assessment by both patients
and relatives and indeed by doctors themselves. But this issue
detracts from the central issue that we wish to explore. In
Parsons's terms entry into the sick role involves a crucial transfer
of responsibility. The patient is seen as not being responsible
for his illness nor for his own treatment. The doctor intervenes
precisely in order to provide the treatment, and the patient recip-
rocates by carrying out his instructions. Passivity-dependence and
activity-dominance are built into this reciprocal role structure
from its inception. However, and this is a crucial point, Mechanic
correctly cautions us against accepting that the medical profession
is solely responsible for determining entry to the sick role. He
points out that whether symptoms are acted upon depends on their
'visibility' as indicators of deviancy. The person defined as
mentally ill is brought into the hospital primarily as the result
of lay decisions. But the laymen involved usually presume that
the patient is in hospital as a result of medical decisions and
expert knowledge. By making the doctor responsible for admission,
the patient and his family members are able to evade the reality
of the painful things that they may have suffered, and it places
the doctor in a position of pseudo-authority which is likely to
impair his effectiveness in treatment.

Scott (1973) graphically explores how the cultural defence of
medical intervention is brought into effect when, through the pains
and threats of their interpersonal conflicts, family members reach
a threshold and suddenly see the behaviour of one member of their
family as being beyond understanding. The patient's behaviour is
construed as unpredictable and the hospital then has to admit the
patient. The relatives and the patient usually assume that this
is an obligation not open to question. Admissions on this basis
usually mean that the hospital staff are forced to draw a line
which rigidly divides the ill from the well. Relationships between
the patient and relatives become severed and disconnected. Also
those aspects of the patient's behaviour that are threatening to
his relatives are seen by them as forms of disturbance in the
patient. Obviously, this then allows relatives to not see themselves as part of the treatment process, since to be involved with
treatment would mean a violation of the cultural view of mental
illness.

It is not only relatives who deny their agency in the admission
process. Scott claims, on the basis of his clinical experience at
Napsbury Hospital, that patients do not see themselves as responsible for being in hospital. They typically attribute their admission to the agency of others since they know that the role of
the mental patient is that he is not responsible for his actions.

Admission for patients by crisis usually represents an escape
from an intolerable interpersonal situation, as it is for the
relatives. But discharge is equally problematic. As Scott says,
'time and again it has been very evident that patients do not
want to leave hospital, they want refuge but this cannot be
admitted' (Scott, 1973).

Although the cases we monitored at the Porchester unit were
admissions by referral from outpatient clinics rather than directly
from GPs, they conformed to the pattern outlined by Scott. In the
cases of Mrs Smith and Mrs Wright, family members initiated the
patients' hospitalisation process. In both cases the patient was
seen as displaying behaviour that could not be tolerated within
the family setting. For example, Mr Wright sought psychiatric help
for his wife because he construed her overt spiritualist behaviour
as unacceptable within the family setting. Moreover, in these
cases both patients denied any agency in being admitted into hospital.

In all three cases the therapists were placed in a position of
total responsibility by family members and patients. This meant
that it was virtually impossible to gain the active participation
of both patients and family members in the treatment process. For
example, in the case of Mrs Davis the patient saw the medical staff
as endowed with magical cures. It took virtually the length of her
admission to persuade her that this was not the case and that treatment demanded her active involvement. Therapists typically encountered difficulty in gaining the participation of spouses in marital
therapy. Frequently they could not understand why they were being
required to join in therapy with their wives when the latter had
been labelled 'ill' and had been hospitalised by medical authority.
This state of affairs was exemplified most clearly in the case of
Mrs Smith. The therapist expected Mr Smith to participate in
marital therapy on an equal basis with his wife. Instead, he acted
as an interpreter of her problems in the two abortive conjoint
sessions that took place after Mrs Smith's first admission. Indeed,
in all three cases the husband construed the medical staff as responsible for the patient's treatment.

Scott's contention that hospital admission represents an escape
from an intolerable interpersonal situation is also borne out by
the evidence contained in the cases we have reported. For example,
in the case of Mrs Davis the patient was seeking refuge from a
problematic relationship with her father. In the case of Mrs Wright
the patient connived with her husband's desire for her to seek
psychiatric help because she sought refuge from an unbearable
marital situation. When asked, at an interview, what being in
hospital meant to her, Mrs Wright replied that, 'It's been wonderful
to be free, in that I've loved being able to join in all sorts of
things without wondering whether Jim would approve, or whether it
would upset the family harmony.'

Our study of Porchester unit, therefore, supports Scott's claim
that the cultural view of mental illness, which is based on the
idea that the behavioural norms applying to physical illness apply
equally to mental illness, is an obstacle in the treatment of
patients and relatives. Scott's work is heavily biased towards
examining the influence of the medical model on the community and

the ways in which patients and family members use it to cope with interpersonal problems. He does discuss the crucial role that hospital staff tend to play in colluding with patients and their relatives over issues relating to hospital admission. However, his analysis does not contain an historical dimension so he fails to point out that the staff's conformity with cultural definitions of mental illness is a direct result of the fact that historically the psychiatric profession was able to establish the medical model as the only legitimate model for construing mental disorder. Lay views of mental disorder became conditioned by the profession's view, so that many contemporary views of mental disorder clearly originated from views which were initially confined to the profession itself.

Scott's ideas were originally developed as a result of his work at Napsbury and it may appear at first sight to have little relevance to the work of the Porchester unit as the members of staff clearly did not accept the medical model in a simple and straightforward way. However, it is clear that the consultants failed to confront the problem of the treatment barrier when admitting patients. By failing to clarify the basis of hospitalisation with patients and family members, the consultants implicitly colluded with their conceptions of the problem and their expectations regarding hospital admission. Almost without exception these were contradictory to those of the staff. As we have seen, this often meant that dislocations occurred in the therapeutic process. Many of the junior members of staff, who were the therapists in the inpatient situation, found it difficult to carry out psychotherapy because patients had been allowed to enter the unit without a realistic discussion with staff about their expectations and the plans of the unit with respect to treatment.

For example, consultants did not inform patients and their relatives during initial interviews that admission was conditional. In all three of our cases discussed, a condition of hospital admission was that the patient's spouse would be required to participate in marital therapy. None of the spouses was fully aware of the necessity for his involvement until his wife had been in hospital for some time. Initially they all resisted participating in marital therapy on an equal basis with their wives. If we refer to Scott's analysis of the treatment barrier we may understand why this was the case. The process of hospitalisation is construed as distinguishing those who are ill, and thus who require treatment, from those who are well. Therefore it is not hard to see why a spouse reacts passively to marital therapy when his partner has been hospitalised. In the cases we have documented this stance was invoked as a means of avoiding interpersonal conflicts.

At a practical level the senior staff in the unit handled issues relating to the treatment barrier in very contradictory ways. At decision-making meetings there was much discussion of the significance of patients' interpersonal problems. And yet, in other situations, particularly when patients and relatives were present, there was a tendency to behave towards them as if only the patients were ill. Now it may be argued that such inconsistencies are inevitable in the complex situations that arise in psychiatric units, but this argument can be countered by reviewing the work of units

that have sought to confront and eradicate such problems.   In
practice, these have involved attempts to establish working con-
tracts with both patients and relatives.   The very notion of a
contract between a patient and a doctor immediately confronts
the treatment barrier itself because it assumes that the patient
is an agent and is therefore capable of taking responsibility for
his actions.

THE USE OF CONTRACT-MAKING PROCEDURES

Some recent work by Cooklin (1974) is a particularly interesting
example of this type of approach.   Cooklin utilises a very broad
notion of contract which he views as 'the area of understanding
and agreement between the patient and ward staff about how they
perceive themselves, and each other and the job in hand'.   In
practice Cooklin includes a wider spectrum of persons involved in
the contract-making process, for example the patient's 'significant
others' (typically his immediate family) and the referring agent
(typically a GP).   In Scott's terms the employment of a contract-
making procedure is an attempt to make patients and their families
share the responsibility for their problems and the purpose of
hospitalisation with members of staff.   Cooklin studied the introduction of contract-making procedures into an acute female admission ward situated in a large mental hospital and university
department of psychiatry complex.   The ward was the only one with
a small lockable section, since it was responsible for admitting
the most problematic cases.   A significant proportion of its
patients admitted in crises were transient in the city and therefore
had no roots in the local community.
     Within the mental hospital itself the ward was seen as a dumping
ground for patients that other units could not cope with.   The
difficulties of the unit were amplified by the fact that it had a
high teaching commitment and patients were therefore likely to be
interviewed by students as well as staff.
     There was a high rate of staff turnover and patient turnover,
and there was a high case load of personality disorders.
     These factors combined to make the ward a highly confusing and
unsatisfactory therapeutic setting.   For example, staff often complained of being unable to be involved with patients' distress,
especially that of the personality-disordered group.   The validity
of their treatment was often questioned and compared negatively
with the clear-cut treatment of the psychotic group of patients.
     Cooklin cites three factors that provided the impetus for the
ward to reappraise the goals of admission.   First, there were
divisions between staff and patients which hindered the development
of milieu therapy.   Second, there was staff dissatisfaction.
Third, the staff found the medical model conceptually inadequate
in coping with patients' problems, especially problems in living.
     Initial discussions were held by staff in order to identify the
ward's problems and its needs.   The discussions concluded that it
was necessary to: (1) improve communication between the staff group
in order that those staff members involved in the treatment process
other than the admitting doctor should know the purpose and

significance of admission; (2) improve communications between
staff and patient groups; (3) clarify the goals of inpatient treatment; (4) improve the management of 'acting out' and demanding
patients.

To these ends a procedure was established so that there was
always a staff-patient contract conference held within forty-eight
hours of admission.   The staff were represented on an interdiscip-
linary basis so that all of the helping professions within the ward
were represented at each conference.   A specially designed record
card was introduced - this documented six different sets of information:

1 the overt and suggested covert reasons for the patient's
   referral;
2 the patient's stated needs;
3 the patient's needs as seen by the referring agent;
4 the patient's needs as seen by the ward staff;
5 the primary referral source;
6 the patient's previous inpatient, outpatient and day-patient
   treatment, and his length of psychiatric history.

The degree of agreement achieved on these issues between staff and
patient was rated and recorded on the card, and the staff also
predicted what the patient might gain from the admission and its
appropriate duration.

The information for the record card was derived from the conference, in which the patient (and sometimes relatives of the
patient) was interviewed.   After the initial meeting the staff met
on their own to fill out the record card.   If there were any areas
of conflict or misunderstanding evident between the staff and
patient they would meet again, and then the degree of agreement
would be assessed.

Initially many patients were hostile to the contract-making
conference.   For example, some patients claimed that they had been
sent to the hospital because they were ill and that it was unfair
to ask them what they wanted.   Some of the psychotic patients
became more incomprehensible and others relinquished their symptoms.
During the early months staff did not carry out contract-making
conferences with all patients admitted into the ward.   They excused
themselves on the grounds of pressures of work, or on the grounds
that some patients were too psychotic.   But Cooklin points out that
the fact that the proportion of patients seen by the conference
increased as the months went by indicated that the staff initially
lacked confidence and were suspicious of the functions of the
conference.

The effects of the introduction of contract-making meetings in
the ward are crucial to our argument.   For example, there was an
increased recognition by staff of the adult and healthy part of
the patients.   This encouraged patients to enter treatment alliances
relevant to the very limited goals possible in a ward under such
pressure.   The meetings themselves created a forum in which patients
and staff could establish real and shared responsibility for forms
of treatment.   In addition, there was a redefinition of the function
of inpatient treatment, particularly for crisis admission.   In the
project 25 per cent of patients stated that they sought admission
for purposes of asylum and 50 per cent complained of problems in

their living situation. By recognising and accepting patients'
needs for asylum, staff were able to make a more constructive use
of this function of hospitalisation. This in turn led to an
increase in staff confidence and an increase in participation by
both staff and patients. For example, junior staff complained
less about senior staff since their actions in relation to patients
were less mysterious. Ward management became easier, and use of
the locked part of the ward declined during the period of the
study as the project led to widespread use of contract-making
conferences.

The success of Cooklin's work must, of course, be treated with
caution as such innovations are notoriously subject to Hawthorne
effects. Fortunately, some of Scott's own work at Napsbury
supports Cooklin's findings.

Scott's own approach to overcoming the treatment barrier at
Napsbury mental hospital was essentially similar to that of the
Edinburgh project. Over a two-year period Scott's team set out
to challenge the culturally accepted role of mental patient. At
ward meetings, staff did not accept patients' denials of agency.
They asked patients what they wanted from being in hospital. They
remained unresponsive to psychotic modes of explanation and thus
were sometimes able to undercut these within one session and reveal
more significant issues usually of an interpersonal nature.

Scott's team also made it a condition of admission that relatives attend at least one ward meeting soon after the patient had
been admitted. Relatives, like patients, regularly avoided issues
concerning the situation that led to admission since they typically
attributed the decision to admit the patient to the doctor concerned. Nevertheless, staff persisted in eliciting from relatives
the real reasons that lay behind the patient's admission, thereby
making them share responsibility for the hospitalisation process.

Until Scott's approach to the treatment barrier had been adopted,
the ward was characterised by recurrent bed pressure crises, over-
crowding, violence, squabbling and tension. However, after the
adoption of Scott's approach, the ward underwent considerable
changes. Breakages became much rarer and the use of sedatives
dropped; more significantly, the average length of stay by patients
declined significantly and progressively although the admission and
readmission rates remained approximately the same. The reduction
of the inpatient load freed staff to go into the community and
hence deal with problems before they became too acute.

Scott's method for dealing with the problem of the treatment
barrier has led to other community-based approaches. In particular,
Dr D. Wallbridge, a colleague of Scott's at Napsbury, has successfully demonstrated that it is possible to gain the co-operation
of patients, family members, GPs and social workers in forming
contractual agreements with respect to the purpose of hospital admission before the patient enters hospital. The findings of
Wallbridge's study are as yet unpublished, as are those of a project
taking place at York Clinic, Guys Hospital (1976). Although this
project is still in its infancy, it also seems to demonstrate the
efficacy and value of a contract-making approach towards the treatment of mental disorder.

STRUCTURE, DECISION-MAKING AND THERAPEUTIC OUTLOOK

It is obvious that, if a contract-making approach is to be employed
within a hospital setting, the therapeutic team must be highly
organised. Indeed, recent publications from the Department of
Health and Social Security which have discussed this matter have
stressed the important role that the therapeutic team must play in
the development of comprehensive psychiatric services (DHSS, 1971,
1975). However, the discussion of the nature of teamwork has been
limited and vague. There has been a marked failure to appreciate
the relationship between the internal structure of the therapeutic
team and its functions of diagnosis and treatment within a hospital
setting. Instead, these publications have stressed the value of a
multi-disciplinary approach to treatment, the roles and responsibilities of individual team members, and the relationship between
the specialist therapeutic team, which is typically hospital-based,
and the primary care team, which consists of GPs, health visitors
and home nurses.
    Our study of Porchester unit demonstrated that there was often
a discontinuity between decisions established at ward rounds and
the day-to-day treatment of the patient. Moreover, decision-making
was often heavily biased by interventions from senior medical staff
who had virtually no day-to-day contact with patients. This often
led junior members of staff to act on their own initiative and
ignore decisions which they saw as arbitrary and unhelpful to
patients who were their major responsibility. These difficulties
are obviously related to the structure of the therapeutic teams
involved, but other factors are also significant.

THE ANALYSIS OF COMPLEX ORGANISATIONS

In order to facilitate our discussion it is helpful to examine
Perrow's (1965) method of analysing complex organisations. Perrow
is a systems analyst who views hospitals as examples of complex
organisations which process inputs (in their case, patients) in
such a way that they are materially changed (cured) as a result
of passing through them. Hospitals are therefore assumed to
function in similar ways to factories, schools or any other organisation that produces a definable product. His perspective is to
focus on the work performed on the basic material that is to be
altered rather than focusing on the interaction of organisational
members or the function of the organisation for society.
    Perrow argues that three major factors influence the functioning
of such organisations: first, the cultural system, which sets
legitimate goals; second, technology, which determines the means
available for reaching these goals; and third, the social structure
of the organisation in which specific techniques are embedded in
such a way that achievement of goals is allowed.
    Perrow's use of the term 'technology' is very specific, and it
would be misleading to use the term without exploring his definition of it. Perrow defines technology as 'A technique or complex
of techniques employed to alter "materials" (human or non-human,
mental or physical) in an anticipated manner' (1965, p.915).
He elaborates this definition in the following way:

1 Some knowledge of a non-random cause-and-effect relationship is required; that is, the techniques lead to the performance of acts that, for known or unknown reasons, cause a change under specified conditions.

2 There is some system of feedback such that the consequences of the acts can be assessed in an objective manner.

3 It is possible to secure repeated deomonstrations of the efficacy of the acts.

4 There is an acceptable, reasonable and determinant range of tolerance; that is, the proportion of successes can be estimated, and even though the proportion is small, it is judged high enough to continue the activity.

5 Finally, the techniques can be communicated sufficiently that most persons with appropriate preliminary training can be expected to master the techniques and perform them under acceptable limits of tolerance.

Having presented his definition, we can now explore the relationship between the three variables that he used in his analysis. Perrow argues that these variables are in fact interdependent. For example, structure can operate in such a way as to inhibit changes in goals and technology or indeed to bring them about. Likewise, technology can modify values by demonstrating the potentialities of the material that is to be altered. Cultural values or belief systems may encourage a search for new techniques or indeed prevent a proliferation of them.

The interdependence of these variables has been evident in the development of psychiatry. Over the centuries there have been enormous variations in the cultural definition of the mentally ill which have significantly influenced the type of techniques employed in coping with mental disorder. Depending on the prevailing cultural definition, the mentally ill have been variously exorcised, treated with physical treatments, psychoanalysed, etc. Significantly, the introduction of the new physical treatment techniques in the 1930s affected the social structure of hospitals. For example, the introduction of insulin coma treatment in the 1930s resulted in the formation of highly integrated and co-ordinated treatment teams owing to the life-threatening aspects of the treatment. The structure of psychiatric units is a reflection of this heritage, as we have already argued in a previous chapter.

However, although we shall make use of Perrow's method of analysing organisations, it is necessary to broaden it, especially with respect to the relationship between structure and technology. Perrow's account is limited because it does not take into consideration the influence of class relations and sex roles on the structure and technology of organisations.

THE INFLUENCE OF SOCIAL STRUCTURE ON ORGANISATIONS

Navarro (1975), in a critique of Illich's work, 'Medical Nemesis', provides this additional dimension for our argument. He has criticised the assumption that technological knowledge determines the division of labour and social relations inherent in an organisation. He argues that such an assumption begs the question of why technological knowledge is distributed in the way that it is and why technology is frequently a vehicle for human oppression and not of liberation. Indeed, Navarro's view is that it is precisely social relations (who controls what, and how that control takes place) that determine the type of organisation to be chosen and the type of technology to be used. In a capitalist society the need for the employer to control the process of work determines the existence of a highly fragmented division of labour and the use of technologies that are compatible with hierarchical structures. He therefore sees technology as reinforcing the already existing hierarchical and potentially fragmentary division of labour. The hierarchies that exist in work situations are therefore determined primarily by the class and sex roles existent in society and not by technological innovations.

Navarro illustrates these views by an analysis of the responsibility held by the members of multi-disciplinary health teams. Within the health team there is a well defined hierarchical order. The physician or psychiatrist is typically a man from an upper middle-class background; below him, the supportive nurses, most often women, come from lower middle-class backgrounds; and at the bottom the attendants, auxiliaries and service workers are most frequently women who are from working-class backgrounds. Navarro claims that, although there have been vast advances in medical technology during the twentieth century, this structure has remained unchanged. According to him, what explains this hierarchical division of labour is the class backgrounds and sex roles of the individuals concerned. Technology and access to technological knowledge merely reinforce this hierarchy. In this respect the acquisition of technological knowledge through education and training is viewed by Navarro as the mere legitimation of the existing class and sex hierarchical distribution of power and responsibilities.

If we turn to the social structure of Porchester unit, it can be seen that there was a straightforward relationship between the class background and sex of the members of staff and the positions they held in the staff hierarchy. The senior medical posts were held by men from either upper middle-class or middle-class backgrounds. The psychiatric social workers were all women from middle-class backgrounds, while the nursing staff were from lower middle-class backgrounds (and were predominantly women). The service workers were again predominantly female but were from working-class backgrounds.

Navarro's analysis helps to illuminate some aspects of the unit's functioning, but it is still necessary to examine the complex relationship between the structure of the therapeutic teams and the 'technology' employed by the members of staff in the treatment of patients. The crucial point here is that the structure of the therapeutic teams was similar to the hierarchical structures to be found in other branches of medicine. This is entirely to be expected, given the history of psychiatry and its adherence to the medical model. But we must avoid being simplistic about this issue. A striking feature of the Porchester unit's method of functioning concerned its eclecticism. Although physical and drug forms of treatment were used, the unit generally espoused psychotherapeutic forms of treatment. In addition, psychotherapeutic skills were not distributed among team members in such a way that the form of hierarchy embodying the medical model could be justified. For example, one of the senior psychiatric social workers was probably better trained as a psychotherapist than any of the consultants, and other social workers had greater skills and experience than the more junior psychiatric staff.

The medical model, and the treatment technologies based upon it, is conducive to creating a high degree of division of labour, but nevertheless the medical profession retains its overall control over any treatment. It retains its control because of its historically established rights and because many of its activities are legally sanctioned, so that no other profession can have equal power. But a crucial question is raised at this point. What happens when psychotherapeutic forms of treatment are introduced into psychiatric settings? Are such therapies compatible with the complex division of labour associated with the medical model?

Perrow argues that mental hospital settings that do not involve the intensive use of dyadic psychotherapy are doomed to be ineffective. He particularly attacks all forms of milieu therapy, since he insists that they have failed to produce an effective form of treatment despite claims to the contrary. More traditional hospital settings fail equally because they are suited only for achieving custodial goals - they lack effective treatments, and their modes of functioning often relate more to the needs of the staff than to the needs of the patients.

Perrow argues, without exploring the issue in any detail, that outpatient clinics are likely to be effective settings for psychotherapy. By inference from other parts of his general argument it is possible to establish why he holds this view. In essence, he argues that hospital settings are counter-therapeutic because they do not utilise effective treatments. The social structure of the hospital also militates against effective treatment (although Perrow claims, incorrectly and naively in our opinion, that a basic change in treatment technology can cause a change in social structure so that the hospital can become effective). We would argue that the introduction of a potentially effective form of treatment, namely psychotherapy, into a hospital setting that reflects an alien treatment technology is essentially problematic. The dyadic relationship between the psychotherapist and patient is immediately diluted by a whole series of other relationships. Elsewhere we have pointed out that the social structure of the unit was very complex. Patients inevitably had to relate to a whole series of staff members - psychiatrists, social workers, occupational therapist and nurses. Since the unit was engaged in training students, patients also met medical students, social work students and occasionally psychology students. They also had to experience the trauma of being interviewed in the presence of students - a situation that Raphael's patients also found very difficult to accept.

Given the complexity of their experiences in the unit it is difficult, therefore, to establish what features of the situation were actually therapeutic. Supporters of milieu therapy or administrative psychiatry would argue that we have missed the point - that the very setting in all its complexities is the therapy. But

we insist that Perrow's reading of such situations is nearer the
truth. His views are summed up in the following extract:
    there is no doubt that there is a technology for control, care
    and custody in both large and small hospitals, and no doubt it
    could be improved. Cure is another thing, however.... In the
    case of individual psychotherapy, there is reason to believe
    most of the conditions for techniques of cure are met, though
    opinions vary widely. In the case of large mental hospitals,
    it is argued ... that these conditions are not met: although
    some people get well, by and large they do so unpredictably and
    as a result of mysterious processes such as 'spontaneous re-
    mission', the phlogiston of administrative psychiatry. In the
    case of intensive elite hospitals, where individual psychotherapy
    is used, it is argued that individual psychotherapy is the only
    appropriate technology that has been devised, and the claims
    for cure on other bases, such as through creating a therapeutic
    milieu, are misleading.
Needless to say, the Porchester unit cannot be considered to be
equivalent to the elite hospitals reviewed by Perrow. Although
the unit was very well staffed (in numerical terms), it functioned
as a crisis intervention unit and therefore admitted patients with
widely differing problems, social backgrounds, personal needs, etc.
The day-to-day running of the unit was maintained by nurses and
junior staff with very differing experiences but all of them lacked
extensive training in psychotherapeutic techniques. Given the
complexity of the patient input and the lack of staff skills, it is
not surprising that therapeutic initiatives with patients were
often inconsistent. However, another structural feature of the
unit contributed to these difficulties.

DECISION-MAKING AND THE STAFF HIERARCHY

As we have already noted in Chapter 5, the structure of the therapeutic teams was such that the consultant, who had least contact
and knowledge of the patient, played the dominant role in contributing to decision-making processes. Although he was not
personally involved in inpatient therapy, he was responsible for
the patient's admission to the unit, for establishing a diagnosis,
and for directing the treatment programme devised for the patient.
In practice, the senior house officers and the psychiatric social
workers carried the burden of undertaking psychotherapy although
nursing staff and occupational therapists also had a large amount
of contact with the patient. We would argue that this type of
structure is essentially problematic when psychotherapy is the
main method of therapy. The structure, as we have already argued,
was more compatible with the diagnostic and treatment techniques
of general medicine.
    One of the characteristics that distinguishes general medical
practice from psychiatry is its diagnostic precision. Mechanic
(1969) has stated that:
    the usefulness of a diagnostic disease model depends on its
    level of confirmation, which in turn depends on the reliability
    of the diagnosis (the amount of agreement among practitioners

in assigning the diagnostic label) and its utility in predicting
the course of the condition, its etiology and how it can be
treated successfully.
Unlike psychiatric diagnosis, diagnosis in ordinary medical practice is more reliable because a considerable amount is known about
the nature of many conditions. A second distinguishing feature of
ordinary medical practice is that, when a diagnostic category is
applied to a patient's illness, the physician's understanding of
the illness and the course of treatment he adopts usually follow
from the diagnosis. Moreover, in ordinary medical practice symptoms can be identified, and the course of treatment can be monitored
by judicious use of the props of medical technology.

We do not wish here to appear naive and underestimate the importance either of subjective factors in these processes or of exercising sound judgment in ordinary medical practice. There is little
doubt that the latter ability is a highly valued part of the
physician's professional skill. For example, in most branches of
medicine there are cases where a variety of treatments are seen as
acceptable alternatives. The final choice of equally plausible
treatments may be based on the treatment 'philosophies' of the
physicians involved rather than on more objective criteria.
Measurement techniques such as X-rays yield data that must be
interpreted, and hence even such 'objective' data are susceptible
to the frailties of human judgment. Nevertheless, it is true to
say that there are greater possibilities for diagnostic agreement
among practitioners and greater possibilities for using objective
tests as a basis for making diagnoses.

If we return to the structure of the therapeutic teams of the
Porchester unit it may be seen that this structure is consistent
with the diagnostic and treatment techniques employed in ordinary
medicine. A hierarchical structure and a high degree of division
of labour would have been compatible with a state of affairs in
which treatment decisions and diagnoses were supported by independent methods of observation. Treatment decisions and diagnoses
would theoretically vary little between members of staff, regardless of the nature of their involvement in the therapeutic process,
since they would have access to information that was not solely
dependent on an individual's judgment.

It must be evident from our presentation of the case history
material that the unit's members of staff rarely, if at all, made
use of 'objective' information when deciding on the nature of a
patient's problem and the courses of treatment to adopt. Assessments and treatment decisions were made by the consultants, who
rarely had any day-to-day contact with patients. This meant that
their decisions were rarely based on the two types of knowledge
that many theorists (including Carl Rogers) consider to be vital
and necessary for effective psychotherapy, i.e. objective and
phenomenological knowledge. Rogers himself argues that there are
three kinds of knowing - subjective, objective and interpersonal
(Pervin, 1970):

In subjective knowing we know something from our own internal
frame of reference. In objective knowing, what we know has
been checked against the observation of others. In interpersonal
knowing, we use our own empathic skills to understand the

phenomenal field of another person. This last type of knowing
is called phenomenological knowledge and according to Rogers,
it represents a legitimate and necessary part of the science
of psychology.
From our study of the unit it may be seen that the hierarchical
team structure and its division of labour inhibited the consultants
from employing phenomenological knowledge when directing the treatment of inpatients. On the basis of Rogers's definition of
'knowing', we feel that the acquisition of this type of knowledge
is important for making assessments and treatment decisions. It
may be argued that the absence of phenomenological knowledge on
the part of the consultants in the cases we have documented lead
them to make decisions which were not always in the best interests
of the patients. For example, in the case of Mrs Davis the consultant instructed his SHO to discharge the patient immediately,
although she had agreed with Mrs Davis that she should spend a
weekend at home before leaving the unit permanently. The SHO rejected the consultant's instruction because she predicted on the
basis of her relationship with the patient that such a change in
plan would cause Mrs Davis considerable distress. In our opinion
the consultant's distance from the therapeutic situation meant
that he could not appreciate the significance that both the SHO
and the patient attached to their agreement.
    Of course it can be maintained that it is unrealistic to expect
consultant psychiatrists to establish close contact with inpatients
because they have many other pressing responsibilities; so long as
some form of objective method of assessment is employed in monitoring the progress of treatment, this is a sufficient basis on
which it may be directed. We have already stated that no such
methods were used by the unit's staff. The nearest they came to
employing an 'objective' method was inter-subjective agreements on
behalf of the junior staff arrived at by having close day-to-day
contact with the patient and observing his behaviour. However,
even when there was unanimity among the junior team members regarding the state of a patient their assessment was rejected sometimes, quite unreasonably, by the consultant. For example, in the
case of Mrs Wright they argued that Mrs Wright ought to be discharged, since by remaining in inpatient care she was being protected from facing up to her marriage. Such a state of affairs
was obviously counter-productive because an aim of Mrs Wright's
treatment was to make her confront the state of her marriage realistically. However, against all the evidence, most of which is contained in the chapter on Mrs Wright, the consultant rejected his
junior colleagues' assessment and argued that inpatient care was a
constructive measure in the case of this patient. He felt that by
remaining in hospital Mrs Wright would undergo a process of en-
lightenment about her marriage and therefore would be able to
participate wholeheartedly in marital therapy.

THE TEACHING ROLE OF THE CONSULTANTS

It may be argued that we have misunderstood the nature of the
structure of the therapeutic teams, especially when the training

role of the consultants is considered. Certainly, the teaching commitments of the senior staff were great. They were responsible both for instructing groups of medical students attending two monthly psychiatric firms and for training junior doctors and social workers in the assessment and treatment of mental disorders. The extent of these commitments limited their opportunity for direct clinical contact with patients. In practice the senior medical staff's control of decision-making was justified partly on the basis of their being ultimately legally responsible for the welfare of patients in their care, and partly because of their superior expertise in psychotherapy and other methods of treatment.

The procedure adopted in training SHOs (and to a lesser extent trainee social workers) in psychotherapy involved immersing them in the therapeutic situation. For example, as soon as senior house officers commenced their period of employment in the unit they undertook major responsibility for the treatment of their team's inpatients. Obviously as time progressed the number of patients they treated increased as a result of new admissions. The supervision of trainee therapists consisted of advice and directives regarding individual cases which were communicated by consultants at ward rounds and team meetings and at tutorials which took place once a week on an hourly basis.

Such procedures seem reasonable enough at a common-sense level but through Perrow's eyes we would ask the question, 'Did psychotherapy as practised and taught in the unit constitute a technology?' In order to answer the above question it is essential to return once more to a consideration of Perrow's definition of technology and assess whether the theory and practice of psychotherapy in the unit meet his criteria. It is our contention that the theory and practice of psychotherapy at Porchester unit did not constitute a technology in Perrow's sense since it failed to meet any of his criteria. In particular, at no stage during the period of research did the senior medical staff explicitly formulate or communicate their views of psychotherapy to trainee junior doctors and social workers in ways that conform to Perrow's criteria. Equally, at no stage were objective methods of assessment used to determine (1) whether therapeutic change occured, or (2) whether therapeutic change, if it occurred, was caused by the relationship between the therapist and the patient or by other variables such as the milieu of the unit, chemotherapy, ECT, etc.

In fact, the question of efficacy was not considered as important by the unit. Even such a crude statistic as the re-admission rate to the unit was not established during the period of study, although one of the consultants did subsequently obtain the re-admission rate by getting the Medical Records Department to carry out a survey. Significantly, the unit itself did not maintain a record of the re-admission rate.

However, despite these inadequacies, it is perhaps Perrow's fifth criterion that warrants most discussion. How can psychotherapeutic techniques be communicated 'sufficiently' so that trainees can master them and become tolerably proficient? We would argue that there are essentially several dimensions involved in answering this question. For example, the trainee psychotherapist must be involved in procedures that enhance his self-knowledge and self-awareness. As Karl Jaspers says (1963):

The psychotherapist who has not seen himself can never truly
see through his patient because then he allows the assertion
of alien, ununderstandable drives within himself. The psychotherapist who cannot help himself can never really help his
patient. It is therefore an old demand that the physician
should be the object of his own psychological scrutiny.
At Porchester neither senior medical staff nor trainee therapists
were required to undergo this process of self-discovery and understanding before treating patients. Moreover the junior doctors
and trainee social workers were never observed by their senior
colleagues in the therapeutic situation. Indeed the interior design
of the unit did not cater for this possibility since, for example,
none of the interviewing rooms was provided with one-way mirrors.
This state of affairs compares unfavourably with ordinary medical
practice where the junior doctor acquires many of his skills by
actually observing senior colleagues performing them.

THE LATENT FUNCTIONS OF HIERARCHICAL TEAM STRUCTURES

Inevitably we must conclude that the unit's approach to psychotherapy, when examined in the context of the structure of the
therapeutic teams, was highly problematic. It can be argued that
a hierarchical structure may be put to other uses than those
related to facilitating the training of psychotherapy or the
directing of treatment programmes. To begin with it may enable
the senior medical staff to distance themselves from the treatment
situation and thus avoid demonstrating whether they have the com-
petence to carry out psychotherapy. By adopting this stance they
are able to behave as if they are experts without having to commit
themselves to the scrutiny of their junior colleagues. Instead
of providing detailed and meticulous demonstrations of psychotherapeutic skills involving themselves as models, the consultants
may retreat into the all-too-easy role of being the 'expert ad-
viser'. In ward rounds they therefore may demonstrate their
'scientific' skills by producing instant formulations concerning
aspects of patient's behaviour and by weaving together pieces of
information whose status as evidence is highly questionable. By
virtue of the powerful position they hold in the team hierarchy,
they are therefore able to behave as if they are experts, although
their knowledge of the patients may be often clearly inferior to
that of their junior colleagues. As a result of this state of
affairs patients may become objects of speculation and are not
reviewed in the intimate detail that the uniqueness of their problems and lives deserve.
From another perspective the issues that we are discussing return
us to the issue of eclecticism. To a great extent the senior
medical staff of Porchester unit had moved away from traditional
psychiatric theory and practice. Even when they adopted traditional
methods of treatment these were not construed as ends in themselves
but as adjuncts to psychological forms of treatment. However, they
had failed to develop a consistently psychotherapeutic approach to
their patients. They therefore fell into the trap that Clare's
approach opens up. Patients are undoubtedly complex, and a minority

clearly have organic features that contribute to their symptomatology, but this does not mean that a loose eclectic approach is
required. Various forms of treatment may have to be combined but
these must be subordinated to a general psychotherapeutic approach.
Since senior staff were never involved in the latter there was a
tendency for them to change their treatment tactics. Inevitably
this caused confusion.

Another latent function associated with hierarchical team
structures may be concerned with the professional socialisation
of staff in training. That is to say, trainees are involved in
learning the rules of behaviour relevant to their respective professional roles within a hospital setting. They are being made
aware of the division of labour and their relationship to the
authority structure within this type of setting. Thus senior
members of staff act as role models for trainees. For example,
the consultants through their actions demonstrate to their junior
colleagues that the post of consultant requires the incumbent to
behave primarily as a diagnostician and as a co-ordinator of tasks
performed by other professional groups within the psychiatric
setting. Since their involvement in therapy is never publicly
demonstrated, they fail to provide a concrete model in this crucial
area. Trainee psychiatric social workers are made aware that
although they can expect to have a therapeutic role when trained,
they cannot expect diagnostic and therapeutic autonomy over
patients.

THE MAINTENANCE OF EQUILIBRIUM

Many of the points of criticism that we have made concerning the
unit's functioning are confirmed when we consider the attitudes
of the junior members of staff to the unit in which they worked.
Informally they were often bitter and angry about the way the unit
operated. In particular, they were often highly critical of the
role performed by the consultants. Nevertheless, the junior members
of staff rarely openly challenged the consultants, and even when
conflict arose at the infrequent staff meetings and ward rounds
it was muted. The equilibrium of the unit was maintained in several
ways. To begin with, certain members of staff used informal stra-
tegies to engineer situations that were compatible with their
expectations of their roles. For example, the psychiatric social
workers were often hostile to carrying out psychotherapy on an
inpatient basis since they lacked autonomy and control over the
therapeutic situation. Therefore, they took measures to avoid
therapeutic involvement on this basis. For example, during one
stage of Mrs Smith's admission the consultant thought that the
Smiths should undergo marital therapy. However, he wished to base
his decision on his psychiatric social worker's assessment after
she had interviewed Mr Smith. In fact, she recommended against
marital therapy, reasoning that such a step could be destructive
to the Smiths' relationship. However, when one of us (G.B.) interviewed her after Mrs Smith had been discharged and asked her to
explain her opposition to marital therapy, it transpired that
factors other than the one we have just mentioned played a vital
role in her assessment:

I'm criticising ... the system here and some of the people
involved in it. I think if you're going to offer therapy to
a patient then the person who is going to offer them therapy
should be the person who does the initial assessment and works
out a treatment plan; that it should be left entirely within
their hands with only advice and discussion coming from outside,
and that because the people who admit patients here aren't
necessarily the ones who go on to treat them then there are all
sorts of complications that come into the situation. If Mrs
Smith and her husband had come up to outpatients and had either
seen me straight off, or had seen the consultant very briefly
and then seen me straight off, I think we could probably have
offered the Smiths conjoint therapy.

Junior doctors and social workers adopted other types of strategy.
For example, if they disagreed with a consultant's treatment
decision, where possible they would simply avoid carrying it out.
By taking this step they made judicious use of the therapeutic
teams' division of labour. That is to say, they appreciated the
fact that the consultants did not have day-to-day contact with
inpatients and therefore could not ensure that treatment decisions
were being carried out.

The status quo of the unit was maintained by other means. Apart
from ward rounds and case conferences, staff meetings were very
infrequent. This limited the opportunities for confrontation between junior members of staff and their senior colleagues. Moreover, there was inevitably a high rate of turnover among junior
members of staff. The maximum term of employment of senior house
officers was one year and typically it took them at least six
months to assert themselves in their role. There was also a high
rate of turnover among the social workers, since all four psychiatric social workers who were employed in November 1973 had left
within two years. In all probability the high rate of staff turnover contributed to maintaining the unit's structure and methods
of operation.

Ultimately it was the control that the senior medical staff
exercised over the other employees at Porchester that was the most
significant factor in determining the status quo that reigned over
the unit. In the first place they accommodated those demands of
their junior doctors and ancillary professions that did not threaten
their autonomy. For example, during the period of research, after
the psychiatric social work staff had made representations for
greater therapeutic involvement, they were invited to share responsibility with the junior medical staff for interviewing and assessing the needs of patients who had taken overdoses of medication
and who were patients on the medical wards of a nearby hospital.
But more crucially, the most important aspect of the senior medical
staff's power over the unit's other members of staff was to do with
promotion and future prospects of employment. In particular,
senior house officers and psychiatric social workers depended on
their senior colleagues for references. Thus, it was naturally in
their interests to maintain conflict-free relationships with the
consultants.

From the preceding discussion it may be seen that, although
junior members of staff attempted to obtain whatever extension they

could to their roles, they never sought to challenge and change
the unit's structure and methods of operation. Our conclusions
in this respect are similar to those outlined by Nigel Goldie
(1976) in a paper with the significant title, 'The Division of
Labour Among the Mental Health Professions - A Negotiated or an
Imposed Order?' The main focus of Goldie's paper is to consider
the nature of the division of labour between psychiatrists, clinical
psychologists and social workers, and more particularly the nature
of the social structure within hospital settings. One of the main
problems that his research discovered was that, although in an
objective sense there were marked differences in the power held
by those groups, social workers and clinical psychologists tended
to deny that such differences in any way limited their 'freedom'
and 'autonomy'. His paper seeks to reconcile the objective features of social structure with subjective ones.

Interestingly, Goldie confirms our observation that ancillary
staff such as social workers used the social structure of the unit
to avoid carrying out decisions of consultants with which they
disagreed. As Goldie (1976) points out,

Many social workers drew attention to how they were able to
ignore, re-interpret, or modify requests made to them by doctors, or as one of them observed, 'It is very easy to manipulate
the situation here.' This was especially the case where the
social workers only saw the consultants infrequently.... The
significant aspect of this information being ... the choice of
tactical means of resistance, thereby avoiding a direct confrontation with the psychiatrist.

However, Goldie's main finding is concerned with the way in which
social workers and clinical psychologists accommodate themselves
to the objective facts regarding their position in the power structure of hospital settings. Both groups claimed complete freedom
and autonomy to organise their work, and yet they realised that
this freedom was limited by the power of the psychiatrists. At a
practical level they emphasised the need to work within realistic
limits precisely in order to maintain autonomy over these limited
areas of work. Most of the clinical psychologists and social
workers studied by Goldie accepted these limitations on their
actions because they assumed that it was the psychiatrists' legal
responsibility for patients that affected what they themselves
could do. As Goldie states, 'legal responsibility remains as a
continual reminder to the staff of their inferior position'
(Goldie, 1976).

Goldie considers the limitations that ancillary staff imposed
on their activities as a significant factor in maintaining the
status quo in hospital settings. This argument is as follows
(Goldie, 1976):

That they may have imposed boundaries around themselves, after
experiencing disapproval, or in anticipation of it, is an
interesting example of the way control and stability are often
maintained within institutions that seek to win the moral
involvement of their members.

The status quo was also maintained by the lay staff endeavouring
to gain acceptance from particular psychiatrists in order to gain
freedom to perform certain functions, like the practising of

certain kinds of therapy.   However, as Goldie says, 'recognition is generally only afforded by particular psychiatrists, and is dependent on them sharing the same assumptions about not only the nature of mental illness, but also each other's role' (Goldie, 1976).

In the Porchester unit there were no clinical psychologists, but the working relations between the psychiatrists and social workers did conform to the pattern outlined by Goldie.   Admittedly, the social workers had a great deal of autonomy, but this was largely because of the vacuum created by the fact that the senior medical staff did not participate in therapy on a day-to-day basis. In the final analysis, as we have attempted to demonstrate, the consultants effectively controlled the decision-making process but they were prepared to give social workers autonomy in exercising their therapeutic skills.   But it is, of course, eminently imagin-able, and this is the substance of Goldie's analysis, that the consultants could legitimately seek to reorganise the work of the social workers so that their therapeutic role would be severely curtailed.

SOCIAL CHANGE AND THE FUTURE OF PSYCHIATRY

In this chapter we have explored the problem of the treatment barrier and sought to establish that contract-making procedures provide a fruitful area for research and innovation.   We have examined the hierarchical structure of treatment teams and attemp-ted to demonstrate the implications of such a structure.   However, we do not seek to provide panaceas for these problems - contract-making procedures may go some way towards solving some of the very real moral dilemmas that therapists working in NHS settings have to face, but more fundamental changes concerned with the role of the psychiatric profession can occur only within the context of basic social change.

Our analysis is based partly on Waitzin and Waterman's (1974) examination of the exploitation of the sick role in capitalist societies.   They argue that

the sick do not suffer in isolation from the broad socio-political structures in which they live.   There are numerous interconnections between medicine and the broader social system of which medicine is a part.   In all societies, health care is a service provided by one group of people (health workers) to another (patients).   Societies differ greatly, however, in the ways they organise this service.   The organisational forms which govern the treatment of the sick reflect broad normative principles within a society; the normative framework within which health workers and patients interact may be called the society's medicocivil structure.

Since the nature of the medical service of a society is dependent on the way the broader society is structured, Waitzin and Waterman argue that modification of the medical services or aspects of the medical services can take place only with 'More general socio-political reorganisation' (Waitzin and Waterman, 1974).

If we examine the relationship between the sick role, which is

a principle feature of the treatment barrier, and the broader
society, we may understand why the introduction of a contract-
making procedure is dependent on changes in the sociopolitical
structure. Parsons' (1951b) view of the sick role is most relevant
in the context of this discussion. In his analysis, illness is one
form of deviance and thus is viewed as a problem requiring social
control. As such, the sick role acts as a limitation on the dissatisfaction and frustration caused by personal troubles which may
result from the roles society imposes on individuals. Parsons himself indicates the social and political implications of the sick
role in his own work (Parsons, 1951b):

> The criminal, being extruded from the company of 'decent' citi-
> zens can only by coercion be prevented from joining up with his
> fellow criminals.... The conditional legitimation of the sick
> person's status, on the other hand, places him in a special
> relation to people who are not sick, to the members of his
> family and to the various people in the health services, parti-
> cularly physicians. This control is part of the price he pays
> for his partial legitimation, and it is clear that the basic
> structure resulting is that of the dependence of each sick
> person on a group of non-sick persons rather than of sick persons
> on each other. This in itself is highly important from the point
> of view of the social system since it prevents the relevant
> motivations from spreading through either group formation or
> positive legitimation. It is especially important that the moti-
> vational components, which cannot be expressed in the deviant
> behaviour itself, in this case tend to tie the sick person to
> non-deviant people, rather than to other deviants....
>   But again, the sick role not only isolates and insulates, it
> also exposes the deviant to reintegrative forces.

Parsons's conservative standpoint allows him to contemplate the
sick role with equanimity. He recognises it as merely one of
several deviant routes that individuals may take as a response to
personal crises. However, as Waitzin and Waterman (1974) argue,

> The sick role becomes a convenient tool to maintain the status
> quo. For individuals who encounter oppressive qualities of the
> social roles (familial, occupational, etc.) which are part of
> the objective conditions under which they must live, the sick
> role permits temporary deviance from the usual role expectations.
> It also isolates the deviant and prevents the group formations
> which would be needed for fundamental social change. In this
> sense, the sick role cools out the opposition.

It must be noted that if this characterisation of the sick role as
a means of social control is correct, then doctors are agents of
social control. By being responsible for 'certifying' illness,
physicians are limiting deviance and preserving social stability.
Moreover, they are deflecting the attention of patients away from
the social and economic injustices that trouble them in their
everyday life. On the basis of this discussion, we would argue
that general change in the psychiatrist-patient relationship, from
one characterised by the sick role and a superordinate-subordinate
relationship to one characterised by contract-making and shared
responsibility, is dependent on alterations in the social structure
of society.

The same is true with respect to the introduction of more egalitarian staff structures in psychiatric settings. As Navarro (1975) argues, in a discussion of the role and function of the health team,

The joint provision of (the) care by the patient himself, his family and all members of the team is seriously handicapped in our class-structured society, where roles and functions are not distributed according to the need for them, but primarily according to the hierarchical structure prevalent in our society, dictated by its class structure and class relations.

It may appear that we are implicitly adopting a nihilistic standpoint which assumes that the status quo cannot be changed because of the historical and socio-political factors that we have examined throughout this book. This is not our position. We certainly wish to avoid creating new panaceas, but on the other hand we do seek to establish methods of relating to clients that avoid the dominating social control element that characterises so much of psychiatric practice.

Much of the literature of anti-psychiatry, particularly that associated with the work of Laing and Szasz, is manifestly irrelevant to this task. Laing's therapeutic communities function outside the NHS, while Szasz, of course, would never contemplate working within a system of state medicine in the first place. We would not decry the many forms of self-help groups that have been developed over the past few years. They are undoubtedly capable of providing rich experiences and new insights into ways of helping people in crisis. But the mushrooming of such groups only serves to allow the NHS to operate in its traditional ways. The Free School movement is an interesting parallel in this respect, since no matter how superior and adventurous the teaching may be in such schools, the state system continues, producing mis-educated children in its relentless and machine-like way. In practice, Free Schools may be little more than safety valves that allow the state system to work even more effectively.

How then can critics of the present system proceed without becoming nihilists? We are far from knowing the answer, but we can at least begin to elaborate our position by considering how other critics have tackled the same task. In Britain the heritage of treating mental health problems as political ones runs very deep, and Peter Sedgwick, lecturer in politics at Leeds University, has attempted to establish a framework for approaching such questions. In his now famous article, 'Mental Illness is Illness', he argues the following point which serves as a useful starting point for our discussion (Sedgwick, 1972):

It may surprise some readers to hear that I, as a revolutionary socialist and Marxist, am so desirous of stimilating effective reforms in the mental health field. But, the evolution of transitional demands on the existing social and political structure is essential. Just as the revolutionary exposes and pressurises Parliamentary 'democracy' by demanding consistent democracy; just as he exposes and fights the courts of bourgeois 'justice' by demanding consistent justice: so he must expose and combat the evils of our anti-therapeutic institutions of 'psychistry' by demanding consistent psychiatry. A transitional

demand, in Trotsky's classic conception, is one which is placed
on the system in the full knowledge that the system cannot grant
it: the failure of the system to deliver its declared pledges
will then expose its reactionary character before the masses.
In the present era, which is characterised by mass demands for
adequate medical treatment, all demands for public health provision (including the demand for mass psychiatric services) are
transitional in quality. The revolutionary can enter a united
front with reformists to place new pressures on the social
order: if the system really can grant all that it claims to be
able to do, the Marxist will have no quarrel with it, or with
the reformists and liberals who expect it to carry out its pro-
mises. If (as the Marxist expects) the system cannot deliver
the goods, then his liberal or reformist allies will become
radicalised, and may even join the ranks of his Marxist comrades.
So a united front is always possible, and indeed must always be
sought, between revolutionaries and reformers. But no united
front and no dialogue is possible between revolutionaries and
cynics. Cynics are, quite simply, people who have no hope:
and therefore have no capacity to express any demands for the
future. The sociological critics of the 'mental illness' concept are, as ideologues, deeply cynical: if they do have hope,
or any possibility of formulating demands in the mental health
field, such hope is not made manifest through the ideas contained
in their books and articles. And the cynic cannot really be a
critic; the radical who is only a radical nihilist, or a radical
tragedian, is for practical purposes the most adamant of conservatives.

We would agree with Sedgwick's argument in favour of transitional
demands, but his position cannot be fully understood unless one
knows that he assumes that there is an essential continuity between
mental and physical illness. This issue need not detain us here,
however, as we have argued against it throughout the book. However,
it is crucial to note that Sedgwick is extraordinarily uncritical
of the methods of current psychiatry - he insists that:

> I myself am perfectly happy to see as many mentally ill persons
> as possible treated, fully and effectively, in this society; for
> no matter how many may become adjusted through expert techniques,
> the workings of capitalism will ever create newer and larger
> discontent.

In demanding the allocation of more resources for the treatment of
mental disorder and in demanding that psychiatry should be 'consistent', Sedgwick clearly fails to examine both the content and
the ideological framework of such services. He seems to assume
that to demand more services for the mentally disordered is equivalent to demanding more general hospitals, more intensive care
units, more doctors, etc. What he fails to estimate is the social
control function of psychiatric services. To him such services
make for 'adjustment'; this is apparently a goal in itself, and
yet Sedgwick claims to be a 'modern, engaged' Marxist!

Sedgwick is not alone in adopting this position. MIND (the
National Association for Mental Health) also tends merely to demand
more services although the organisation is at least assured that in
making such a demand some attention has to be paid to the quality

of the services. In particular, the National Association for Mental Health (NAMH) has demanded that psychiatrists should at least be trained in psychotherapy. The organisation has also financed some pioneering work investigating the ways in which the 1959 Mental Health Act invades the liberties of the citizen. But these initiatives remain isolated and the NAMH generally operates in such a way that it feeds the illusion that health issues are above politics.

Clearly, there must be a political struggle for better services, but it is also imperative that workers within the psychiatric services unite in order to fight for the democratisation of the structures in which they work. At the same time the utilisation of contract-making procedures will begin to confront the use of psychiatric service as means of social control. But such procedures must also confront patients' and families' use of the sick role as a legitimated means of escaping from crisis. In many cases the type of contract established with the patients will simply be one of providing asylum because the difficulties that the patient confronts are overwhelming (acute housing difficulties, and situations involving the use of personal violence, would be obvious examples). But in other cases the contract established would attempt to prevent the types of manipulation that families use in electing certain members as 'mentally ill' when the whole family structure is under pressure.

However, the successful confrontation of such forms of manipulation is not the end of the process. The psychiatric services are in general obsessed by both bed occupancy rates and discharge rates, but there is no reason to assume that the rapid discharge of a patient or the avoidance of admission in the first place is consistent with adequate therapy. Contract-making procedures are largely meaningless without the development of community-based organisations that actually provide substantive assistance to the individuals that require them. Whether such agencies would themselves avoid becoming agencies of social control would depend precisely on their methods of operation, but there are sufficient examples both in Britain and the USA to indicate that it is perfectly possible to develop such organisations without converting them into vehicles for the depoliticisation of mental health problems.

To many readers our conclusions may appear desultory. At the height of a severe economic crisis it is difficult to write about health issues without appearing banal and irrelevant, since the impact that unemployment has upon mental health is well known. Brenner's (1973) meticulous documentation of the relationship between business cycles and size of resident population in mental hospitals in the USA is a sufficient reminder that economic factors are of paramount importance in determining the extent of mental disorder within a population. He shows that the number of patients in such hospitals increases as the business cycle downturns. In Britain active attempts to decrease the size of hospital populations may apparently negate the generality of his finding, but it is essential that a similar analysis should be carried out using patient contacts with psychiatric services rather than bed occupancy as the main statistic.

However, it is implicit in our position that the struggle should be carried out on a number of fronts simultaneously. We would therefore conclude by arguing that it is also crucial that the problem of the efficacy of the psychiatric services should be investigated. We have insisted that the efficacy of current treatments in psychiatry is more apparent than real. Drugs may control symptoms but this is not to say that they provide any form of cure. We would therefore argue that the old policy introduced by the Tavistock Clinic in the 1930s - 'No research without therapy, no therapy without research' - should be fought for within the NHS. Needless to say, this policy applies equally to both psychiatry and physical medicine.

References

CHAPTER 1 THE RISE OF THE PSYCHIATRIC PROFESSION

BOTT, E. (1976), Hospital and Society, 'Br. J. Med. Psychol.',
49, 97-140.
BMA (1974, unpublished), Draft reply to the DHSS concerning the
Foster Report.
BMJ (1969), cited by Ewins, (1974).
CLARE, A. (1976), 'Psychiatry in Dissent', London, Tavistock.
EWINS, D. (1974), 'The Origins of the Compulsory Commitment
Provisions of the Mental Health Act (1959)', unpublished MA thesis,
University of Sheffield.
FOUCAULT, M. (1967), 'Madness and Civilization', London, Tavistock.
ILLICH, I. (1975), 'Medical Nemesis', London, Calder & Boyars.
JONES, K. (1970), 'A History of the Mental Health Services',
London, Routledge & Kegan Paul.
MECHANIC, D. (1969), 'Mental Health and Social Policy', Englewood
Cliffe, Prentice Hall.
NAMH (1974), 'MIND Report on Psychotherapy', London.
PARSONS, T. (1951), 'The Social System', Chicago, Free Press.
RUSSELL DAVIS, D. (1970), Depression as Adaptation to Crisis,
'Br. J. Med. Psychol.', 43, 109-16.
SEMMEL, B. (1960), 'Imperialism and Social Reform', London, Allen
& Unwin.
SMAIL, D. (1973), Clinical Psychology and the Medical Model, 'Bull.
Br. Psychol. Soc.', 26, 211-14.
WAITZIN, H. and WATERMAN, B. (1974), 'The Exploitation of Illness
in a Capitalist Society', New York, Bobbs-Merrill.
WALTON, H.J. and DREWERY, J. (1966), Psychiatrists as Teachers
in Medical School, 'Brit. J. Psychiat.', 112, 839-46.

CHAPTER 2 CONCEPTUAL FRAMEWORKS IN MEDICINE AND PSYCHIATRY

BARR, J. (1912), What Are We? What Are We Doing? Whence Do We
Come? and Whither Do We Go?, 'Brit. Med. J.', 2, 157-63.
BOCKOVEN, J.S. (1956), Moral Treatment in American Psychiatry,
'J. Nerv. Ment. Dis.', 124, 167-94.

BURY, M. (1974), 'The Social Organisation of Mental Subnormality', unpublished MA thesis, University of Bristol.

CAPLAN, R. (1969), 'Psychiatry and the Community in 19th Century America', New York, Basic Books.

CLARE, A. (1976), 'Psychiatry in Dissent', London, Tavistock.

EYSENCK, H.J. (1975), 'The Future of Psychiatry', London, Methuen.

HENDERSON, D.K. and GILLESPIE, R.D. (1927), 'A Textbook of Psychiatry', London, Oxford University Press.

HOFSTADTER, R. (1965), 'Social Darwinism in American Thought', New York, Braziller.

ILLICH, I. (1975), 'Medical Nemesis', London, Calder & Boyars.

JONES, K. (1972), 'A History of the Mental Health Services', London, Routledge & Kegan Paul.

KUHN, T.S. (1962), 'The Structure of Scientific Revolutions', 2nd edn, University of Chicago Press.

LORD, J.R. (1926), 'The Clinical Study of Mental Disorders', London, Adlard.

MAYER-GROSS, W., SLATER, E. and ROTH, M. (1954), 'Clinical Psychiatry', London, Cassell.

MUSTO, D. (1970), History and Psychiatry's Present State of Transition, 'Arch. Gen. Psychiat.' 23, 385-92.

RACHMAN, S.J. and PHILIPS, C. (1975), 'Psychology and Medicine', London, Temple Smith.

RIESE, W. (1944), The Structure of the Clinical History, 'Bull. Hist. Med.', 16, 437-49.

ROSEN, G. (1946), The Philosophy of Ideology and the Emergence of Modern Medicine in France, 'Bull. Hist. Med.', 20, 328-39.

ROSEN, G. (1972), The Evolution of Social Medicine, in Freeman, H.E., et al. (eds), 'Handbook of Medical Sociology', 2nd edn, Englewood Cliffs, Prentice-Hall.

RUSSELL DAVIS, D. (1970), Depression as Adaptation to Crisis, 'Br. J. Med. Psychol.', 43, 109-16.

CHAPTER 3   AN EVALUATION OF PHYSICAL AND PHARMACOLOGICAL TREATMENTS IN PSYCHIATRY

ACKNER, B., HARRIS, A. and OLDHAM, A.J. (1957), Insulin Treatment of Schizophrenia - a Controlled Study, 'Lancet', 2, 607-11.

ALEXANDER, F.G. and SELESNICK, S.T. (1967), 'The History of Psychiatry', London, Allen & Unwin.

BARTON, R. (1959), 'Institutional Neurosis', Bristol, Wright.

BOURNE, H. (1953), The Insulin Myth, 'Lancet', 2, 964-8.

BREWER, C. (1975), E.C.T. - Forty Years On, 'New Behaviour', 9 October, 50-2.

CLARK, D.H. (1964), 'Administrative Therapy', London, Tavistock.

COCHRANE, A.L. (1972), 'Effectiveness and Efficiency', London, Nuffield Provincial Hospitals Trust.

COOPER, A.B. and EARLY, D. (1961), Evolution in the Mental Hospital, 'Brit. Med. J.', 1, 1600-3.

EVANGELAKIS, M.G. (1961), De-Institutionalization of Patients, 'Dis. Nerv. System', 22, 26-32.

FLEMMING, G.W.T.H. (1944), Prefrontal Leucotomy, 'J. Ment. Sci.', 90, 486-500.

GRYGIER, P. and WATERS, M.A. (1958), Chlorpromazine Used with an Intensive Occupational Therapy, 'A.M.A. Arch. Neurol. and Psychiat.', 79, 697-705.

HORDERN, A. and HAMILTON, M. (1963), Drugs and Moral Treatment, 'Brit. J. Psychiat.', 109, 500-9.

ILLICH, I. (1975), 'Medical Nemesis', London, Calder & Boyars.

JONES, K. (1972), 'A History of the Mental Health Services', London, Routledge & Kegan Paul.

KLASS, A. (1975), 'There's Gold in Them Thar Pills', Harmondsworth, Penguin.

LANCET (1944), A Place for the Mentally Ill, 'Lancet', 2, 147-8.

McCOWEN, P. and WILDER, J. (1975), 'Life Style of 100 Psychiatric Patients', London, Psychiatric Rehabilitation Association.

McKEOWN, T. and LOWE, C.R. (1966), 'An Introduction to Social Medicine', Oxford, Blackwell.

MESZAROS, A.F. and GALLAGHER, D.L. (1958), Measuring Indirect Effects of Treatment on Chronic Wards, 'Dis. Nerv. System', 19, 167-72.

MORGAN, H.G. et al. (1975a), The Urban Distribution of Non-Fatal Deliberate Harm, 'Brit. J. Psychiat.', 126, 319-28.

MORGAN, H.G. et al. (1975b), Deliberate Self-Harm, 'Brit. J. Psychiat.', 127, 564-74.

ODEGARD, O. (1964), Pattern of Discharge from Norwegian Psychiatric Hospitals Before and After the Introduction of Psychotropic Drugs, 'Amer. J. Psychiat.', 20, 772-8.

OHE (1975), 'Medicines Which Affect the Mind', London, Office of Health Economics.

OLDHAM, A.J. and BOTT, E. (1971), The Management of Excitement in a General Hospital Ward by High Dosage Haloperidol, 'Acta Psychiat. Scand.', 47, 369-76.

PERROW, O. (1965), Hospitals, Technology, Structure and Goals, in March, J.G. (ed.), 'Handbook of Organizations', Chicago, Rand McNally.

POWLES, J. (1973), On the Limitations of Modern Medicine, 'Sci. Med. & Man', 1, 1-30.

RICHARDS, M.P.M. (1975), Innovation in Medical Practice: Obstetricians and the Induction of Labour in Britain, 'Soc. Sci. and Med.', 9, 595-602.

SOMMER, C. and WEINBERG, J. (1944), Techniques and Factors Reversing the Trend of Population Growth in Illinois State Hospitals, 'Amer. J. Psychiat.', 100, 456-61.

CHAPTER 4   THE ORIGINS OF PSYCHIATRIC UNITS IN GENERAL HOSPITALS

BENNETT, A.E. et al. (1956), 'The Practice of Psychiatry in General Hospitals', New York, Architectural Record.

BILLINGS, E.G. (1941), The Value of Psychiatry in General Hospitals, 'Hospitals', 15, 30-4.

BMJ (1936), The Training of the Neurologist and the Psychiatrist, 'Brit. Med. J.', 2, 395-6.

BMJ (1943a), Psychiatry in the General Hospital, 'Brit. Med. J.', 1, 637.

BMJ (1943b), Psychiatry at the Cross-Roads, 'Brit. Med. J.', 2, 331-2.

EDELSTON, H. (1950), letter in 'Lancet', 1, 133.
HAUN, P. (1950), 'Psychiatric Services in General Hospitals',
London, Oxford University Press.
JONES, K. (1972), 'The History of the Mental Health Services',
London, Routledge & Kegan Paul.
KASANIN, J. (1937), Function of the Psychiatrist in a General
Hospital, 'Lancet', 2, 1518-21.
'LANCET' (1936), Observation Wards, 'Lancet', 2, 798-9.
'LANCET' (1937), Referred to the Psychiatrist, 'Lancet', 2, 1496-7.
'LANCET' (1938), Psychiatric Clinics in General Hospitals, 'Lancet',
1, 850-1.
'LANCET' (1945), The Psychiatric Services - Joint Recommendations,
'Lancet', 1, 763-5.
'LANCET' (1950), Mechanism and Purpose, 'Lancet', 1, 27.
LEEPER, R.R. (1931), Some Reflections on the Progress of Psychiatry,
'J. Ment. Sci.', 77, 683-91.
LORD, J.R. (1929), The Evolution of the Nerve Hospital as a Factor
in the Progress of Psychiatry, 'J. Ment. Sci.', 75, 307-15.
PENTREATH, E.U.H. and DAX, E.C. (1937), Mental Observation Wards,
'J. Ment. Sci.', 83, 347-56.
REES, R.T. and SHEPLEY, W.H. (1943), Psychiatric Treatment in
General Hospitals, 'Brit. Med. J.', 1, 735.
SANDS, D.E. (1943), Treatment of Psychiatric Patients in General
Hospitals, 'Brit. Med. J.', 1, 628-30.
SPENCER, A.M. (1943), Psychiatry in General Hospitals, 'Brit. Med.
J.', 2, 54.
WALK, A. (1964), Mental Hospitals, in Poynter, F.L. 'ed.), 'The
Evolution of Hospitals in Britain', London, Pitman.

CHAPTER 5   THE ASCENDANCY OF PSYCHIATRIC UNITS IN GENERAL HOSPITALS

BAKER, A.A. (1958), Breaking Up the Mental Hospital, 'Lancet',
2, 253-4.
BAKER, A.A. (1961), Pulling Down the Old Mental Hospital, 'Lancet',
2, 656-7.
BARTON, R. (1960), 'Institutional Neurosis', Bristol, Wright.
BENADY, D.R. and DENHAM, J. (1963), Development of an Early
Treatment Unit from an Observation Ward, 'Brit. Med. J.', 2,
1569-72.
COCHRANE, A.L. (1972), 'Effectiveness and Efficiency', London,
Nuffield Provincial Hospitals Trust.
COPAS, J.B., FRYER, L. and ROBIN, A. (1974), 'Treatment Settings
in Psychiatry', London, Kimpton.
DUNKLEY, E.W. and LEWIS, E. (1963), North Wing - a Psychiatric
Unit in a General Hospital, 'Lancet', 1, 156-9.
EYSENCK, H.J. (1975), 'The Future of Psychiatry', London, Methuen.
FREEMAN, H.L. (1960), Oldham and District Psychiatric Services,
'Lancet', 1, 218-2.
GARRATT, F.N., LOWE, O.R. and McKEOWN, T. (1958), Institutional
Care of the Mentally Ill, 'Lancet', 1, 612-14.
GOFFMAN, E. (1961), 'Asylums - Essays on the Social Situation of
Mental Patients', New York, Anchor.
GRANT-SMITH, R. (1922), 'The Experiences of an Asylum Patient',
London, Allen & Unwin.

HERSHENSON, D.B. (1961), Toward a Science of Ergology, 'J. Counselling Psychol.', 16, 458-69.

HOENIG, J. (1968), The De-segregation of the Psychiatric Patient, 'Proc. Roy. Soc. Med.', 61, 115-20.

HOENIG, J. and HAMILTON, M.W. (1966), A New Venture in Administrative Therapy, 'Amer. J. Psychiat.', 123, 270-9.

HOENIG, J. and HAMILTON, M.W. (1969), 'The De-segregation of the Mentally Ill', London, Routledge & Kegan Paul.

JONES, K. (1960), 'Mental Health and Social Policy, 1845-1959', London, Routledge & Kegan Paul.

JONES, K. (1972), 'The History of the Mental Health Services', London, Routledge & Kegan Paul.

KEDDIE, J.T.C. (1955), 'Proc. Roy. Soc. Med.', 48, 745-6.

KREITMAN, N. (1962), Psychiatric Orientation among Psychiatrists, 'Br. J. Med. Psychol.', 46, 75-81.

'LANCET' (1962), Psychiatry in General Hospitals, 'Lancet', 1, 1107.

LEYBERG, J.T. (1959), A District Psychiatric Service. The Bolton Pattern, 'Lancet', 2, 282-4.

LITTLE, J.C. (1974), 'Psychiatry in a General Hospital', London, Butterworth.

LOMAX, M. (1921), 'The Experiences of an Asylum Doctor', London, Allen & Unwin.

McKEOWN, T. (1958), The Concept of a Balanced Hospital Community, 'Lancet', 1, 701-4.

MORRIS, V. (1959), 'Mental Illness in London', London, Maudsley Monograph.

PALLIS, D.J. and STOFFELMAYER, B.E. (1973), Social Attitudes and Treatment Orientation among Psychiatrists, 'Br. J. Med. Psychol.', 46, 75-81.

QUERIDO, A. (1955), The Amsterdam Psychiatric First Aid Scheme and some Proposals for New Legislation, 'Proc. Roy. Soc. Med.', 48, 741-4.

RAPHAEL, W. (1974), 'Just an Ordinary Patient', London, King Edward's Fund for London.

ROYAL COLLEGE OF PSYCHIATRISTS (Scottish Division) (1973), 'The Future of Psychiatric Services in Scotland'.

SNAITH, R.P. and JACOBSON, S. (1965), The Observation Ward and the Psychiatric Emergency, 'Brit. J. Psychiat.', 111, 18-26.

TREACHER, A. (in preparation), Mental Illness Statistics During War-Time - Myth and Reality.

WALTON, H.J. and DREWERY, J. (1966), Psychiatrists as Teachers in Medical Schools, 'Brit. J. Psychiat.', 112, 839-46.

WHO (1953), Expert Committee on Mental Health - Third Report, 'World Hlth. Org. Techn. Rep. Ser.', 73.

WOODSIDE, M. (1968), Are Observation Wards Obsolete? 'Br. J. Psychiat.', 114, 1013-18.

CHAPTER 10 CONCLUSION

BRENNER, M.H. (1973), 'Mental Illness and the Economy', Cambridge, Mass., Harvard University Press.

COOKLIN, A.I. (1974), Exploration of the Staff-Patient 'Contract' in an Acute Female Admission Ward, 'Br. J. Med. Psychol.', 47, 331-5.

DHSS (1971), Hospital Services for the Mentally Ill, London, Department of Health and Social Security.

DHSS (1975), Better Services for the Mentally Ill, London, Department of Health and Social Security.

GOLDIE, N. (1976), 'The Division of Labour Among the Mental Health Professions - a Negotiated or an Imposed Order?', BSA conference, April 1976.

JASPERS, K. (1963), 'The Nature of Psychotherapy', Manchester University Press.

MECHANIC, D. (1962), Some Factors in Identifying and Defining Mental Illness, 'Ment. Hyg.', 46, 66-74.

MECHANIC, D. (1969), 'Mental Health and Social Policy', Englewood Cliffs, Prentice Hall.

NAVARRO, V. (1975), The Industrialisation of Fetishism or the Fetishism of Industrialisation: a Critique of Ivan Illich, 'Soc. Sci. and Med.', 9, 351-63.

'NEW PSYCHIATRY' (1976), Contract to Cure, 'New Psychiatry', 3(1), 6.

PARSONS, T. (1951a), Illness and the Role of the Physician: a Sociological Perspective, 'Am. J. Orthopsychiat', 21, 452-60.

PARSONS, T. (1951b), 'The Social System', Chicago, Free Press.

PARSONS, T. (1952), Illness, Therapy and the Modern, Urban American Family, 'J. Soc. Illness', 8131-44.

PERROW, C. (1965), Hospitals, Technology, Structure and Goals, reprinted in March, J.G. (ed.), 'Handbook of Organisations', Chicago, Rand McNally, 1975.

PERVIN, L.A. (1970), 'Personality: Theory, Assessment, and Research', Chichester, John Wiley.

SCOTT, R.D. (1973), The Treatment Barrier: Part 1, 'Br. J. Med. Psychol.' 46, 45.

SEDGWICK, P. 'Mental Illness is Illness', National Symposium on Deviance, York, 1972.

WAITZIN, H. and WATERMAN, B. (1974), 'The Exploitation of Illness in a Capitalist Society', New York, Bobbs Merrill.